Ion-Selective Microelectrodes

and Their Use in Excitable Tissues

Ion-Selective Microelectrodes
and Their Use in Excitable Tissues

Edited by

Eva Syková, Pavel Hník, and Ladislav Vyklický

Czechoslovak Academy of Sciences
Prague, Czechslovakia

Plenum Press · New York and London

Library of Congress Cataloging in Publication Data

Main entry under title:

Ion-selective microelectrodes and their use in excitable tissues.

Proceedings of a symposium organized by the Czechoslovak Academy of Sciences as a satellite symposium to the 28th International Congress of Physiological Sciences and held July 8-11, 1980, in Prague, Czechoslovakia.
   Bibliography: p.
   Includes index.
   1. Electrodes, Ion selective—Congresses. 2. Nerve tissue—Congresses. 3. Muscle—Congresses. I. Syková, Eva. II. Hník, Pavel. III. Vyklický, Ladislav. IV. Československá akademie věd. [DNLM: 1. Microelectrodes—Congresses. 2. Ions—Metabolism—Congresses. 3. Nervous system—Physiology—Congresses. WL 102 I68 1980]
QP519.9.E43I67   599.01'8   81-1625
ISBN 0-306-40723-X   AACR2

Proceedings of a symposium on Ion-Selective Microelectrodes and Their Use in Excitable Tissues, organized by the Czechoslovak Academy of Sciences as a satellite symposium to the 28th International Congress of Physiological Sciences and held July 8—11, 1980, in Prague, Czechoslovakia

© 1981 Plenum Press, New York
A Division of Plenum Publishing Corporation
233 Spring Street, New York, N.Y. 10013

PREFACE

The Symposium on "Ion Selective Microelectrodes and Their Use in Excitable Tissues" was held in Prague from July 8-11, 1980. It was organized by the Institute of Physiology of the Czechoslovak Academy of Sciences as a satellite symposium of the XXVIII International Congress of Physiological Sciences in Budapest. Sixty participants met for three days in the historical setting of the Strahov Monastery.

The informal and relaxed atmosphere of the scientific sessions, together with the social programme made the meeting a success and helped to cement old friendships and to form new ones. The organizers were happy to welcome as participants representatives from most of the laboratories working with ion-selective microelectrodes (ISMs) in the world. Neurophysiological research with liquid ion-exchanger ISMs in the Prague laboratory was started as early as 1971 due to the fact that one of us (P.H.) had the opportunity of learning the technique directly from Dr.J.L. Walker in Salt Lake City. It was thanks to his patience and, later, his courtesy in providing us with the liquid ion-exchanger for potassium and silicone that we were able to get a start in what turned out to be, in a year or so, very strong international competition.

This volume contains the papers presented at the Symposium. It is divided according to the actual sessions with names of the chairmen, who helped the organizers to make the Symposium a real success. We should like to express our grateful appreciation to them for being so patient and helpful.

It is almost impossible to name all members of the organizing committee who should receive credit for the success of an international meeting of this kind. The editors of this volume wish to thank Plenum Press for their help in preparing the Proceedings for camera-ready printing. Some of the contributors have used figures previously published elsewhere. Thanks are hence due to the publishers, editors and authors who have generously given their permission for their use.

E. Syková
P. Hník
L. Vyklický
October 1980

CONTENTS

SESSION I
ELECTROCHEMISTRY OF THE ISM AND
IONOPHORES FOR THE ISM

THEORY OF ION-SELECTIVE ELECTRODES

Jiří Koryta

J. Heyrovský Institute of Physical Chemistry
and Electrochemistry,
Czechoslovak Academy of Sciences,
Opletalova 25, 110 00 Prague 1,
Czechoslovakia

Ion-selective electrodes are potentiometric sensors containing an electrochemical membrane as an essential component. Besides the glass electrode which was discovered by Cremer and by Haber and Klemensiewicz at the beginning of the century and introduced to practical potentiometry particularly by MacInnes and Dole, the ion-selective electrodes in a narrow sense of the word date from the sixties with the basic contributions of Pungor, Frant and Ross, Simon and their co-workers (for the review of the history of ion-selective electrodes, see Koryta 1975).

We have two classes of ion-selective electrodes, the electrodes with fixed-site membranes and those with liquid membranes, both of them playing a major role in biomedical analysis (Koryta, 1980). However, at present, only the liquid-membrane systems have an important, sometimes even unique, position in electrophysiological studies of excitable cells and tissues owing to their comparatively easy miniaturization. Consequently, this review will be exclusively concerned with the basic aspects of the liquid membranes.

Ion-selective microelectrodes should have the following properties: their impedance should not be too high, they should have a short response time and high selectivity (related, of course, to the particular composition of the biological fluid under investigation).

There are two principal types of liquid-membrane systems, those based on hydrophobic ion-exchangers and those using electroneutral ion-carriers. Both these groups do not entirely differ as will be shown later.

3

A liquid membrane is a layer of an organic ("oil") solvent immiscible with water both its surfaces contacting an aqueous solution. When the membrane is confined to a polymer matrix it retains its property of a homogeneous liquid phase though of a rather complicated shape. Most probably the matrix has little importance for the ion-exchanging properties of the membrane while it can significantly influence the transport in the membrane. At these two interfaces there occur ion-transfer processes which result in an equilibrium or a steady state. The ions transferred across these interfaces are then transported to the bulk of the membrane phase.

The transport inside the membrane was discussed in detail by Sandblom et al. (1967a, b) and Walker et al., (1968). Since, in my opinion, the interfacial properties determine the basic characteristics of the membrane this paper will only deal with the properties of the interface water/membrane solvent (oil phase).

The basic contribution to this problem was made by Nernst and Riesenfeld (1902) who studied the ion transfer at the interface water/phenol with a single salt distributed among these phases under conditions of electrical current flow as well as in equilibrium. Further contributions to the problem were made by Beutner (1913), Bonhoeffer et al.(1953) and, particularly, by Karpfen and Randles (1953). These results can be summarized in the following way: Between the aqueous (w) and the organic (o) phase an electrical potential difference is established (the Nernst-Donnan potential) depending on the activity of the common ion I,

$$\Delta_o^w \varphi = \varphi(w) - \varphi(o) = (\mu_i^{0,o} - \mu_i^{0,w}) / (zF) +$$

$$+ (RT/zF)\ln[a_i(o)/a_i(w)] =$$

$$= \Delta G_{tr,i}^{0,o \rightarrow w} /(zF) + (RT/zF)\ln[a_i(o)/a_i(w) =$$

$$= \Delta_o^w \varphi_i^0 + (RT/zF)\ln[a_i(o)/a_i(w)], \qquad (1)$$

where the φ's are inner electrical potentials, μ_i^0's standard chemical potentials and a_i's activities of the ion I in each phase. These activities are defined, for example, on the molar scale; in the case of limiting dilution they approach molar concentrations (units mol. dm^{-3}). The quantity $\Delta G_{tr,i}^{0,o \rightarrow w}$ is the standard Gibbs energy of transfer from the organic to the aqueous phase for the ion I. In order to attribute a definite value to this quantity, an extrathermodynamic approach has to be used, for example, the "TATB assumption" stating that the standard transfer Gibbs energies of tetraphenylarsonium cation and of tetraphenylborate anion are equal for any pair of solvents (Parker 1969). On the basis of this assumption scales of standard Gibbs transfer energies and of standard electrical potential differences $\Delta_o^w\varphi^o$ can be composed(Gavach and Henry, 1974; Koryta et al., 1977a).

In the case of a single electrolyte BA which is distributed between both phases

$$\begin{array}{c|c} w & o \\ \hline BA & BA \end{array}$$

according to the partition coefficient a distribution potential (Karpfen and Randles, 1953) is established. This potential depends entirely on the standard Gibbs free energies of the ions B^+ and A^- while it is independent of their final concentrations. In the case of the membrane of an ion-selective electrode at least three types of ions are needed, for example, the determinand B_1^+, the ion-exchanging anion A_2^- and the hydrophilic anion A_1^-. Due to its hydrophobicity, the ion-exchanging ion is practically confined to the organic phase in the system

$$\begin{array}{c|c} w & o \\ \hline B_1A_1 & B_1A_2 \end{array}$$

while the hydrophilic anion A_1^- prevents the salt B_1A_1 from entering the membrane. Thus equation (1) describes the situation at one of the interfaces of the ion-selective electrode. The total membrane potential, which is measured potentiometrically, pertains to the system

$$\begin{array}{c|c|c} w(1) & o & w(2) \\ \hline B_1A_1 & B_1A_2 & B_1A_1 \end{array}$$

where 1 denots the aqueous phase under investigation and 2 the inner solution of the ion-selective electrode. The membrane potential is then given by the simple relationship

$$\Delta\varphi_M = \varphi(w1) - \varphi(w2) = (RT/F)\ln[a_{B_1^+}(2)/a_{B_1^+}(1)] \tag{2}$$

Since $a_{B_1^+}(2)$ is a constant, the membrane potential shows a <u>Nernstian response</u> towards the ion B_1^+ in the outer solution. This result is not basically changed when, due to a low permittivity of the membrane solvent, the ion-pairs are formed between B_1^+ and A_2^- in the membrane.

When an ion in the outer solution has the standard Gibbs transfer energy comparable with the determinand it enters the membrane and is exchanged, in part, for the ion B_1^+ present in the membrane. Under these conditions the potential between the outer solution and the membrane, $\Delta_o^w\varphi$, decreases because the activity $a_{B_1^+}(o)$ diminishes.

A non-equilibrium situation ensues in the membrane connected with the transport of the interferant B_2^+ into the bulk of the membrane and of the determinand to the interface. If they diffuse with the same velocity, no diffusion potential is formed in the membrane and the membrane potential is given by the Nikolsky equation

$$\Delta\varphi_M = - (RT/F)\ln \left[(a_{B_1^+}(1) + K_{B_1B_2}^{Pot} \, a_{B_2^+}(1))/a_{B_1^+}(2) \right] \qquad (3)$$

where the selectivity coefficient $K_{B_1B_2}^{Pot}$ is given by equation

$$K_{B_1B_2}^{Pot} = \exp[(\Delta G_{tr,B_1^+}^{o,w \to o} - \Delta G_{tr,B_2^+}^{o,w \to o})/[RT]]. \qquad (4)$$

The Gibbs transfer energies $\Delta G_{tr,i}^{o,w \to o}$ are given by the difference of the solvation Gibbs energies and thus, they represent a quantitative measure of the hydrophobicity or hydrophility of the ion concerned. The ion-pair formation in the organic phase acts, to a certain degree, in favour of the exchange of a more hydrophobic determinand present in the membrane for a less hydrophobic interferant. The less hydrophobic cation will be, most probably, smaller in size in comparison with the determinand and the ions with a smaller crystallographic radius are more inclined to ion-pairing than the larger ones.

The original treatment of the case of ion-selective electrodes based on neutral ion-carriers such as valinomycin, macrotetrolides, crown polyethers or acyclic substances introduced by Simon and co-workers (for the review, see Meier et al., 1980) would require the presence of a hydrophilic anion A_1^- in the membrane when the salt B_1A_1 is extracted with a subsequent complex formation with the ion-carrier. Various other approaches based on different assumptions have also been worked out (Boles and Buck, 1973; Perry et al., 1976; Thomas et al., 1977). However, following the suggestion made by Morf et al.,(1974), all difficulties connected with the anion problem are removed by using a hydrophobic counterion such as tetraphenylborate in the membrane phase. The concentration of this counterion determines, at the same time, the concentration of the determinand in the membrane phase, so that the whole problem is reduced to the preceding case, equation (2). With macrocyclic ligands like valinomycin which perfectly trap the cations in their internal cavity the complex of the neutral carrier with the determinand and with the interferant exhibits the same interaction with the membrane medium. In this case the selectivity coefficient is simply given by the ratio of the stability constants of the interferant and of the determinand with the carrier (Ciani et al., 1969).

The difficulties connected with the high resistance of the ion-exchanger solution containing neutral carriers can also be removed by using a hydrophobic counterion in the membrane phase. However, the use of a coaxial-type ion-selective microelectrode makes it possible to work with membrane solutions of rather low conductivity (Ujec et al., 1978, 1979).

In the case of usual types of ion-selective electrodes the response-time depends on a number of factors, including the transport of the determinand to the surface of the membrane, the surface processes at the surface and, eventually, the transport in the membrane phase. In view of the microporous structure of the surface in the case of the solid and plastic-film based membranes this problem is often quite complicated. However, in the case of liquid-membrane ion-selective microelectrodes the problem of the transport in the aqueous phase can be completely removed in the immersion experiment (Vyskočil and Kříž, 1972) or completely controlled in the iontophoretic experiment (Lux and Neher, 1973). Thus, in the absence of an interferant we have to deal with the comparatively simple situation when the electrode having an initial membrane potential $\Delta\varphi_i$ depending on an equilibrium concentration of the determinand is brought into contact with another concentration of the determinand in the analysed solution c_s. The rate with which the potential $\Delta\varphi$ shifts from the value of $\Delta\varphi_i$ to the resulting equilibrium value $\Delta\varphi_f$ depends on the rate of charging the electrical double-layer formed at the interface membrane/aqueous solution and on the rate of transfer of the determinand ion across this interface.

The kinetics of ion-transfer across the interface of two immiscible electrolyte solutions (ITIES) under flow of electrical current is being intensively studied (Gavach and Henry, 1974; Koryta et al., 1977a; 1980). It could be shown that this process follows identical laws as electrode kinetics at metallic electrodes (Koryta, 1979). The electrical double-layer formed at ITIES has a capacity comparable to that of the double-layer at the interface mercury/aqueous electrolyte (Gavach et al., 1977; Samer and Hájková, 1980). Thus, the rate of potential change is described by a simple equation where the rate of charging the double-layer is put equal to the rate of ion transfer across the interface

$$v_c = v_t.$$ (5)

The quantity v_c is given by equation for the charging current

$$v_c = - C\frac{d\eta}{dt}$$ (6)

where C is the capacity of the interface and the overpotential η is given by the difference $\Delta\varphi - \Delta\varphi_f$. For the transfer kinetics we use the basic equation of electrochemical kinetics (Vetter, 1961; Cammann and Rechnitz, 1976; Koryta et al., 1977b)

$$v_t = j^o \exp\left[\frac{\alpha F \eta}{RT} - \exp\left(-\frac{(1-\alpha)\ F\eta}{RT}\right)\right] \tag{7}$$

where j^o (A cm^{-2}) is the exchange current density, α is the charge transfer coefficient and F, R and T have the usual significance. The different signs before α and $(1 - \alpha)$ than in usual electrochemical kinetics are connected with the definition of $\Delta\varphi = \varphi(w) - \varphi(o)$ where $\varphi(w)$ and $\varphi(o)$ are the electrical potentials of the aqueous and of the membrane phase. Furthermore, the electrical current connected with the transfer of positive ions from the outer aqueous phase into the membrane is considered positive. For small values of η (when $[\Delta\varphi_f - \Delta\varphi_i] \ll \frac{RT}{F}$) equation (7) can be linearized,

$$v_t \simeq j^o F \eta / (RT). \tag{8}$$

By combining (5), (6) and (8) we obtain a simple differential equation

$$- C\ (d\eta\ /dt) = j^o F \eta\ /(RT). \tag{9}$$

The response-time τ will be defined as the time interval during which the overpotential η changes from its initial value $\eta_i \equiv \Delta\varphi_i$ to the final value $\eta_f = 0.05\,\eta_i$ (τ_{95}). By solution of (9) we obtain

$$\tau_{95} = \frac{RT}{F} \cdot \frac{C}{j^o} \ln \frac{\eta_i}{\eta_f} = \frac{RT}{F^2} \cdot \frac{C}{k^o c_s^\alpha (1-\alpha)} \ln \frac{\eta_i}{\eta_f}, \tag{10}$$

$$\tau_{95} = \frac{3.0\ RT}{F^2} \cdot \frac{C}{k^o c_m^\alpha c_s (1-\alpha)}, \tag{11}$$

where k^o(cm.s^{-1}) is the standard rate constant of ion transfer and c_m and c_s the concentrations of the determinand in the membrane and in the outer solution (mol.cm^{-3}), respectively.

Table 1. Parameters of the charge transfer reaction

Ion	α	$k^o/(\text{cm.s}^{-1})$
tetraethylammonium	0.35	$2.2\text{x}\ 10^{-3}$
tetrapropylammonium	0.27	$2.3\text{x}\ 10^{-3}$
tetrabutylammonium	0.23	$5\ \ \text{x}\ 10^{-3}$
Cs^+	0.46	$5.5\text{x}\ 10^{-2}$

While the values of k^o for the ion transfer across the interface water/membrane solvents are not known, some information can be obtained from the values of these constants measured at the interface water/ nitrobenzene (Gavach et al., 1975; Samec et al., 1979) which are listed in Table 1.

Thus, for 10 mmol/l membrane electrolytes and mmol/l determinands in the outer aqueous phase and for the values of C equal to $10 - 20$ μF cm^{-2} the values of τ_{95} are of the order of milliseconds which is comparable with the results found with ion-selective microelectrodes (Lux and Neher, 1973; Ujec, 1980).

REFERENCES

Beutner, R., 1913, Neue Erscheinungen der Elektrizitätserregung, welche einige bioelektrische Phänomene erklären, Z. Elektrochem., 19:319.

Boles, J.H., and Buck, R.P., 1973, Anion responses and potential functions for neutral carrier membrane electrodes, Anal. Chem., 45:2057.

Bonhoeffer, K.-F., Kahlweit, M., and Strehlow, H., 1953, Ueber elektrochemische Analogien zwischen nichtwässrigen Elektrolytlösungen und Ionenaustauschern, Z. Elektrochem., 57:614.

Cammann, K., and Rechnitz, G.A., 1976, Exchange kinetics at ion-selective membrane electrodes, Anal. Chem., 48:856.

Ciani, S., Eisenman, G., and Szabo, G., 1969, A theory for the effects of neutral carriers such as the macrotetralide actin antibiotics on the electric properties of bilayer membranes, J. Membrane Biol., 1:1.

Gavach, C., D´Epenoux, B., and Henry, F., 1975, Transfer of tetra-N-alkylammonium ions from water to nitrobenzene - chronopotentiometric determination of kinetic parameters, J. Electroanal. Chem., 64:107.

Gavach, C., and Henry, F., 1974, Chronopotentiometric investigation of the diffusion overvoltage at the interface between two non-miscible solutions, J. Electroanal. Chem., 54:361.

Gavach, C., Seta, P., and D´Epenoux, B., 1977, The double layer and ion adsorption at the interface between two non-miscible solutions. Part I. Interfacial tension measurements for the water-nitrobenzene tetraalkylammonium bromide systems, J. Electroanal. Chem., 83:225.

Karpfen, F.M., and Randles, J.A.B., 1953, Ionic equilibria and phase-boundary potentials in oil-water systems, Trans. Farady Soc., 49:823.

Koryta, J., 1975, Ion-selective Electrodes, Cambridge University Press, Cambridge.

Koryta, J., 1980, Ed.:"Medical and Biological Applications of Electrochemical Devices", J. Wiley and Sons, Chichester.

Koryta, J., 1979, Electrochemical polarization phenomena at the interface of two immiscible electrolyte solutions, Electrochim. Acta, 24:293.

Koryta, J., Vanýsek, P., and Březina, M., 1977a, Electrolysis with electrolyte dropping electrode II. Basic properties of the system, J. Electroanal. Chem., 75:211.

Koryta, J., Vanýsek, P., Khalil, M.W., Mareček, V., and Samec, Z., 1977b, A mechanistic tool for liquid-membrane ion-selective electrode investigation: Polarization of the liquid-liquid interface, in: Ion Selective Electrodes, Proceedings of the Conference of Ion-Selective Electrodes, Budapest, Pungor, E.,ed., Akadémiai Kiadó, Budapest.

Koryta, J., Březina, M., Hofmanová, A., Homolka, D., Hung, L.Q., Khalil, W., Mareček, V., Samec, Z.,Sen, S.K., Vanýsek, P., and Weber, J., 1980, A new model of membrane transport: electrolysis at the interface of two immiscible electrolyte solutions, Bioelectrochem. Bioenerget., 7:61.

Lux, H.D., and Neher, E., 1973, The equilibration time course of $[K^+]_o$ in cat cortex, Exp. Brain Res., 17:190.

Meier, P.C., Ammann, D., Morf, W.E., and Simon, W., 1980, Liquid-membrane ion-selective electrodes and their biomedical applications, in: Medical and Biological Applications of Electrochemical Devices, Koryta, J., ed., Wiley and Sons, Chichester,p.13

Morf, W.E., Kahr, G., and Simon, W., 1974, Reduction of the anion interference in neutral carrier liquid-membrane electrodes responsive to cations. Anal.Lett., 7:9.

Nernst, W., and Riesenfeld, E.H., 1902, Ueber elektrolytische Erscheinungen an der Grenzfläche zweier Lösungsmittel, Ann. Physik, 8(4):602.

Parker, A.J., 1969, Protic-dipolar aprotic solvent effects on rates of bimolecular reactions, Chem. Revs., 69:1

Perry, M., Löbel, E., and Bloch, R., 1976, The mechanism of polymeric valinomycin-based potassium specific electrodes, J. Membrane Sci., 1:233.

Samec, Z., and Hájková, D., 1980, private communication.

Samec, Z., Mareček, V., and Weber, J., 1979, Charge transfer between two immiscible electrolyte solutions. Part II. The investigation of Cs^+ ion transfer across the nitrobenzene/water interface by cyclic voltammetry with IR drop compensation, J. Electroanal. Chem., 100:841.

Sandblom, J., Eisenman, G., and Walker, J.L., 1967a, Electrical phenomena associated with the transport of ions and ion pairs in liquid ion-exchange membranes I. Zero current properties. J. Phys. Chem., 71:3862.

Sandblom, J., Eisenman, G., and Walker, J.L., 1967b, Electrical phenomena associated with the transport of ions and ion apirs in liquid ion-exchange membrane II. Nonzero current properties, J. Phys. Chem., 71:3871.

Thomas,A.P., Viviani-Nauer, A., Arvanitis, S., and Simon, W., 1977, Mechanism of neutral carrier mediated ion transport through ion-selective bulk membranes, Anal. Chem., 49:1567.

Ujec, E., 1980, private communication.

Ujec, E., Keller, O., Pavlík, V., and Machek, J., 1978, Electrical parameters of a coaxial, low-resistance, potassium-selective micro-electrode, Physiol. bohemoslov., 27:570.

Ujec, E., Keller, O., Machek, J., and Pavlík, V., 1979, Low impedance coaxial K^+ selective microelectrodes, Pflügers Arch., 382:189.

Vetter, K.J., 1961, "Elektrochemische Kinetik", Springer-Verlag, Berlin, p.122.

Vyskočil, F., and Kříž, N., 1972, Modifications of single and double-barrel potassium specific microelectrodes for physiological experiments, Pflügers Arch., 337:265.

Walker, J.L., Eisenman, G., and Sandblom, J., 1968, Electrical phenomena associated with the transport of ions and ion pairs in liquid ion-exchange membrane III. Experimental observations in a model system, J: Phys. Chem., 72:978.

NEW ION SELECTIVE LIQUID MEMBRANE MICROELECTRODES

D. Ammann, F. Lanter, R. Steiner, D. Erne
and W. Simon

Swiss Federal Institute of Technology
Department of Organic Chemistry
CH-8092 Zürich, Switzerland

INTRODUCTION

Certain natural (Štefanac and Simon, 1967) and synthetic (Morf et al., 1979) lipophilic ligands for cations (ion carriers, ionophores) made a wide range of microelectrodes with different selectivities available. Especially the development of electrically neutral ionophores led to clear improvements in selectivities and detection limits. Here we report on the present possibilities in the use of ion-selective liquid membrane microelectrodes.

LIQUID MEMBRANE MICROELECTRODES AND THEIR APPLICATIONS

A selection of relevant liquid membrane microelectrode systems with examples of their application is given in Table 1, along with the optimized membrane compositions (column 2; see also Figure). The following information may be of use:

Li^+-Electrode

The most severe limitation in its applications is the rather poor discrimination of Na^+ and K^+. The electrodes have selectivity factors $\log K_{LiNa}^{Pot}$ and $\log K_{LiK}^{Pot}$ of about -1.3 and -2.3 (Thomas et al., 1975), respectively. For most extracellular studies the Li^+-levels of interest will be near the detection limit; thus, their feasibility becomes questionable.

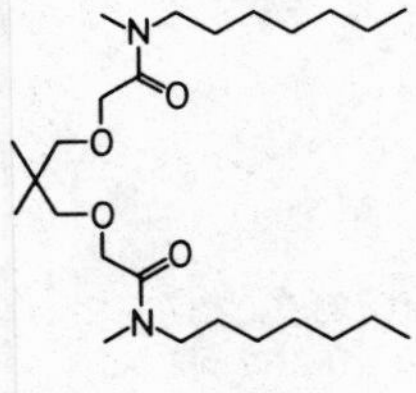

Fig. 1. Constitutions of the membrane components discussed

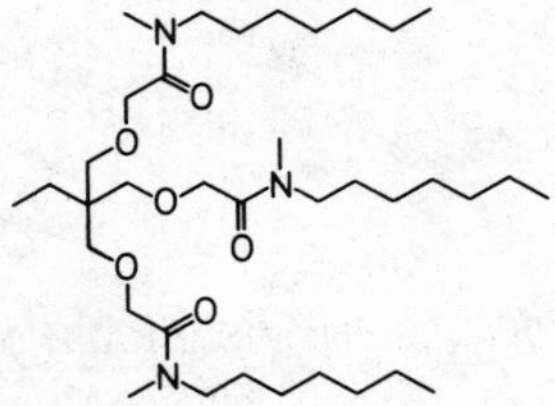

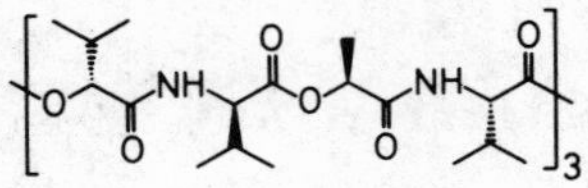

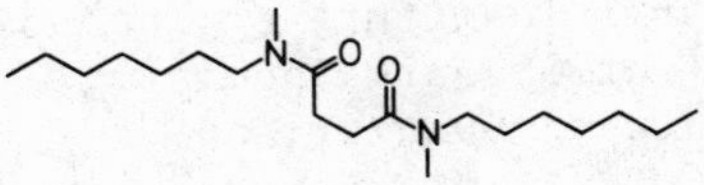

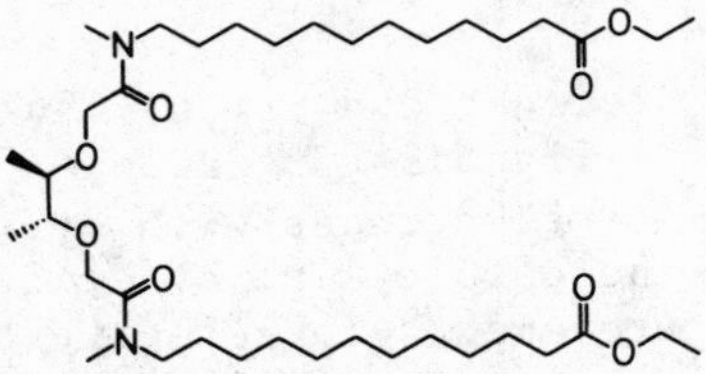

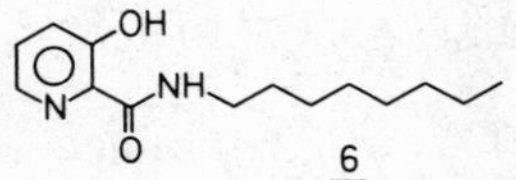

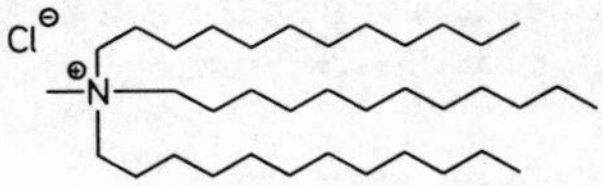

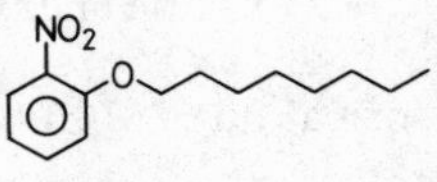

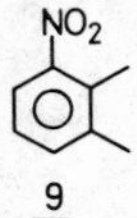

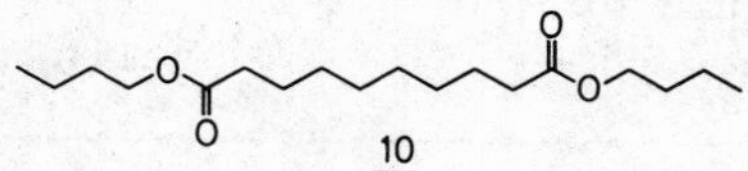

Fig. 1. (continued).

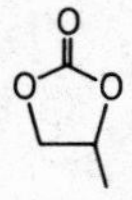

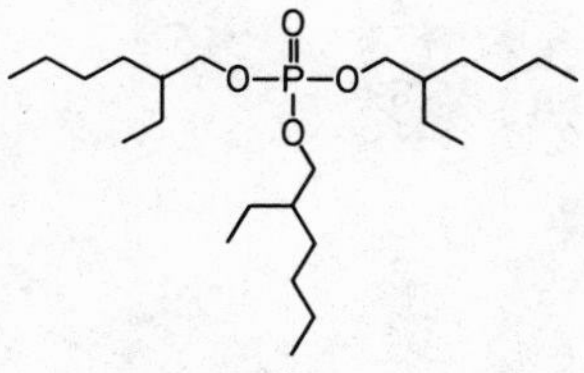

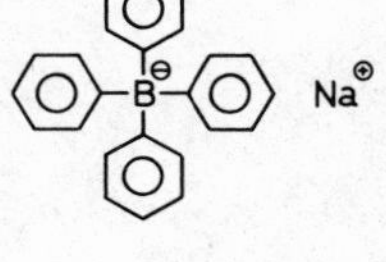

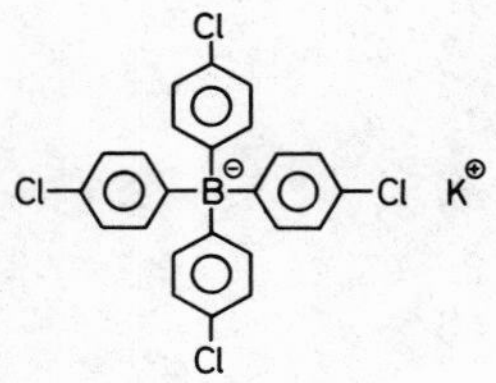

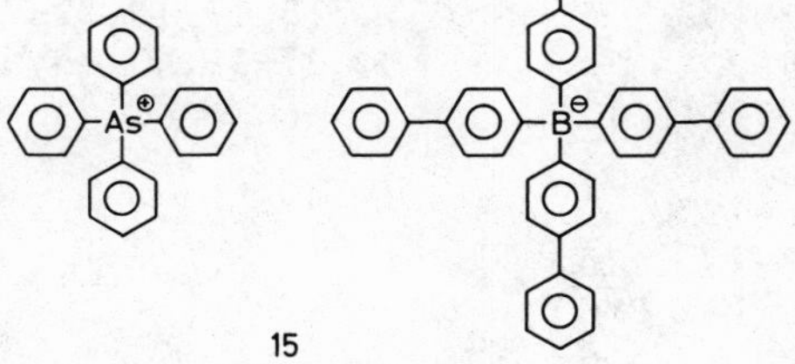

Table 1. Liquid Membrane Microelectrodes and Their Applications

Microelectrode [References]	Composition of ion-selective liquid wt.-%		Representative examples of applications	
			extra-cellular	intra-cellular
Li^+ 52	9.7%	$\underline{1}$		52
	85.5%	$\underline{12}$		
	4.8%	$\underline{13}$		
Na^+ 50	10.0%	$\underline{2}$		28
	89.5%	$\underline{8}$		
	0.5%	$\underline{13}$		
Na^+ 41	10.0%	$\underline{2}$		41
	89.0%	$\underline{9}$		
	1.0%	$\underline{14}$		
K^+ 59	5.0%	$\underline{3}$		59
	2.0%	$\underline{14}$		
	25 0%	$\underline{9}$		
	68			
Mg^{2+} 31	20.0%	$\underline{4}$		31
	1.0%	$\underline{13}$		
	79.0%	$\underline{11}$		
Ca^{2+} 45	10.0%	$\underline{5}$	4,7,8,17-19,21-23,26,	3,10,11,20,24
	89.0%	$\underline{8}$	30,37-39,40,49,51	34,46,47
	1.0%	$\underline{13}$		
Ca^{2+} 55	6-12%	$\underline{5}$		35, 1
	3-7%	$\underline{15}$		
	10-13%	PVC		
	68-81%	$\underline{8}$		
H^+ 15	20.0%	$\underline{6}$		
	1.0%	$\underline{13}$		
	79.0%	$\underline{8}$		
Cl^- 43	33.0%	$\underline{7}$		
	67.0%	$\underline{8}$		

Na^+-Electrode

Although Na^+-selective glass (e.g. $NASS_{11-18}$) have been described (Eisenman, 1967) which have a sufficiently high selectivity with respect to K^+ for intracellular studies, the corresponding microelectrodes have not found wide acceptance in practice (Kessler et al., 1967). Elevated glass transition temperatures led to technical problems in the preparation of microelectrodes (Lavallée et al., 1969). The most often used recessed-tip glass microelectrodes for Na^+ (Thomas, 1976) suffer from disadvantages such as the volume of this recess (Thomas, 1976), and therefore the possibility of tip blockage (Thomas, 1976), and sluggish response (Thomas, 1976). A repeated reactivation of the glass is necessary (Thomas, 1976).

Microelectrodes based on liquid ion exchanger sidestep these drawbacks (Walker, 1971; Kraig and Nicholson, 1976). The original neutral-carrier based system (Steiner et al., 1979) led to microelectrodes that permit reliable intracellular studies of Na^+ activities (Khuri, 1978). Extracellular measurements with this electrode are prone to interference due to the rather poor Na^+/Ca^{2+}-selectivity ($\log K_{NaCa}^{Pot} = 0.2$) (Steiner et al., 1979). A modification of the membrane composition (O'Doherty et al., 1979) relating this ionophore ($\underline{2}$ in Figure 1) yields electrodes that feature lowered resistance and substantially increased interference by Ca^{2+} ($\log K_{NaCa}^{Pot} = 0.5$).

K^+-Electrode

The classical, widely used (Walker, 1971) membrane system based on $\underline{14}$ (Figure 1, CORNING 477317) suffers from high interference by Na^+ ($\log K_{KNa}^{Pot} = -1.9$)(Oehme and Simon, 1976) and lipophilic cations such as acetyl choline ($\log K_{KAcetyl\ choline}^{Pot} = 3.7$) (Oehme and Simon, 1976). With valinomycin as carrier, electrodes can be proposed that are superior in terms of these interferences ($\log K_{KNa} = -3.5$)(Oehme and Simon, 1976) ($\log K_{KAcetyl\ choline}^{Pot} = -2.5$) (Oehme and Simon, 1976, but a one-hundred-fold increase of resistance is incurred. Through variation of membrane components, valinomycin based microelectrodes with slightly reduced resistance but identical selectivity behavior have been realized (Wuhrmann, 1979). They have been used with success (Coles and Tsacopoulos, 1977; Wuhrmann, 1979).

Mg^{2+}-Electrode

Although it has been proposed to use Erichrome Blue SE as indicator dye for the spectrophotometric determination of magnesium in cells (Brinley and Scarpa, 1975), at present only little is known about the concentration of ionized magnesium in living cells. Recently, the development of a new class of synthetic neutral carriers ($\underline{4}$ in Figure 1) (Erne et al., in preparation) enabled the preparation of liquid membrane microelectrodes with sufficient selectivity for intracellular Mg^{2+}-activity studies (Lanter et al., 1980). Single barrelled microelectrodes with a tip diameter of about 1 μm have a membrane resistance of ~$3.10^{10}\Omega$ and response times below 10 s. For intracellular Mg^{2+} studies potassium is the most severe interfering ion (log K_{MgNa}^{Pot} = -1.1; log K_{MgK}^{Pot} = -1.4; log K_{MgCa}^{Pot} = +1.1) and therefore an appropriate calibration procedure has to be chosen (Weingart and Hess, in preparation).

Ca^{2+}-Electrode

Due to the vanishingly small intracellular Ca^{2+}-activities ($a_{Ca} \leq 10^{-6}$mol l^{-1}) as compared to Na^+-, K^+-, and Mg^{2+}-activities, extreme specifications as to selectivities of a Ca^{2+}-selective micro-electrode are required. Sensors based on electrically charged organo-phosphates (Brown et al., 1976) are a rather poor proposition for intracellular applications because of Mg^{2+}-interference (Ammann et al., 1979; Tsien and Rink, 1980). In contrast, Ca^{2+}-selective neutral carrier microelectrodes (Simon et al., 1978) show outstanding se-lectivities, a low detection limit and are today widely used for extra- as well as intracellular Ca^{2+}-activity determinations (see Table 1). Improvements in respect to selectivity and stability of the neutral carrier microelectrode have been realized by incorporating the salt 15 instead of 13 into the Ca^{2+}-selective membrane that in addition contains poly(vinylchloride)(Tsien and Rink, 1980).

H^+-Electrode

Glass electrodes with outstanding selectivity for H^+ are avail-able; however, the reduction of the active membrane to a size of about 1 μm still poses some technical problems (Thomas, 1978). Double barrel-led versions are even more difficult to prepare (Khuri, 1976; Levy and Coles, 1977). Liquid membrane electrodes would overcome this. Synthe-tic H^+-carriers (see 6 in Figure 1) which induce adequate select-ivity in solvent polymeric membranes for intra- as well as extra-cellular work have been realized (Erne et al., 1979). The same is true for the corresponding microelectrodes (Erne et al., 1979). At present the most severe limitation seems to be their high electric resistance ($10^{12}\Omega$ for a tip diameter of 2.5 μm).

Cl^--Electrode

Microelectrodes based either on classical anion exchangers (Wal-ker, 1971) or on solid state membranes (Walker and Brown, 1977) have been used for intra- and extracellular measurements. An exchanger with similar specifications to the ion selective liquid CORNING No. 477 315 (DeLaat et al., 1974; Silver, 1975; Deisz and Lux, 1978) can be obtained by preparing a saturated solution of 7 in 8 (see Table 1 and Figure 1) . As a rule, exchangers of this type show a high preference of lipophilic anions relative to Cl^-.

ACKNOWLEDGEMENT

This work was partly supported by the Swiss National Science Foundation.

REFERENCES

1. Alvarez-Leefmans, F.J., Rink, T.J., and Tsien, R.Y., 1980, Intracellular free calcium in Helix aspersa neurones, J. Physiol. (Lond.), 306:24P.

2. Amman, D., Meier, P.C., and Simon, W., 1979, Design and use of calcium-selective microelectrodes, in: "Detection and Measurement of Free Ca^{2+} in Cells", C.C. Ashley and A.K. Campbell, eds., Elsevier/North-Holland Biomedical Press, Amsterdam, New York, Oxford.

3. Ashley, C.C., Rink, T.J., and Tsien, R.Y., 1978, Changes in free Ca during muscle contraction measured with an intracellular Ca-selective electrode, J. Physiol. (Lond.), 280:27P.

4. Bosher, S.K., and Warren, R.L., 1978, The very low calcium content of cochlear endolymph, an extracellular fluid, Nature, 273:377.

5. Brinley, F.J., Jr., and Scarpa, A., 1975, Ionized magnesium concentration in axoplasm of dialyzed squid axons, FEBS Letters, 50:82.

6. Brown, H.M., Pemberton, J.P., and Owen, J.D., 1976, A calcium-sensitive microelectrode suitable for intracellular measurement of calcium(II) activity, Anal. Chim. Acta, 85:261.

7. Bruggencate, G., ten, and Steinberg, R., 1978, Effects of ouabain and adenosine on extracellular Ca^{2+} and K^+ as measured with ion-selective microelectrodes in cerebellar cortex, Naunyn-Schmiedeberg's Arch. exp. Path. Pharmak., Suppl. to 302:R55.

8. Bruggencate, G., ten, Steinberg, R., Stöckle, H., and Nicholson, C., 1978, Modulation of extracellular Ca^{2+}- and K^+-levels in the mammalian cerebellar cortex, in: "Iontophoresis and Transmitter Mechanisms in the Mammalian Central Nervous System", R.W. Ryall and J.S. Kelly, eds., Elsevier/North-Holland Biomedical Press, Amsterdam, New York.

9. Coles, J.A., and Tsacopoulos, M., 1977, A method of making fine double-barreled potassium-sensitive microelectrodes for intracellular recording, J. Physiol. (Lond.), 270:12P.

10. Coray, A., Fry, C.H., Hess, P., McGuigan, J.A.S., and Weingart, R., 1980, Resting calcium in sheep cardiac tissue and in frog skeletal muscle measured with ion-selective microelectrodes, J. Physiol. (Lond.), in press.

11. Dahl, G., and Isenberg, G., 1980, Decoupling of heart muscle cells: correlation with increased cytoplasmic calcium activity and with changes of nexus ultrastructure, J. Membr. Biol., in press.

12. Deisz, R.A., and Lux, H.D., 1978, Intracellular chloride concentration and postsynaptic inhibition in crayfish stretch receptor neurons, Arzneim.-Forsch./Drug Res., 28:870.

13. DeLaat, S.W., Buwalda, R.J.A., and Habets,A.M.M.C., 1974, Intracellular ionic distribution, cell membrane permeability and membrane potential of the Xenopus egg during first cleavage, Exp. Cell Res., 89:1.

14. Eisenman, G., 1967, "Glass Electrodes for Hydrogen and Other Cations," M. Dekker Inc., New York.

15. Erne, D., Ammann, D., and Simon, W., 1979, Liquid membrane pH electrode based on a synthetic proton carrier, Chimia, (Switzerland) 33:88.

16. Erne, D., Stojanac, N., Ammann, D., Hofstetter, P., Pretsch, E., and Simon, W., Helv. Chim. Acta, in preparation.

17. Gardner-Medwin, A.R., and Nicholson, C., 1977, Measurements of extracellular potassium and calcium concentration during passage of current across the surface of the brain, J. Physiol. (Lond.), 275:66P.

18. Heinemann, U., Lux, H.D., and Gutnick, M.J., 1977, Extracellular free calcium and potassium during paroxysmal activity in the cerebral cortex of the cat, Exp. Brain Res., 27:237.

19. Heinemann, U., Lux, H.D., Gutnick, M.J., 1978, Changes in extracellular free calcium and potassium activity in the somatosensory cortex of cats, in: "Abnormal Neuronal Discharges," N. Chalazonitis and M. Boisson, eds., Raven Press, New York.

20. Hess, P., and Weingart, R., 1980, Intracellular free calcium modified by pH_i in sheep cardiac Purkinje fibres, J. Physiol. (Lond.), in press.

21. Heuser, D., Astrup, J., Lassen, N.A., Nilsson, B., Norberg, K., and Siesjo, B.K., 1977, Are H^+ and K^+ factors for the adjustment of cerebral blood flow to changes in functional state: a microelectrode study, in: "Cerebral Function Metabolism and Circulation," D.H. Ingvar and N.A. Lassen, eds., Acta neurol. scand., 56 (Suppl.) 64:216

22. Heuser, D., 1978, The significance of cortical extracellular H^+, K^+ and Ca^{2+} activities for regulation of local cerebral blood flow under conditions of enhanced neuronal activity, in: "Cerebral Vascular Smooth Muscle and its Control," Ciba Foundation Symp. 56, Elsevier Excerpta Medica, Amsterdam.

23. Heyer, C.B., and Lux, H.D., 1978,Unusual properties of the Ca-K system responsible for prolonged action potentials in neurons from the snail Helix pomatia, in: "Abnormal Neuronal Discharges," N. Chalazonitis and M. Boisson, eds., Raven Press, New York.

24. Hofmeier, G., and Lux, H.D., 1978, Time course of intracellular free calcium and related electrical effects after injection of $CaCl_2$, Pflügers Arch.ges. Physiol., Suppl. to 373:R47.

25. Kessler, M., Clark, L.C., Jr., Lübbers, D.W., Silver, I.A., and Simon, W., 1976, "Ion and Enzyme Electrodes in Biology and Medicine", Urban and Schwarzenberg, Munich, Berlin, Vienna.

26. Kessler, M., Höper, J., Schäfer, D., and Strehlau, R.,1977, Measurements of extracellular and of interstitial cation activity (pK, pNa, pCa) with ion-selective electrodes, Bibliotheca Anatomica, 15:237.

27. Khuri, R.N., 1976, Intracellular potassium in single cells of renal tubules, in: "Ion and Enzyme Electrodes in Biology and Medicine," M. Kessler, L.C. Clark, Jr., D.W. Lübbers, I.A. Silver, and W. Simon, eds., Urban and Schwarzenberg, Munich, Berlin, Vienna.

28. Khuri, R.N., 1978, Intracellular electrochemical potentials of K^+, Na^+, Cl^-, HCO_3^- and H^+ in cells of renal tubules, Arzneim.-Forsch./Drug Res., 28:880.

29. Kraig, R.P., and Nicholson, C., 1976, Sodium liquid ion exchanger microelectrode used to measure large extracellular sodium transients, Science, 194:725.

30. Kraig, R.P., and Nicholson, C.,1978, Extracellular ionic variations during spreading depression, Neurosci., 3:1045.

31. Lanter, F., Erne, D., Ammann, D., and Simon, W., 1980, Anal. Chem., in preparation.

32. Lavallée, M., Schanne, O.F., and Hebert, N.C., 1969, "Glass microelectrodes", Wiley and Sons, Inc., New York, London, Sydney, Toronto.

33. Levy, S., and Coles, J.A., 1977, Intracellular pH of Limulus ventral photoreceptor measured with a double-barrelled pH microelectrode, Experientia, 33:553.

34. Lux, H.D., and Hofmeier, G., 1978, Kinetics of the calcium-dependent potassium current in Helix neurons, Pflügers Arch. ges. Physiol., Suppl. to 373:R47.

35. Marban, E., Rink, T.J., Tsien, R.W., and Tsien, R.Y., 1980, Free calcium in ferret ventricular muscle at rest and in contracture, measured with ion-sensitive microelectrodes, J. Physiol. (Lond.), in press.

36. Morf, W.E., Ammann, D., Bissig, R., Pretsch, E., and Simon,W., 1979, Cation Selectivity of Neutral Macrocyclic and Nonmacrocyclic Complexing Agents in Membranes, in: "Progress in Macrocyclic Chemistry, Volume 1," M. Izatt and J.J. Christensen, eds., John Wiley and Sons, New York, Chichester, Brisbane, Toronto.

37. Nicholson, C., Steinberg, R., Stöckle, H., and ten Bruggencate, G., 1976, Calcium decrease associated with aminopyridine-induced potassium increase in cat cerebellum, Neurosci. Lett., 3:315.

38. Nicholson, C., ten Bruggencate, G., Steinberg, R., and Stöckle, H., 1977, Calcium modulation in brain extracellular microenvironment demonstrated with ion-selective micropipette, Proc. Natl. Acad. Sci., 74:1287.

39. Nicholson, C., ten Bruggencate, G., Stöckle, H., and Steinberg, R., 1978, Calcium and potassium changes in extracellular microenvironment of cat cerebellar cortex, J. Neurophysiol., 41:1026.

40. Nicholson, C., 1979, Brain cell micro-environment as a communication channel, in: "The Neurosciences Fourth Study Program," F.O. Schmitt, and F.G. Worden, eds., MIT Press, Cambridge,Mass.

41. O'Doherty, J., Garcia-Diaz, J.F., and Armstrong W. McD., 1979, Sodium-selective liquid ion-exchanger microelectrodes for intracellular measurements, Science, 203:1349.

42. Oehme, M., and Simon, W., 1976, Microelectrode for potassium ions based on a neutral carrier and comparison of its characteristics with a cation exchanger sensor, Anal. Chim. Acta, 86:21.

43. Oehme, M., 1977, Beitrag zur Entwicklung ionenselektiver Mini- und Mikroelektroden und zu deren Messtechnik, Thesis No. 5953, Swiss Federal Institute of Technology, Zurich.

44. Silver, I.A., 1975, Measurement of pH and ionic composition of pericellular sites. Phil. Trans. R. Soc. Lond. B., 271:261.

45. Simon, W., Ammann, D., Oehme, M., and Morf, W.E., 1978, Calcium-selective electrodes, Ann. N.Y. Acad. Sci., 307:52.

46. Sokol, J.H., Lee, C.O., and Lupo, F.J., 1979, Measurement of the free calcium ion concentration in sheep cardiac Purkinje fibres with neutral carrier Ca^{2+}-selective microelectrodes, Biophys. J. 25:143a.

47. Sonnhof, U., Bührle, Ch.Ph., and Richter, D.W., 1980, The action of glutamate upon the motoneuron's membrane investigated by measuring extra- and intracellular ion activities K^+, Ca^{2+}, Na^+, J. Physiol. (Lond.), in press.

48. Štefanac, Z., and Simon, W., 1967, Ion specific electrochemical behavior of macrotetrolides in membranes, Microchem. J., 12:125.

49. Steinberg, R., and Bruggencate G.,ten, 1978, Dependence of extra-cellular Ca^{2+} upon active transport mechanism in cerebellar cortex, Pflügers Arch., Europ. J. of Physiol., Suppl. to 373:R68.

50. Steiner, R.A., Oehme, M., Ammann, D., and Simon, W., 1979, Neutral carrier sodium ion-selective microelectrode for intracellular studies, Anal. Chem., 51:351.

51. Stöckle, H., Bruggencate, G.,ten, Nicholson, C., and Steinberg, R., 1977, Rhythmic modulation of extracellular Ca^{2+}- and K^+-levels in the cerebellar cortex related to climbing fibre activity, Pflügers Arch., Europ. J. of Physiol., Suppl. to 368:R37.

52. Thomas, R.C., Simon, W., and Oehme, M., 1975, Lithium accumulation by snail neurones measured by a new Li^+-sensitive microelectrode, Nature, London, 258:754.

53. Thomas, R.C., 1976, "Ion and Enzyme Electrodes in Biology and Medicine", M. Kessler, L.C. Clark, Jr., D.W.Lübbers, I.A. Silver and W. Simon, eds., Urban and Schwarzenberg, Munich, Berlin, Vienna.

54. Thomas, R.C., 1978, "Ion-sensitive intracellular microelectrodes", Academic Press, London, New York, San Francisco.

55. Tsien, R.Y., and Rink, T.J., 1980, Calcium selective microelectrodes are much improved by a new poly(vinylchloride)-gelled sensor, Science, in press.

56. Walker, J.L.,Jr., 1971, Ion-specific liquid ion exchanger microelectrodes, Anal. Chem., 43:89A.

57. Walker, J.L., and Brown, H.M., 1977, Intracellular ionic activity measurements in nerve and muscle, Physiological Reviews, 57:729.

58. Weingart, R., and Hess, P., in preparation.

59. Wuhrmann, P., Ineichen, H., Riesen-Willi, U., and Lezzi, M., 1979, Change in nuclear potassium electrochemical activity and puffing of potassium-sensitive salivary chromosome regions during Chironomus development, Proc. Natl. Acad. Sci. USA, 76:806.

SENSITIVITY OF K^+-SELECTIVE MICROELECTRODES TO pH AND SOME BIOLOGICALLY ACTIVE SUBSTANCES

N. Kříž and Eva Syková

Institute of Physiology
Czechoslovak Academy of Sciences
Vídeňská 1083, 142 20 Prague 4, Czechoslovakia

INTRODUCTION

Direct measurements of ion concentration changes in vivo became possible after the development of ion-selective microelectrodes (ISM) with a liquid ion-exchanger located in the shank of a glass micropipette tip (Walker, 1971). For potassium ISM, an organic resin Corning code 477317 was used as the ion-exchanger. This ion-exchanger employs 1-2-dimethyl-3-nitrobenzen for dissolving 2g/100 ml potassium tetrakis (p-chlorophenyl)borate (Baum and Wise, 1971). The relative selectivities of Corning ion-exchanger for some cations were first shown by Wise et al.(1970). The selectivities of the K^+-electrode for some interferring ions with respect to the principal ion were also determined by Moody and Thomas (1971), Walker (1971), Khuri et al. (1972) and others. Electrode potentials were measured in mixtures of constant ionic strength and appropriate selectivity constants were calculated – $K_{K,Ca} = 0.002$, $K_{K,H} = 0.025$, $K_{K,Na} = 0.02$, which are valid for ionic strength 0.1 mol.1^{-1} (Walker, 1971).

Recently, the ISM method was studied in more detail and microelectrodes were modified for different kinds of biological experiments (Khuri et al., 1972; Vyskočil and Kříž, 1972; Neher and Lux, 1973; Kříž et al., 1974). For review see Hník et al.(1980).

In all experiments using direct measurements of potassium concentration, changes in living tissues with ISM, the limited specificity of the Corning ion-exchanger must be considered. The limited specificity for potassium ions led us to study the selectivity of these electrodes for biological purposes in more detail.

MATERIAL AND METHODS

For our experiments we used either single or double-barrel ISMs. Their preparation was described in detail previously (Vyskočil and Kříž, 1972; Kříž et al., 1974). The ion-selective channel was filled with a column of liquid K^+-exchanger Corning code 477317 to a distance of 200-300 μm from the tip (approximately the previously siliconing part of tip) and the remaining volume of this channel was filled with 0.5 mol.1^{-1} KCl. In the case of double-barrel microelectrode the reference channel was injected with 0.15 mol.1^{-1} NaCl. The impedance of ISM electrodes was 100-500 MΩ.

Before each measurement, the ISMs were calibrated in a set of standard KCl solutions in the range of 1-100 mmol.1^{-1} K^+ with a stable content of 150 mmol.1^{-1} Na^+ as background, to give a solution of ionic composition as close as possible to that of the extracellular fluid. The sensitivity of potassium ISM to Na^+ in competition with K^+ is given by the value of selectivity constant $K_{K,Na}$ = 0.012 (Moody and Thomas, 1971; Vyskočil and Kříž, 1972) (compare with value $K_{K,Na}$ = 0.02, Walker, 1971). The limited selectivity of potassium ISM therefore causes a deviation from linearity in the calibration curve when plotted on a semilogarithmic scale at low K^+ concentrations – this applies below approximately 8 mol.1^{-1} K^+ (Kříž et al., 1974). Individual calibration curves were drawn for each electrode before and after the experimental measurements.

The recording technique was similar to that previously described (Kříž et al., 1974). The potassium ISM responses to changes in potassium concentration were recorded differentially between the reference and ion-selective microelectrodes by means of a DC differential, high-impedance preamplifier (R_{imp} 10^{14} Ω). The electrode responses were registered on a linear ink recorder (Labora EZ 5).

The selectivity of potassium ISM was tested against these drugs: acetylcholine chloride (Berlin-Chemie), ammonium chloride (Lachema), bicuculline (Sigma), choline chloride (Merck), γ-aminobutyric acid (Sigma), glycine (NBC), hydrochloride acid (Lachema), insulin (neutral-Zn, SPOFA), L-DOPA (SPOFA), L-glutamic acid (Mann), noradrenaline (SPOFA), picrotoxin (Fluka AG), serotonin (Koch-Light), sodium hydroxide (Lachema) and tetraethylammonium bromide (Lachema). All the drugs used for testing were dissolved either in freshly redistilled water or in saline containing 3 mmol.1^{-1} K^+ and 150 mmol.1^{-1} Na^+. For the pH experiments, we used sets of solutions with different H^+ activity prepared by combination of HCl or NaOH solutes, respectively.

RESULTS

The sensitivity of potassium selective microelectrodes to changes in H^+ activity

The sensitivity of potassium ISM to changes in H^+ activity was tested in the range 10^{-12} to 10^{-1} mol.1^{-1} in solutions prepared by the addition of HCl or NaOH to redistilled water (record A in Fig. 1). At least two factors influence the shape of curve A besides pH: a) the addition of NaOH increases the concentration of sodium ions to which the electrodes are also sensitive, b) the total ionic strength of the solution is altered during each addition of HCl or NaOH.

Subsequent measurements were therefore performed in a suitable electrolyte medium in which the total ionic strength was maintained constant (curve B in Fig. 1) by adjusting the amount of NaCl added

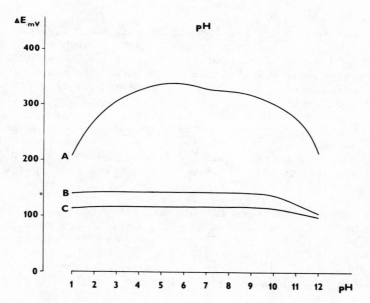

Fig. 1. The effect of changes in H^+ activity on the potential of the potassium selective microelectrode. pH measurements were performed with 10 microelectrodes; the results obtained with one of the electrodes: A - ISM in solutions of various pH, prepared by addition of HCl or NaOH to pure redistilled water. B - the sodium content was maintained constant to maintain the total ionic strength at 0.15 mol.1^{-1} (in the pH range 3-12 with 1 % accuracy). C - pH measurements in solutions with a stable composition of 3 mmol.1^{-1} K^+ and 150 mmol.1^{-1} Na^+, ionic strength 0.153 mol.1^{-1}.

into the medium. The ionic strength 0.15 mol.1^{-1} was held constant with a 1 % accuracy which can be maintained only in the pH range of 3.0 to 12.0. Curve C represents the pH measurements in solutions with a stable content of 3 mmol.1^{-1} K^+ and 150 mmol.1^{-1} Na^+, – with a total ion strength of 0.153 mol.1^{-1}. Thus, if the total ionic strength is maintained constant, the potential of the potassium ISM is not affected by changes in H^+ activity over the range of pH 2 to 9.

The sensitivity of potassium selective microelectrode to some biologically active substances

A group of biologically active substances was tested and classified according to their effect on the potassium ISM potential.

Glycine, γ-amino butyric acid, insulin. The first group of drugs included glycine, γ-amino butyric acid GABA and insulin. These drugs had no effect on the potassium ISM potential even in the following highest concentrations: glycine: 1 mol.1^{-1}, GABA: 0.1 mol.1^{-1}, insulin: 1 unit/ml.

Picrotoxin and bicuculline. Picrotoxin had no effect on the potassium ISM potential even in the highest concentration employed, namely 2×10^{-3} mol.1^{-1}. Bicuculline in the highest concentration used for testing, 2×10^{-4} mol.1^{-1}, caused a potential change of ISM 2-3 mV. This potential shift had a stable incremental value under different potassium concentrations.

L-DOPA, L-glutamic acid, noradrenaline. Several drugs had only a barely perceptible effect on the potassium ISM potential, especially in solutions containing 3 mmol.1^{-1} K^+ and 150 mmol.1^{-1} Na^+. This effect is seen more clearly if a drug solution is prepared in redistilled water.

Fig. 2 shows the results obtained after testing L-DOPA. As may be seen, the effect of L-DOPA on ISM potential was detectable at concentrations above 10^{-4} mol.1^{-1}. The action of L-glutamic acid on the ISM potential is shown in Fig. 3. Its interaction could be observed above 10^{-5} mol.1^{-1}. The effect of noradrenaline on the ISM potentil was observed from a concentration of 6×10^{-5} mol.1^{-1} upwards (Fig.4).

Serotonin, acetylcholine, choline. Serotonin and choline derivates were most effective in producing significant changes of potassium ISM membrane potential. The results obtained with serotonin are shown in Fig.5. Serotonin in redistilled water solutions substantially change the ISM potential above a concentration of 10^{-5} mol.1^{-1}. The potential decreased in the concentration range from 10^{-5} mol.1^{-1} to 10^{-3} mol.1^{-1} with a slope of 75 mV per 10 fold concentration increase.

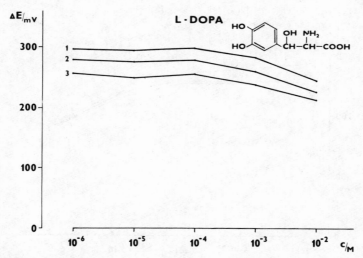

Fig. 2. The effect of various concentrations of L-DOPA on the potential of potassium selective microelectrodes. 1,2,3 - results from three different electrodes. In 1) 296 mV, in 2) 279 mV and in 3) 257 mV potential in redistilled water.

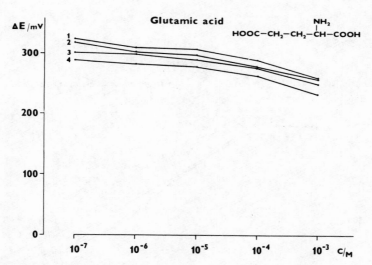

Fig. 3. The effect of various concentrations of L-glutamic acid on the potential of potassium selective microelectrodes. 1,2, 3,4 - results from four different electrodes. In 1) 324 mV, in 2) 318 mV, in 3) 302 mV and in 4) 289 mV potential in redistelled water.

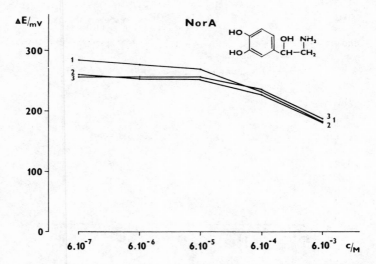

Fig. 4. The effect of various concentrations of noradrenaline on the potential of a potassium selective microelectrode. 1,2,3 - results from three different electrodes. In 1) 284 mV, in 2) 260 mV and in 3) 256 mV potential in redistilled water.

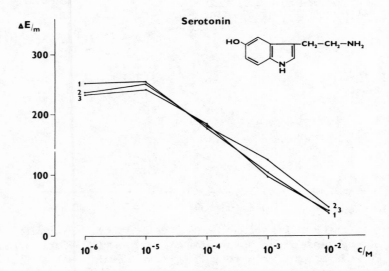

Fig. 5. The effect of various concentrations of serotonin on the potential of potassium selective microelectrodes. 1,2,3 - results from three different electrodes. In 1) 252 mV, in 2) 237 mV and in 3) 233 mV potential in redistilled water.

The results for choline and acetylcholine are shown in Fig. 6 and Fig. 7. The solid lines are used for results obtained with three different electrodes in aqueous solution. When aqueous solutions of these drugs are used, the potential is altered above concentrations of 10^{-6} mol.1^{-1}. In the region of 10^{-5}mol.1^{-1} to 10^{-4} mol.1^{-1} the potential rapidly falls with a slope of about 100 mV and 180 mV per 10-fold change in concentration for choline and acetylcholine, respectively. The broken lines represent experiments where these drugs were dissolved in saline solution; the ISM potential was affected above the concentration about 5×10^{-5} mol.1^{-1}.

Ammonium chloride, tetraethylammonium bromide

The results of the responses of potassium ISM to ammonium ions NH_4^+ are shown in Fig. 8. The solid lines depict NH_4^+ measurements in redistilled water with three electrodes. The same electrodes were used for calibration in potassium solutions within the same range of concentrations – broken line. We compared the potentials obtained with electrodes in NH_4^+ and K^+ solutions and calculated the selectivity constant for NH_4^+, namely $K_{K,NH_4} = 0.27$, which is valid for the NH_4^+ tested concentration range.

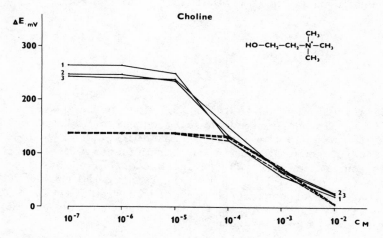

Fig. 6. The effect of various concentrations of choline on the potential of potassium selective microelectrodes. 1,2,3 – results from three different electrodes. Solid line – experiments using choline solutions in redistilled water. Broken line – results obtained with the same electrode using choline solutions in 3 mmol.1^{-1} K^+ and 150 mmol.1^{-1} Na^+.

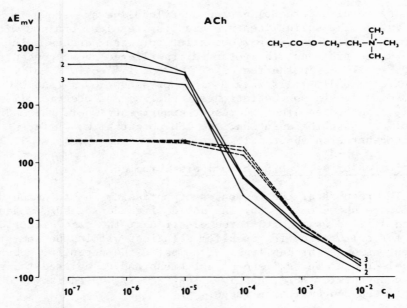

Fig. 7. The effect of various concentrations of acetylcholine on
the potential of potassium selective microelectrodes. 1,2,3
– results from three different electrodes. Solid line – the
response of ISM to ACh in aqueous solutions. Broken line-
results obtained with the same electrode in ACh solutions
containing 3 mmol.1^{-1} K$^+$ and 150 mmol.1^{-1}Na$^+$.

The selectivity constant for NH$_4$$^+$ concentrations from 1 to 10
mmol.1^{-1} was also determined in solutions with a stable content of
150 mmol.1^{-1} Na$^+$. In the upper section of Fig. 8 an example of such
evaluation is shown. The solid curve represents electrode calibration
in an aqueous solution of NH$_4$$^+$. The broken curve corresponds to
electrode calibration in solutions containing 150 mmol.1^{-1} Na$^+$, whereas the potassium concentration was changed from 1 to 10 mmol.1^{-1}.
The selectivity constant K_{K,NH_4} was the same as that calculated from
aqueous solutions of NH$_4$ and K$^+$.

The effect of tetraethylammonium (TEA) on the potential of potassium ISM is shown in Fig. 9. Measurements were made with three
different electrodes in TEA solutions containing 3 mmol.1^{-1} K$^+$ and
150 mmol.1^{-1} Na$^+$ as back round. The ISM potential was affected from
the concentration of 10^{-3} mol.1^{-1} upwards and fell rapidly down to
reverse values at the inflection point of about 10^{-2} mol.1^{-1}.

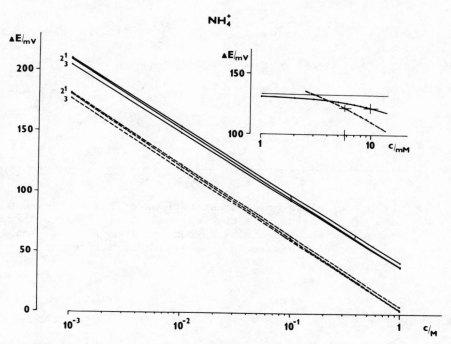

Fig. 8. Changes in the potential of potassium selective microelectrodes evoked by various ooncentrations of ammonium ion. 1, 2 3 - results from three different electrodes. Solid line - results obtained with NH_4^+ solutions prepared in redistille water. Broken line - results obtained with NH_4^+ solutions containing 3 mmol.1^{-1} K^+ and 150 mmol.1^{-1}. Upper insert - shows an example of the evaluation of the selectivity constant for ammonium ions. Solid curve - calibration of ISM obtained in aqueous solutions of 1-10 mmol.1^{-1} NH_4^+. Broken curve - calibration of the same electrode in solutions containing potassium in the concentration range from 1 to 10 mmol.1^{-1} with 150 mmol.1^{-1} of Na^+ as background.

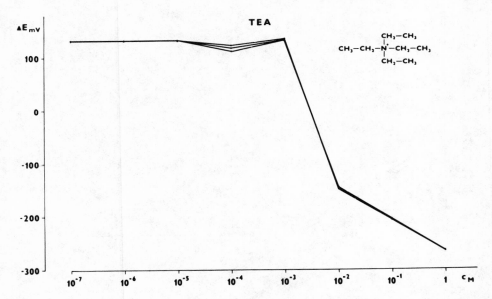

Fig. 9. The effect of various concentrations of TEA on the potential of potassium selective microelectrode. TEA solutions
prepared with a stable background of 3 mmol.l^{-1} K$^+$ and 150
mmol.l^{-1} Na$^+$. Measurements were made with three microelectrodes.

DISCUSSION

We tested such biologically active substances, the concentration
of which may be altered even under physiological conditions. For
example, during muscle work local pH changes occur. We therefore
studied the sensitivity of ISM to pH changes. The influence of H$^+$
activity changes on the ISM potential was mentioned by Walker (1971).
He tried to evaluate this influence by calculating the selectivity
constant - $K_{K,H}$ = 0.025 valid for constant ionic strength 0.1 mmol.l^{-1}
and $K_{K,H}$ = 0.016 for ionic strength 1.0 mmol.l^{-1}. In experiments of
Khuri et al., 1972 in the salt standards used the effect of pH was
found to be negligible between pH 5 and 8. In our experiments the
potential of ISM was not affected by changes in H$^+$ activity within
the range of pH 2 to 9, if the total ionic strength was maintained
constant 0.15 mol.l^{-1} by adding Na$^+$. In the presence of K$^+$ (3 mmol.l^{-1}
K$^+$, 150 mmol.l^{-1} Na$^+$, total ionic strength 0.153 mol.l^{-1}) we obtained the same results. Our results are in good agreement with the findings of Moody and Thomas (1971) valid for 100 mmol.l^{-1} K$^+$ solutions.

The element common to the whole group of active drugs tested is
the presence of the NH-group, which is located at various sites in

Table 1. Concentration of some biologically - active substances in the central nervous system

Compound	Part of brain - animal	Concentration nmol/g wet	References
Acetylcholine	Whole brain		Collier,B. et al.,
	- mouse	13.9	(1972)
	- rat	18.9	Cambell,L.B. et al. (1970)
Ammonia	One hemisphere		Kandera, J. et al.
	- rat	986	(1968)
		1940	Shaw, R.K. and Heine, J.D. (1965)
	Whole brain		Tews,J.K. and Stone,
	- mouse	430	W.E. (1965)
Dopamine	Whole brain		Welch, B.L. and Welch
	- mouse (excl. bulb.olfact.)	4.88	A.S. (1968)
	- rat	4.37	Häggendal, J.(1967)
GABA	One hemisphere		Kandera,J. et al.
	- rat	2330	(1968)
		1520	Shaw, R.K. and Heine, J.D. (1965)
	Whole brain		Agrawal, H.C. et al.
	- mouse	2520	(1968)
	- cat	1370	Himwich, W.A. and Agrawal,H.C. (1969)
Glutamic acid	One hemisphere		Kandera, J. et al.
	- rat	11570	(1968)
		9260	Shaw, R.K. and Heine, J.D. (1965)
	Whole brain		Agrawal,H.C. et al.,
	- mouse	11500	(1968)
	- cat	7870	Himwich, W.A. and Agrawal, H.C. (1969)
Glycine	One hemisphere		Kandera, J. et al.
	- rat	629	(1968)
		830	Shaw,R.K. and Heine, J.D. (1965)

Table 1 - continued

Compound	Part of brain - animal	Concentration n mol/g wet	References
	Whole brain - mouse - cat	1610 780	Agrawal,H.C. et al. (1968) Himwich,W.A. and Agrawal,H.C. (1969)
Choline	Whole brain - mouse One hemisphere - rat	29.2 8.7	Gibson,G.E. and Blass, J.P. (1976) Mann,S.P. and Hebb,C. (1977)
Noradrenaline	Brain - mouse (excl. bulb.olfactor.) - rat	2.70 1.95	Welch,B.L. and Welch,A.S. (1968) Häggendal,J. (1967)
Serotonin	Brain - mouse - rat	4.77 1.42	Valzelli, L. (1967) Bertaccini, G. (1959)

different molecules in the simple form or with various substituents. It has been reported in the literature that the sensitivity of potassium ISM (Corning resin) to NH_4^+ by comparison with K^+ ions is given by the value of the selectivity constant $K_{K,NH_4} = 0.023$ (Moody and Thomas, 1971). The sensitivity of the electrode is twice as great for NH_4^+ as for Na^+ $K_{K,Na} = 0.012$. From our measurements it follows that the sensitivity of potassium ISM to NH_4^+ is much higher than previously reported. The value of the selectivity constant determined from both series of experiments performed in redistilled water or in saline solutions, is the same - namely K_{K,NH_4^+} 0.27, which is 10 times higher than that quoted by Moody and Thomas 1971 and in good agreement with the finding of Wise et al. (1970).

This relatively high sensitivity to NH_4^+, however, cannot explain the potential change in the presence of serotonin (containing NH_2 and NH groups) above concentration of 10^{-5} mol.1^{-1}, which is higher than the theoretical Nernstian relationship. A similar situation occurs with other molecules containing a quaternary nitrogen N^x for example: choline, acetylcholine and TEA. The sensitivity of potassium ISM to these substances is so high that above a certain concentration the electrode ceases to function as an ISM sensitive to K^+ and the membrane potential value shifts up to very high values with the reverse polarity. From the physico-chemical point of view, this potential change of ISM cannot only be an electrochemical response induced by changes in drug concentration and one could expect some physical interaction with the ion-exchanger membrane. At higher concentrations, choline and acetylcholine probably form stronger complexes with the ion-exchanger molecule than K^+. This is supported by the fact that the potassium selective microelectrode membrane is based on an analogous principle as the ion-selective electrode resin for various choline esters (Baum, 1972).

It is possible to assume that each molecule containing N^x could affect the potential of the potassium ISM. From the molecular configuration and position of the NH-group it is possible to predict the intensity of the interaction. According to the literature (Neher and Lux, 1973), the extent of interaction between an active drug molecule and the ISM membrane depends on the carbon chain length of the substituent. But according to our experiments this can only be an approximate guide. We can thus conclude that after using the ISM in solutions of choline and acetylcholine at concentrations up to 10^{-2} $mol.1^{-1}$ these substances may be removed from the ISM membrane, while after addition of TEA 10^{-3} $mol.1^{-1}$ the principal function of the ISM membrane - namely its selective response to a change in K^+ concentration - becomes inoperative.

We tested the sensitivity of ISM to convulsive drugs bicuculline and picrotoxin which are used in pharmacological and physiological experiments in the central nervous system (CNS). There is no quaternary N^x in the molecules of picrotoxinin or picrotin, which in an equimolecular mixture form picrotoxin ($C_{30}H_{34}O_{13}$), and also no effect on the potential of the ISM, even at a concentration of $2x10^{-3}$ $mol.1^{-1}$. But bicuculline which has a nitrogen group ($C_{20}H_{17}N O_6$), caused a slight potential change at the highest concentrations ($2x10^{-4}$ $mol.1^{-1}$). This potential shift of 2-3 mV had stable increment values for different potassium concentrations.

Furthermore, we should stress one more point. We also tested a few drugs from the large number of those which might influence the potassium ISM membrane potential. Nevertheless, we can conclude that especially the substances with N^x or NH_2 groups could influence the ISM sensitivity for potassium. In Table 1 a short survey is given of substances tested with several examples of their concentrations in the CNS of the mouse and rat. It is evident that some of them (glutamic acid, ammonia) in physiological concentration can interfer during detection of potassium concentration changes. It is therefore necessary to take this possibility into account during experiments with potassium ISM (Corning resin) not only in the CNS but in all tissues where such biologically active substances could be present as synaptic transmitters or where changes in their concentration could occur.

REFERENCES

Agrawal, H.C., Davis, J.M., and Himwich, W.A., 1968, Developmental changes in mouse brain: weight, water content and free amino acids, J. Neurochem., 15:917.

Baum, G., 1972, The influence of hydrophobic interaction on the electrochemical selectivity ratios or liquid membrane responsive to organic ions, J. Phys.Chem., 76:1872.

Baum, G., and Wise, W.M., 1971, U.S.Pat.no. 3,598,713, Aug. 10.

Bertaccini, G., 1959, Effect of convulsant treatment on the 5-hydroxytryptamine content of brain and other tissues of the cat, J. Neurochem., 4:217.

Cambell, L.B., Hanin, I., and Jenden, D.J., 1970, Gas chromatographic evaluation of the effects of some muscarinic and antimuscarinic drugs on acetylcholine and choline levels in the rat, Biochem. Pharmacol., 19:2053.

Gibson, G.E., and Blass, J.P., 1976, Impaired synthesis of ACh in brain accompanying mild hypoxia and hypoglycemia, J. Neurochem., 27:37.

Häggendal, J., 1967, The effect of high pressure air or oxygen with and without carbon dioxide added on the catechol amine levels of rat brain, Acta physiol.scand., 69:147.

Himwich, W.A., and Agrawal, H.C., 1969, Amino Acids, Table I, in: "Handbook of Neurochemistry I, Chemical Architecture of the Nervous System", Abel Lajtha, ed., Plenum Press, New York.

Hník, P., Syková Eva, Kříž, N., and Vyskočil, F., 1980, Determination of ion activity changes in excitable tissues with ion-selective microelectrodes, in: Medical and Biological Applications of Electrochemical Devices, J. Koryta, ed., John Wiley & Sons Ltd., New York.

Kandera, J., Levi, G., and Lajtha, A., 1968, Control of cerebral metabolite levels. II. Amino acid uptake and levels in various areas of the rat brain, Arch. Biochem.Biophys., 126:249.

Khuri, R.N., Hajjar, J.J., and Agulian, S.K., 1972, Measurement of intracellular potassium with liquid ion-exchange microelectrodes, J. Appl.Physiol., 32:419.

Kříž, N., Syková, E., Ujec, E., and Vyklický, L., 1974, Changes of extracellular potassium concentration induced by neuronal activity in the spinal cord of the cat, J. Physiol.(Lond.), 278:1.

Mann, S.P., and Hebb, C., 1977, Free choline in the brain of the rat, J. Neurochem., 28:241.

Moody, G.J., and Thomas, J.D.R., 1971, Table 29, in: "Selective Ion Sensitive Electrodes", Merrow, G. Britain,

Neher, E., and Lux, H.D., 1973, Rapid changes of potassium concentration at the outer surface of exposed single neurons during membrane flow, J.gen.Physiol., 61:385.

Shaw, R.K., and Heine, J.D., 1965, Ninhydrin positive substances present in different areas of normal rat brain, J. Neurochem.,12:151

Tews, J.K., and Stone, W.E., 1965, in: Progress in Brain Research, Horizons in Neuropsychopharmacology, W.A.Himwich and J.P.Schade, eds., Elsevier, Amsterdam.

Valzelli, L., 1967, Excerpta Medica International Congress Ser.No.129, in: Proc. 5th Int.Cong.of Neuro-psycho-pharmacology, Washington (1966).

Vyskočil, F., and Kříž, N., 1972, Modifications of single and double-barrel potassium specific microelectrodes for physiological experiments, Pflüg.Arch., 33⁻ 265.

Walker, J.L.,Jr., 1971, Ion specific liquid ion exchanger microelectrodes, Analyt.Chem., 43:89A.

Welch,B.L., and Welch, A.S., 1968, Greater lowering of brain and adrenal catecholamines in group-housed than in individually-housed mice administered DL-α-methylthyrosine, J.Pharm.Pharmacol.,20:244

Wise, W.M., Kurey, M.J., and Baum, G., 1970, Direct potentiometric measurement of potassium in blood serum with liquid ion-exchange electrode, Clin.Chem., 16:103.

DOUBLE-BARREL ION SELECTIVE [K^+, Ca^{2+}, Cl^-] COAXIAL MICROELECTRODES (ISCM) FOR MEASUREMENTS OF SMALL AND RAPID CHANGES IN ION ACTIVITIES

E. Ujec, O.Keller, N. Kříž, V. Pavlík and J. Machek

Institute of Physiology
Czechoslovak Academy of Sciences
Vídeňská 1083, 142 20 Prague 4, Czechoslovakia

INTRODUCTION

Double-barrel liquid ion-exchanger microelectrodes (ISM) are used at present to measure concentration changes in biological tissues (Lux et al., 1972; Vyklický et al., 1972; Vyskočil et al., 1972; Hník et al., 1972; Lux and Neher, 1973; Oehme et al., 1976). The ISM (K^+, Ca^{2+}, Cl^-) have a longitudinal resistance (R_e) from 200 MΩ to 2 GΩ.

The transfer properties of the ISM can be substantially improved by reducing the longitudinal resistance (R_e) of the ion sensitive channel and by adjusting its geometry to that of the reference barrel. This was achieved by employing a thin micropipette as the reference barrel and by introducing a similar thin micropipette coaxially into the column of the ion exchanger in the thicker ion-sensitive barrel. It was assumed that by reducing the distance between the inner and outer tips, the longitudinal resistance (R_e), as well as the electrical time constant (τ_e) and the noise level (N) will be substantially reduced.

ELECTRICAL AND ELECTROCHEMICAL PRINCIPLES OF ISCM

The thin micropipette was introduced under visual control into the column of the ion-exchanger by means of a horizontal micromanipulator. Ramp pulses applied to this channel were used for assessing R_e and τ_e during coaxial insertion (Fig. 1 - inset).

The exponential relationship between the longitudinal resistance (R_e) and the intertip distance (d_{o-i}) of the inner and outer micro-

41

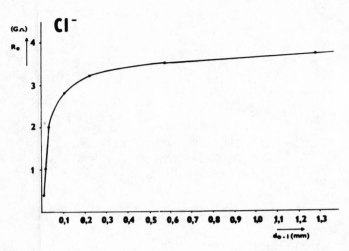

Fig. 1.   Exponential relationship between the R_e of Cl^- liquid ion-
          exchanger (Corning code 477315) and the distance between
          the tip of the outer and the tip of the inner micro-
          pipettes (d_{o-i}) of the ion sensitive ISCM channel.

pipette was found for the K^+, Cl^- and Ca^{2+} sensitive microelectrodes
and is demonstrated for a Cl^- electrode (Fig. 1). Graphical extrapolation (Ujec et al., 1980) of this relationship is in agreement
with the equation:

$$R_e = R_o + R_i$$

i.e. the total longitudinal resistance of the ion-selective channel
R_e equals the sum of the ion-exchanger resistance between the outer
and inner tips R_o and of the longitudinal resistance of the inserted
micropipette R_i.

     In arrangement with this relationship, the shortening of the
ion-exchanger columns reduced the resistance of microelectrodes
filled with a) Simon's Ca^{2+} synthetic neutral carrier from 0.5 -
1 GΩ to 40-100 MΩ ; b) Cl^- sensitive Corning code 477315 from
2,5 - 4 GΩ to 200-500 MΩ ; c) K^+ sensitive Corning code 477317 from
150 - 600 MΩ to 10-60 MΩ .

     The decrease of the resistance from 2 GΩ to 200 MΩ reduced
the noise level from 3 mV (pp) to 0.6 mV (pp), in both the Cl^- and
Ca^{2+} exchangers. The reduction of R_e in the potassium ISCMs and
calcium ISCMs from 200 MΩ to 20 MΩ decreased the noise level from
0.6 mV to less than 100 μV (pp).

     The fidelity of the measurements of the fast changes in ionic
activities is ensured by the proper relationship of constants in-

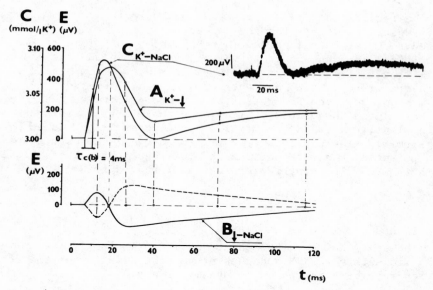

Fig. 2. K^+ transient evoked by peripheral stimulation (somatosensory cortex of the cat) which proves the relationship $C_{K^+-NaCl} = A_{K^+-\downarrow} + B_{\downarrow-NaCl}$.

herent in the system. The electrical time constant τ_e of the ion selective channel must be smaller than the time constant of the ion-concentration change τ_c, and this τ_c must be smaller than the time constant of the ion-concentration change as measured in the biological preparation $\tau_{c(b)}$ (Oehme et al., 1976), so that

$$\tau_e \ll \tau_c < \tau_{c(b)}$$

The electrical time constants measured by the Ramp-system were shorter than 100 µs for all three ion-exchangers tested. The concentration time constants τ_c were measured iontophoretically (Ujec et al., 1973) and also in flowing solutions (Ujec et al., 1979; 1980). For the K^+ exchanger $\tau_c = 1.5$ ms; for the Ca^{2+} exchanger $\tau_c = 7$ ms and for the Cl^- exchanger $\tau_c = 5$ ms. The most rapid $\tau_{c(b)}$ measured in our experiments with the potassium ISCM was 4 ms (Fig. 2).

The records demonstrate the high fidelity of the transfer properties of the recording system.

The records in Fig. 2 were taken with a potassium ISCM from the somatosensory cortex of the cat evoked by a single electrical pulse applied to a peripheral nerve. In the right hand column of Fig. 2 the original records are shown which were redrawn and are shown in the left half of the figure. The upper curve (C_K^+ – NaCl) is a differential record of the K^+ concentration change. The middle (A_K^+ – ↓) is a monopolarly recorded potential difference between the ion-sensitive barrel and the ground, which means that it represents the sum of the electrical field potential and the potential produced by the potassium transient. The lower curve ($B_↓$ – NaCl) represents the evoked field potential measured between the reference channel of the ISCM and the ground. The graphical solution of the equation is:

$$C_K^+{}_{-NaCl} = A_K^+{}_{-↓} + B_{↓-NaCl}$$

If this equation is expressed as $-B_{↓-NaCl} - A_K^+{}_{-↓} - C_K^+{}_{-NaCl}$ it can be seen that B – (broken curve) mirrors exactly the curve of the field potential B and thus proves the fidelity of the ion activity recording in the whole dynamic range.

CONCLUSION

The ISCM is characterized not only by a rapid response and reduced noise level but also by similar transfer properties of the thin reference channel and the coaxially inserted inner micropipette. The tenfold reduction of the longitudinal resistance (R_e), the fivefold decrease of the electrical time constants (τ_e) and noise level (N) brought the values of these parameters of the ion-sensitive channel close to those of the reference channel so that the resolving power of the ISCMs increased five times.

Given the electrical transfer properties of the ISCM are optimally set, the response time also depends on the diffusion processes on the interfaces of the microelectrodes (see Koryta, this volume). This circumstance finds its practical expression in a different time constant of the concentration changes (τ_c) as measured with different ion exchangers (Ca^{2+}, Cl^-, K^+). The new type of microelectrodes (ISCM) made it possible to record rapid and small K^+ activity changes in the order of tens of $\mu mol.l^{-1}$ in the frog dorsal root ganglion (Ujec et al., 1979) and in the somatosensory cortex of the cat (Keller et al., present volume).

REFERENCES

Hník, P., Vyskočil, F., Kříž, N., and Holas, M., 1972, Work-induced increase of extracellular potassium concentration in muscle measured by ion-specific electrodes, Brain Res., 40:559.
Lux, H.D., Neher, E., and Prince, E., 1972, K^+-activity determinations in cat cortex, Pflügers Arch., (Suppl.),332:177.

Lux, H.D., and Neher, E., 1973, The equilibrations time course of $[K^+]_o$ in cat cortex, Exp. Brain Res., 17:190.

Oehme, M., Kessler, M., and Simon, W., 1976, Neutral carrier Ca^{2+} -microelectrode, Chimia, 30:204.

Ujec, E., Kříž, N., Syková, E., and Vyklický, L., 1973, The changes of the K^+ concentration in a model of an extracellular space in CNS, Physiol. bohemoslov., 22:443.

Ujec, E., Keller, O., Machek, J., and Pavlík, V., 1979, Low impedance coaxial K^+ selective microelectrodes, Pflügers Arch., 382:189.

Ujec, E., Keller, O., Kříž, N., Machek, J., and Pavlík V., 1980, Low impedance coaxial ion selective double barrelled microelectrodes for biological measurements, Bioelectrochemistry and Bioenergetics, 7:363.

Vyklický, L., Syková, E., Kříž, N., and Ujec, E., 1972, Post-stimulation changes of extracellular potassium concentration in the spinal cord of the cat, Brain Res., 45:608.

Vyskočil, F., Kříž, N., and Bureš, J., 1972, Potassium-selective microelectrodes used for measuring the extracellular brain potassium during spreading depression and anoxic depolarization in rats, Brain Res., 39:255.

DETERMINATION OF SELECTIVITY COEFFICIENTS OF ION-SELECTIVE MICROELECTRODES

Chin O. Lee

Department of Physiology and Biophysics
Cornell University Medical College
New York, N.Y. 10021

INTRODUCTION

The application of an ion-selective microelectrode to measurements of ion activities requires a determination of its selectivity coefficient, i.e. the ability of a given ion-selective microelectrode to distinguish between the primary ion and the interfering ion. For the measurements of intracellular Na, Ca, Cl, and extracellular K ion activities, it is necessary to determine accurately the selectivity coefficient of each microelectrode because interfering ion activities are much greater than the primary ion activities. In this study we have attempted to evaluate the methods used usually for determining the selectivity coefficients as well as a method modified from others. For this evaluation, selectivity coefficients of recessed-tip and protruded-tip Na^+-selective glass microelectrodes were determined by the various methods and examined.

EQUATIONS FOR DETERMINING SELECTIVITY COEFFICIENTS

Selectivity coefficients of ion-selective electrodes are determined usually by mixture solution method (MSM), fixed interference method (FIM), or separate solution method (SSM). In the MSM, the potential, E of an ion-selective microelectrode is measured with a mixture solution containing the primary ion, A and the interfering ion, B. Thus the selectivity coefficient, k_{AB} is calculated by the following equation:

$$k_{AB} = \left\{ 10^{(E - E_0)/S} - \alpha_A \right\} / (\alpha_B)^{z_A/z_B} \qquad (1)$$

where E_0 is a constant potential of a microelectrode including the potential at phase boundary of the inside of ion-selective microelectrode, the reference electrode potential, and the junction potential. S is an empirical slope of response function (calibration curve) of an ion-selective microelectrode. α_A and α_B are activities of the primary ion, A and the interfering ion, B respectively. z_A and z_B are integers with sign and mangitude corresponding to the charge of the ions A and B respectively. In the FIM*, the potential of an ion-selective microelectrode is measured with solutions of constant level of interfering ion activity, α_B and varying activity of the primary ion, α_A. The potential values obtained are plotted against the activity of the primary ion. The intersection of the extrapolation of the linear portions of this curve will indicate the values of α_A which are to be used to calculate a k_{AB} from the following equation:

$$k_{AB} = \alpha_A / (\alpha_B)^{z_A/z_B} \tag{2}$$

In the SSM, two potentials of an ion-selective microelectrode are measured with each of two separate solutions. One (E_A) is measured with the solution containing the primary ion A at the activity α_A, and the other E_B with that containing the interfering ion B at the activity α_B. Thus a k_{AB} is calculated by the following equation:

$$k_{AB} = \frac{\alpha_A}{(\alpha_B)^{z_A/z_B}} \cdot 10^{(E_B - E_A)/S} \tag{3}$$

A different kind of equation for calculating k_{AB} is introduced:

$$k_{AB} = \frac{1}{(\alpha_B)^{z_A/z_B}} \cdot 10^{(E_B - E_0)/S} \tag{4}$$

This equation has the interfering ion activity (α_B) alone and the potential (E_B) measured with the solution containing the interfering ion. All the parameters in equation (4) were described above.

All the equations shown above are modifications or rearrangements of Nicolsky equation:

$$E = E_0 + S \log \left\{ \alpha_A + k_{AB}(\alpha_B)^{z_A/z_B} \right\} \tag{5}$$

*(IUPAC Recommendations for Nomenclature of Ion-Selective Electrodes, 1976, Pure Appl. Chem., 48:127.)

Each method mentioned above requires different experimental procedures and parameters to determine k_{AB}. For practical purposes, it is desirable that a method be as simple as possible and as accurate as possible. Equation (1) of the MSM requires that α_A and α_B in a mixture solution be known. However it is complicated and difficult to determine accurate ion activities in a mixture solution (Robinson and Stokes, 1965). The ions A and B in a mixture solution may have different activity coefficients. The k_{AB} value may be influenced substantially by a small change in α_A in a mixture solution containing ions A and B where the activity of A ions is much lower than that of ion B. An example may be a mixture solution containing 10 mmol/l NaCl and 150 mmol/l KCl for calibration of a Na^+-selective microelectrode (see RESULTS). In the FIM using equation (2), many potentials are measured with the calibration solutions for obtaining a calibration curve. It is also required to determine the primary ion activities in the mixture solutions. However, the calibration solutions at both ends of the curve become nearly pure solutions containing the primary ion or the interfering ion. This is conceivable because equation (2) is obtained from equation (3) at $E_A = E_B$. In the SSM, equation (3) requires that the potentials E_A and E_B be measured with the pure solution containing the primary ion A and that containing the interfering ion B. However, k_{AB} depends on the interfering ion activity α_B when the slope of a microelectrode response to the interfering ion is not linear or different from that to the primary ion. In this case one may select the pure solutions containing α_A and α_B which are roughly similar to those in a sample solution to be tested. Equation (4) requires the potential (E_B) measured with a pure solution containing the interfering ion activity α_B which is roughly similar to that in the sample solution to be tested. The ion activity coefficients of pure electrolyte solutions are known and can be reliably calculated.

RESULTS

Na^+-selective microelectrodes with recessed-tip and protruded-tip were made from Eisenman's NAS 11-18 glass as described previously (Lee, 1979). In the recessed-tip microelectrodes, insulating micropipettes had tip diameters of about 1 μm or less. To determine selectivity coefficients, potentials of the microelectrodes were measured with the solutions: 10 mmol/l NaCl (γ_{Na} = 0.9023; α_{Na} = 9.023 mmol/l), 100 mmol NACl (γ_{Na} = 0.7785; α_{Na} = 77.85 mmol/l), 10 mmol/l NaCl + 100 mmol/l KCl (γ_{mix} = 0.7555; α_{Na} = 7.555 mmol/l; α_K = 75.55 mmol/l), 10 mmol/l NaCl + 150 mmol/l KCl (γ_{mix} = 0.7280; α_{Na} = 7.28 mmol/l; α_K = 109.2 mmol/l), 100 mmol/l KCl (γ_K = 0.7625; α_K = 76.25 mmol/l), and 150 mmol/l KCl (γ_K = 0.7327; α_K = 109.9 mmol/l). The activity coefficients(γ) of the solutions were calculated by extended Debye-Huckel equation (Robinson and Stokes, 1965). The calculated activity coefficients of the pure solutions are in good agreement with their mean activity coefficients determined ex-

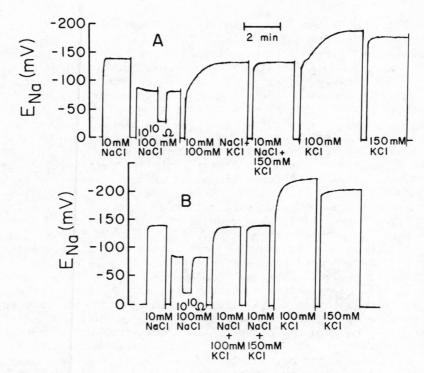

Fig. 1. Potential recordings of the Na$^+$-selective glass micro-
         electrodes with a recessed-tip (A) and a protruded-tip (B).
         The resistances of the microelectrodes were measured in
         100 mmol/l NaCl solution. The resistance values in A and
         B were 1.9 x 10^{10} and 3.2 x 10^{10} ohms respectively. The
         potentials in A and B were measured about 2 and 3 hrs res-
         pectively after the electrodes were filled with 1.5 mol/l
         NaCl.

perimentally ($\gamma_\pm = \gamma_+ = \gamma_-$; MacInnes convention). Ion activities
of the solutions are also shown in the parentheses.

     Fig. 1 shows potential recordings of typical Na$^+$-selective
microelectrodes with a recessed-tip (A) and protruded tip (B). The
microelectrode potentials were measured with the solution shown below
each recording. The recessed-tip microelectrodes had a slow response
time because of the small tip diameter of the insulating micropipette.
Similar results were obtained from 6 recessed-tip and 5 protruded-tip
microelectrodes. Selectivity coefficients of the microelectrodes
used in Fig. 1 were determined by using the measured potentials and
the calculated ion activities of the solutions. Table 1 shows k_{NaK}
values calculated by the equations used in the various methods.

Table 1. Selectivity Coefficients (k_{NaK}) of N^+-selective Glass Microelectrodes Determined by Various Methods

Solutions used	MSM Equ. (1)		FIM Equ. (2)		SSM Equ. (3)		Equ. (4)
	10 mM NaCl + 100 mM KCl	10 mM NaCl + 150 mM KCl	100 mM KCl	150 mM KCl	100 mM NaCl and 100 mM KCl	100 mM KCl	150 mM KCl
k_{NaK}^*	0.036	0.026	0.016	0.019	0.015	0.015	0.016
k_{NaK}^{**}	0.021	0.010	0.007	0.007	0.004	0.004	0.006

The k_{NaK}^* values were obtained from a recessed-tip microelectrode with an exposed-tip length of 70 μm. The k_{NaK}^{**} values were obtained from a protruded-tip microelectrode with an exposed-tip length of 95 μm. The k_{NaK}^* values were greater than the corresponding k_{NaK}^{**} values which is consistent with our previous results (Lee, 1979). In both types of the microelectrodes, the k_{NaK} values determined by the MSM were substantially greater than those determined by other methods. One possible reason for the discrepancy may be the uncertain activity coefficients used for calculating Na ion activities (primary ion) in the mixture solutions (10 mmol/1 NaCl + 100 mmol/1 KCl and 10 mmol/1 NaCl + 150 mmol/1 KCl). In these mixture solutions, Na and K ions may have different activity coefficients. The use of the same activity coefficient for Na and K ions may result in incorrect Na ion activities in the mixture solutions. The k_{NaK} values determined by the FIM were similar to those determined by the SSM and equation (4). These results indicate that FIM, SSM or equation (4) can be used for determining k_{NaK} values of Na^+-selective glass microelectrodes. The experimental procedures for determining k_{NaK} in equation (4) may be simpler than those in other methods. Equation (4) requires the selection of a calibration solution whose interfering ion activity is in similar range to that in the sample solution to be tested. Note that with equation (4) the k_{NaK} (0.015) determined with 100 mmol/1 KCl is similar to that (0.016) determined with 150 mmol/1 KCl. Equation (4) is also convenient for determining selectivity coefficients of Ca^{2+}-selective microelectrodes (Lee and Uhm, 1981).

REFERENCES

Lee, C.O., 1979, Electrochemical properties of Na^+- and K^+-selective glass microelectrodes, Biophysical J., 27:209.

Lee, C.O., and Uhm, D.Y., 1981, Characteristics of Ca^{2+}-selective
    microelectrodes and their application to cardiac muscle cells,
    in: this issue.
Robinson, R.A., and Stokes, R.H., 1965, The Theoretical Interpretation
    of Chemical Potentials (Chapter 9) and The Thermodynamics of
    Mixed Electrolytes (Chapter 15), in: Electrolyte Solutions,
    Butterworth and Co. Ltd., London.

SESSION II
INTRACELLULAR MEASUREMENTS OF IONIC ACTIVITY

INTRACELLULAR POTASSIUM AND CHLORIDE MEASUREMENTS IN SHEEP CARDIAC PURKINJE FIBERS

John L. Walker

Department of Physiology
College of Medicine
University of Utah
Salt Lake City, UT 84108

INTRODUCTION

When liquid ion exchanger, ion selective microelectrodes, with tip diameters of less than 0.5 μm were developed (Walker, 1971), it seemed reasonable to use them to measure intracellular potassium and chloride activities, $a_i(K)$ and $a_i(Cl)$, in sheep cardiac Purkinje fibers. This preparation was chosen for two reasons, it has been a popular preparation for cardiac electrophysiologists so there is a considerable literature describing their electrophysiology and, since they exhibit relatively weak mechanical activity, they are suitable for microelectrode recording.

It was interesting to measure $a_i(Cl)$ because it had been thought to be passively distributed. Hutter and Noble (1961) hypothesize that it is passively distributed with the chloride equilibrium potential, E_{Cl}, being equal to the mean membrane potential, E_M, averaged over the cardiac cycle.

It had also been generally thought that the depolarization of cardiac muscle association with cardiac glycoside intoxication is the result of a decrase in $a_i(K)$ which results in an increase in the potassium equilibrium potential, E_K (Beeler, 1977; Müller, 1963). Since the diastolic membrane potential, E_D, is a function of E_K in sheep cardiac Purkinje fibers (Sheu et al., 1979) an increase in E_K would result in an increase in E_D.

What I have done was to use chloride and potassium microelectrodes to investigate the problem of chloride distribution by measuring $a_i(Cl)$ and to determine if $a_i(K)$ does in fact decrease as a consequence of cardiac glycoside intoxication.

METHODS

Purkinje fibers were dissected from both ventricles of hearts obtained from sheep that had just been exsanguinated. The fibers were transported to the laboratory in chilled Tyrode's solution. A selected fiber was pinned to the bottom of a tissue bath, which was maintained at 37 °C while being perfused with Tyrode's solution. The Tyrode's solution was buffered at pH 7.4 with 5 mM HEPES and gassed with 100% O_2. A stimulator was used to drive the preparation at 1 Hz.

Potassium and chloride electrodes were made by treating the tips of glass micropipets with Siliclad (Clay-Adams) and filling their tips with either potassium liquid ion exchanger (Corning code 477317) or chloride liquid ion exchanger (Corning code 477315) (Walker, 1971). Membrane potentials were measured with 3 M KCl filled micropipets with resistance in the range of 12-15 megohms. The same micro-pipets, tip diameter 0.2-0.3 μm, used for both the ion selective and membrane potential electrodes.

The ion selective electrodes were calibrated by determining their slopes in a series of KCl solutions of known activities. The sodium-potassium selectivity, $k_{K,Na}$, of each potassium electrode was determined by projecting the electrode potential measured in the Tyrode's solution onto the curve used to determine the slope. No selectivity coefficients were measured for the chloride electrodes because the 5 mM HEPES, the only other anion present in the Tyrode's solution, did not make a detectable contribution to the chloride electrode potential.

Intracellular measurements were made with 3 M KCl filled electrodes, potassium electrodes and chloride electrodes. In beating preparations the potentials used for calculation of intracellular ionic activities were the diastolic potentials. The time constants for the ion selective electrodes were sufficiently fast (about 100 msec) for the electrodes to attain constant potentials during diastole. The transmembrane potentials measured with the ion selective electrodes, ΔE, and the KCl filled electrode, E_M, were used in equation 1 to calculate the intracellular ionic activities.

$$a_i(I) = \left[a_o(I) + \sum_J k_{I,J} a_o(J)^{z_I/z_J}\right] \exp\left[\frac{z_I F(\Delta E - E_M)}{nRT}\right]$$

$$- \sum_J {'}k_{I,J}\, a_i(J)^{z_I/z_J} \tag{1}$$

I and J are the principle ions (potassium or chloride) and J are the interfering ions. The subscripts i and o denote inside and outside of the cell, respectively. In all cases activities outside the cell are the activities of Tyrode's solution. $a_i(I)$ (mM) is therefore the intracellular activity of the principle ion; $k_{I,J}$ (dimensionless) is the selectivity coefficient; z (dimensionless) is valence; n (dimensionless) is an empirical constant used to make nRT/F the slope of the ion selective electrode, R, T, and F have their usual meanings. For the chloride electrodes, n = 1. The only correction made for interfering ions was for the contribution of $a_o(Na)$ to the potential of the potassium electrodes in the Tyrode's solution.

Intracellular recordings were not continuous because of the need to calibrate the ion selective electrodes after every series of measurements, and because of changes in the tip potentials of the KCl filled pipets if they were left in the cells for more than a few minutes. The tips of the pipets, one KCl filled and one ion selective, were close together in the preparation, < 1 mm, but they were not known to be in the same cell. Both electrodes were usually in the preparation at the same time. This manner of recording necessitates assuming the preparation is isopotential.

The results of the chloride measurements are presented in Table 1. The values in the table are means and standard deviations. The mean value of $a_i(Cl)$ is approximately four times greater than predicted if $E_{Cl} = E_D$. It is, however, very close to the value predicted by Hutter and Noble (1961) for a sheep Purkinje fiber beating at 1 Hz. Their predicted value was calculated by assuming passive distribution, averaging the membrane potential over the cardiac cycle and setting that average equal to E_{Cl}. The rationale was that net chloride current, I_{Cl}, would be zero under these conditions. To markedly alter the average membrane potential, two preparations were left quiescent for periods of several hours. Under these conditions, if chloride is passively distributed, $a_i(Cl)$ should decrease until $E_{Cl} = E_M$. The results of these experiments are shown in Figure 1. Although there was a slight decrease in $a_i(Cl)$, it was not significant and $a_i(Cl)$ remained constant at 4-5 times the value predicted on the basis of a passive distribution.

Table 1. Intracellular chloride activity, chloride equilibrium potential and membrane potential in sheep cardiac Purkinje fibers.

n	$a_i(Cl)$ (mM)	E_{Cl} (mv)	E_D (mv)
10	17.8 ± 3.8	-47.8 ± 6.0	-89.3 ± 5.5

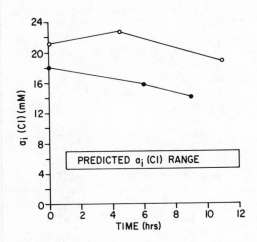

Fig. 1. Intracellular chloride activity in quiescent sheep cardiac Purkinje fibers. Predicted $a_i(Cl)$ assumes $E_{Cl} = E_M$.

The results of the potassium measurements are presented in Table 2. The values in the table are means and standard deviations. As expected, E_D is close to E_K and the quantity $E_D - E_K$ is greater than zero, i.e. E_D is positive with respect to E_K. The relationship between E_D and $a_i(K)$ was examined by plotting E_D as a function of $\log_{10} a_i(K)$. The result is shown in Figure 2. The solid line was calculated by the method of least squares linear regression. The slope of that line is -26.2 mv, which is less than one half of the Nernst slope. For comparison, the dashed line has been drawn through the mean values of E_D and $\log_{10} a_i(K)$ with a Nernst slope.

Considerable difficulty was encountered when trying to follow the time course of $a_i(K)$ changes during exposure of the preparations to the cardiac glyoside, ouabain. The nature of the problem is demonstrated by the experimental results shown in Figure 3. In this

Table 2. Intracellular potassium activity, potassium equilibrium potential and membrane potential in sheep cardiac Purkinje fibers.

n	$a_i(K)$ (mM)	E_K (mv)	E_D (mv)
21	132.3 ± 22.8	-94.0 ± 5.4	-86.7 ± 5.2

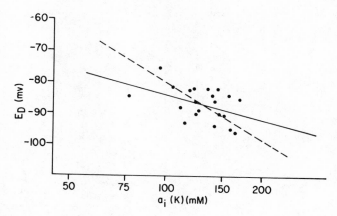

Fig. 2. Diastolic membrane potential as a function of $\log_{10} a_i(K)$ in sheep cardiac Purkinje fibers. The solid line is the least squares linear regression line which has a slope of -26.2 mv. The dashed line had a Nernst slope and is drawn through the mean values of E_D and $\log_{10} a_i(K)$.

experiment, E_D measurements were made in a single preparation with all measurements being made with the same electrode. If the baseline shifted by more than $\pm$ 1 mv after a measurement, that measurement was rejected. The abscissa shows the positions of the measurements relative to one another along the longitudinal axis of the preparation. The numbers accompanying the points give the sequence in which the measurements were made. For the series of fifteen measurements, the mean was -89.0 mv and the standard deviation was 6.1 mv.

To calculate the intracellular activity, it is necessary to combine the measurements made with two electrodes, ΔE and E_D. In the case of $a_i(K)$, the exponential term $(\Delta E - E_D)zF/RT$ (equation 1) is positive which means that variations in ΔE and E_D cause wide fluctuations in the calculated values of $a_i(K)$. As Figure 3 shows, the variation from penetration to penetration, under the best of circumstances, can easily be as large as $\pm$ 5 mV. The best way to overcome this problem is to have both electrodes in the same cell, in which case they should both be "seeing" the same membrane potential. It is, however, possible to obtain useful information by correlating the ΔE and E_D measurements without calculating $a_i(K)$. For measure-

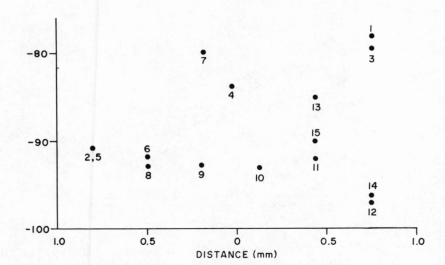

Fig. 3. Diastolic membrane potentials measured in a single sheep cardiac Purkinje fiber. The abscissa shows the relative positions along the fiber, at which the measurements were made. The numbers accompanying the points denote the sequence in which the measurements were made.

ments with the potassium electrode, where $n = 1$ and the only interfering ion considered is the extracellular sodium, equation 1 can be written as shown in equation 2.

$$\Delta E \quad E_D \; - \; \frac{RT}{F} \; \log_e \left[\frac{a_o(K) \; + \; k_{K,Na} \; a_o(Na)}{a_i(K)} \right] \tag{2}$$

Using the definition of the potassium equilibrium potential, E_K, equation 2 can be arranged as shown in equation 3.

$$E_D \; - \; E_K \; = \; \Delta E \; + \; \frac{RT}{F} \; \log_e \left[\frac{a_o(K) \; + \; k_{K,Na} \; a_o(Na)}{a_o(K)} \right] \tag{3}$$

All of the quantities on the right side of equation 3 are known and therefore the difference, $E_D - E_K$, can be obtained from the potassium electrode measurement alone. There should be no error due to variation in the measurement of E_D.

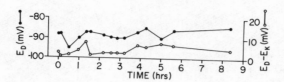

Fig. 4. Diastolic membrane potential (filled circles) and $E_D - E_K$ (open circles) as functions of time in a sheep cardiac Purkinje fiber to which 1×10^{-8} M ouabain was applied at $t = 1.33$ hours.

Figures 4, 5 and 6 show the results of experiments during which ouabain was applied to the preparation. For the experiment shown in Figure 3, the ouabain concentration was 1×10^{-8} M and there was no significant change in either E_D or $E_D - E_K$ over a period of more than six hours. This is one of several experiments, with similar results, that serve as control experiments. In the experiments presented in Figures 4 and 5, the ouabain concentration was 1×10^{-7} M. In both of these experiments, there was a marked membrane depolarization after about one hour. Concurrent with the change in E_D, there was an increase in $E_D - E_K$. Several other experiments had similar results.

DISCUSSION

The results of the experiments in which $a_i(Cl)$ was measured in quiescent preparations indicate that chloride is not passively distributed in sheep cardiac Purkinje fibers. Although no estimate was made of intracellular interference by other anions, estimates made in sheep Purkinje (Vaughan-Jones, 1979) and cat papillary (Spitzer and Walker, 1980) indicate that 3 mM is the upper limit of interference in mammalian cardiac muscle. Even when 3 mM is subtracted from the values shown in Figure 1, $a_i(Cl)$ is not reduced to a value consistent with passive distribution. Vaughan-Jones (1979) has shown that chloride permeability is sufficiently high in sheep Purkinje fibers so that if chloride was passively distributed, $a_i(Cl)$ should have decreased significantly during the time it was quiescent. Furthermore, it has been demonstrated both in sheep Purkinje fibers (Vaughan-Jones, 1979) and cat papillary (Spitzer and Walker, 1980) that when $a_o(Cl)$ is decreased, $a_i(Cl)$ rapidly decreases to a new

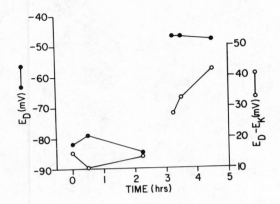

Fig. 5.   Diastolic membrane potential (filled circles) and $E_D - E_K$
(open circles) as functions of time in a sheep cardiac
Purkinje fiber to which 1×10^{-7} M ouabain was applied at
$t = 1.33$ hours.

steady state value. My observations confirm those of Vaughan-Jones
(1979), that $a_i(Cl)$ is too high to be accounted for on the basis of
passive distribution.

In ten preparations both $a_i(Cl)$ and $a_i(K)$ were measured. Linear
regression analysis of the data showed that neither the slope nor
the correlation coefficient were significantly different from zero.
It therefore appears that there is no direct relationship between
the values of $a_i(K)$ and $a_i(Cl)$ in sheep cardiac Purkinje fibers.

In six of the experiments in which ouabain was used, $a_i(Cl)$
measurements were made along with the $a_i(K)$ measurements. In three
of those experiments there was no change in E_D, and either no change
or a slight decrease in $a_i(Cl)$. In the three experiments in which
the preparations depolarized, there was a substantial increase in
$a_i(Cl)$, and E_{Cl} always remained positive with respect to E_D, or E_M
if the preparation became inexcitable. There was not enough data to
treat the results in a quantitative manner, but it is interesting
to note that $a_i(Cl)$ increased during ouabain intoxication while
$a_i Na$ is presumably increasing (Beeler, 1977; Deitmer and Ellis,
1977; Langer, 1977). This is consistent with the idea that co-trans-
port of sodium and chloride, which is dependent upon the sodium
electrochemical gradient, may be the mechanism by which high $a_i(Cl)$
is maintained (Duffey et al., 1978; Russel, 1979; Spring and Kimura,
1978).

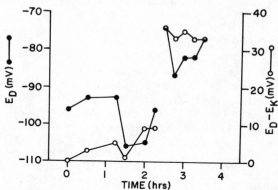

Fig. 6. Diastolic membrane potential (filled circles) and $E_D - E_K$ (open circles) as functions of time in a sheep cardiac Purkinje fiber to which 1×10^{-7} M ouabain was applied at $t = 0.16$ hours.

In the experiments reported here, the slope of the line relating E_D to $\log_{10} a_i(K)$ is -26 mV, which is less than one half of the Nernst slope. At first glance this may seem surprising, but it is consistent with the finding of Sheu et al. (1979) who measured $a_i(K)$ while varying $[K]_o$. They found that above $[K]_o = 12$ mM, E_D parallels E_K; but as $[K]_o$ decreases below 12 mM, E_D deviates progressively further from E_K. In my experiments $[K]_o = 5.4$ mM, well below the point where Sheu et al. (1979) found E_D to begin to deviate from E_K. My finding confirms the fact that at low values of $[K]_o$ the membrane of sheep Purkinje fibers becomes relatively less permeable to potassium and more permeable to some other ion(s).

During the course of the ouabain experiments I found that a series of measurements, in a preparation that was stable for several hours, gave wildly fluctuating values for $a_i(K)$. Since Weidmann (1952) showed that the cells of a Purkinje bundle are electrically well coupled and Imanaga (1974) demonstrated that the dye Procion Yellow, diffuses from cell to cell in a Purkinje bundle, it seemed unlikely that the preparations I was using were not isopotential or that there could be large variations in $a_i(K)$ from cell to cell within a Purkinje bundle. I then carried out the experiment, the results of which are shown in Figure 3, to see how reproducibly the membrane potential can be measured. My conclusion, based on this experiment, is that the potential that is recorded, depends in some way on the manner in which the electrode enters or seals into the cell that is being penetrated.

When making $a_i(K)$ measurements the transmembrane potentials of two electrodes are required and they are combined in an exponential terms whose sign is positive, therefore variability in these measurements can cause large fluctuations in the calculated values of $a_i(K)$. (See Walker and Brown (1977) for a more complete discussion of this problem.) During the ouabain experiments, time did not permit making several measurements with each electrode and using their average values to calculate $a_i(K)$, nor could I record continuously for long periods of time. When I tried to record continuously, the properties of the electrodes changed if their tips remained in the cells for more than 5-15 minutes. This was particularly true of the KCl filled electrodes whose tip potentials and resistances changed markedly, thus rendering the impalements useless.

These problems led to the presentation of the data adopted here, correlating changes in E_D with changes in $E_D - E_K$. In the experiments during which both E_D and $E_D - E_K$ changed by about the same amount, in the same direction, it is clear that E_K must have remained relatively constant. Since the Tyrode's solution, whose potassium activity was constant, was the reference for ΔE measurements, deducing a constant E_K from that measurement implies that $a_i(K)$ was constant. Although the data do not permit more than a qualitative argument, it seems to me that the conclusion is inescapable. The depolarization resulting from ouabain intoxication is not due to a decrease in $a_i(K)$.

The finding that the depolarization associated with ouabain intoxication is not due to a decrease in $a_i(K)$ is a new finding. In the past the depolarization has been thought to be due to a decrease in $a_i(K)$ causing an increase in E_K (Müller, 1963; Beeler, 1977). There are now two other possible causes of the depolarization that must be considered, one of which is indeed an increase in E_K. In the experiments reported here E_K was calculated by using the potassium activity in the bulk (Tyrode's) solution. It is possible that there is increased potassium efflux from the cells resulting in an increased potassium activity in the clefts of the Purkinje fiber during exposure to ouabain. Both of the possibilities can be examined experimentally. Double barrel potassium electrodes can be used to see if there is local extracellular accumulation of potassium during ouabain toxicity. Experiments of this type have already been done. Kunze (1977) used double barrel potassium electrodes to measure changes in $a_o(K)$ in the extracellular space of rabbit atria and Kline and Morad (1978) measured $a_o(K)$ changes in the extracellular space of frog ventricle. The possibility of permeability changes can be investigated by changing the ionic composition of the bathing solution, both during control and application of ouabain, while monitoring E_D. Correlation of solution composition changes with membrane potential changes should reveal any permeability changes that occur. For example, there might be a large increase in sodium permeability relative to the potassium permeability as has been shown to occur in sheep Purkinje fibers exposed to low potassium solutions (Lee and Fozzard, 1979).

CONCLUSIONS

The major conclusions resulting from the experiments described here are:1) intracellular chloride in sheep cardiac Purkinje fibers is not in electrochemical equilibrium and 2) the depolarization associated with ouabain intoxication in sheep cardiac Purkinje fibers is not the result of an increase in E_K due to a decrease in $a_i(K)$. Other conclusions are, there is no direct correlation between $a_i(Cl)$ and $a_i(K)$ in these preparations and when $[K]_o = 5.4$ mM, the diastolic membrane potential is only partially determined by E_K.

ACKNOWLEDGEMENTS

This research was supported by NIH Grants HL 18053 and NS 07938.

REFERENCES

Beeler, G.W., 1977, Ionic currents in cardiac muscle:a framework for glycoside action. Federation Proc., 36:2209.

Deitmer, J.W.,and Ellis, D., 1977, Comparison of the action of various cardiac glycosides on the intracellular sodium activity of sheep heart Purkinje fibres. J. Physiol., 276:27P.

Duffey, M.D., Turnheim, E.K., Frizell,R.A.,and Schultz, S.G., 1978, Intracellular chloride activities in rabbit gallbladder: direct evidence for the role of the sodium-gradient in "energizing" uphill chloride transport. J. Membrane Biol., 42:229.

Hutter, O.F.,and Noble, D., 1961, Anion conductance of cardiac muscle. J. Physiol.,(London) 157:335.

Imanaga, I., 1974, Cell-to-cell diffusion of Procion Yellow in sheep and calf Purkinje fibers. J. Membrane Biol., 16:381.

Kline, R.P.,and Morad, M., 1978, Potassium efflux in heart muscle during activity: extracellular accumulation and its implications. J. Physiol.,(London),280:537.

Kunze, D.L., 1977, Rate-dependent changes in extracellular potassium in the rabbit atrium. Circulation Res., 41:122.

Langer, G.A., 1977, Relationship between myocardial contractility and the effects of digitalis on ionic exchange. Federation Proc., 36:2231.

Lee, C.O.,and Fozzard, H.A., 1979, Membrane permeability during low potassium depolarization in sheep cardiac Purkinje fibers.

Am, J. Physiol., 237:C156.

Müller, von P., 1963, Kalium und Digitalistoxizitat. Cardiologia, 42:176.

Russel, J.M., 1979, Chloride and sodium influx: a coupled uptake mechanism in the squid giant axon. J. Gen. Physiol.,73:801.

Sheu, S.S., Lorth, M., and Lathrop, D.A., 1979, Resting membrane and potassium equilibrium potentials in sheep Purkinje fibers. Biophys. J., 25:198a.

Spitzer, K.W.,and Walker, J.L., 1980, Intracellular chloride activity in quiescent cat papillary muscle. Am. J. Physiol., 238:H87.

Spring, K.R.,and Kimura, G., 1978, Chloride reabsorption by renal proximal tubules of Necturus. J. Membrane Biol., 38:233.

Vaughan-Jones, R.D., 1979, Non-passive chloride distribution in mammalian heart muscle: micro-electrode measurement of the intracellular chloride activity. J. Physiol.,(London),295:83.

Walker, J.L., 1971, Ion specific liquid ion exchanger microelectrodes. Anal. Chem.,43:89A.

Walker, J.L. and Brown, H.M., 1977, Intracellular ionic activity measurements in nerve and muscle. Physiol. Rev. 57:729.

Weidmann, S., 1952, The electrical constants of Purkinje fibers. J. Physiol.,(London),118:348.

INTRACELLULAR ELECTROCHEMICAL POTENTIALS:

SKELETAL MUSCLE vs. EPITHELIAL, STEADY-STATE vs. KINETICS

Raja N. Khuri and Samuel K. Agulian

Faculty of Medicine
American University of Beirut
Beirut, LEBANON

INTRODUCTION

A. Intracellular Electrochemistry

The true internal environment is the cytoplasmic aqueous solution each cell contains within its membrane. The cytosol is the cytoplasmic aqueous solution. Direct and reliable determination of the in-situ ionic composition of the intracellular environment is an essential prerequisite for our understanding of such basic phenomena as transmembrane electrical potentials, enzyme activity and membrane transport.

The first direct intracellular potential measurement was made by Ling and Gerard (1949). Using a fine micropipette filled with salt-bridge solution, they established the intracellular negativity of frog muscle fibers, i.e., determined a transmembrane electrical PD. This marked the beginning of direct intracellular electrophysiology.

The first direct intracellular electrometric determination of a cytoplasmic ionic constituent was made by Caldwell (1954) when he measured the intracellular pH of giant crustacean muscle fibers. Hinke (1959) determined the intracellular potassium and sodium of squid giant axon by means of microelectrodes made of cation-selective glasses. Lev (1964) and Kostyuk et al. (1969) used glass micro-electrodes to determine the intracellular pH, K^+, and Na^+ in single muscle fibers of the frog sartorius. In these studies, the electrical and chemical (ionic) determinations are made by means of separate impalements with two intracellular microelectrodes: one serving as an electrical sensor, the other as a chemical sensor. The chemical

sensing ion-selective microelectrodes consist of electrode glasses
with sealed tips.

The combination of the electrical and the chemical micro-
probes in a double-barreled configuration (Fig. 1) for the simultaneous monitoring of the electrical and chemical ionic potentials
of single cells was achieved by Khuri and co-workers (1971-1972)
when liquid ion-exchangers were employed as the chemical ionic
sensors. This marked the beginning of the direct intracellular
electrochemical approach.

The Intracellular Electrochemical Technique (Khuri, 1971;
Khuri, 1972; Khuri et al., 1972b, 1972c) employs double-barreled
ion-selective, liquid ion-exchange microelectrodes to measure simultaneously the intracellular electrical and chemical potentials of
the same cell. The advantages of using ion-selective microelectrodes
whose sensing element is a liquid ion exchanger are: 1) The degree
of miniaturization that can be achieved, 2) the speed of response,
and 3) the ease with which double-barreled micropipettes can be
fabricated.

Both the electrical and chemical potentials are monitored
on a dual channel electrometer. The first channel monitors the
combined electrical and chemical potentials; the second monitors
only the electrical. In Fig. 2 the electrical component has been
subtracted automatically by using the differential operator of a
dual electrometer, thus yielding a pure sodium ionic potential in
the lower tracing.

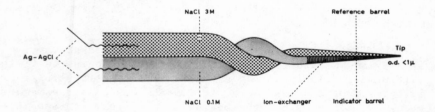

Fig. 1. Double-barreled liquid ion-exchange microelectrode, tool
        for intracellular electrochemical approach. One barrel
        functions as chemical, the other as electrical sensor.

The response time of ion-selective electrodes depends on
several properties of the solution (ionic strength, concentrations,
composition, unstirred layers) and the geometry of the electrode.
Microelectrodes, with their single-pore geometry and very small
area of the outer interface at the tip, have very fast response
times. Liquid ion-exchanger microelectrodes have, in general, much
taster response times than microelectrodes made from ion-selective
glasses, and hence are more suitable for kinetic studies.

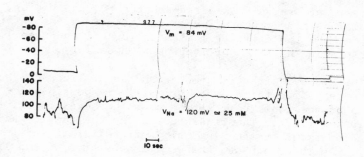

Fig. 2. Steady-state recording of two intracellular potentials: electrical (upper) and ionic potential (lower). Electrical component subtracted automatically by means of differential operator of dual electrometer system.

B. Skeletal Muscle

Skeletal muscle constitutes the major fraction of the total body mass. Therefore, muscle tissue is the major determinant of intracellular fluid ionic composition. Skeletal muscle can serve as the general biologic tissue reference for making comparisons between intracellular ionic compositions.

It is generally accepted that a major portion of cytoplasmic sodium is not free. Since active Na^+ transport is a universal function of virtually all living cells, the low intracellular Na^+ maintains a favorable electrochemical gradient for passive Na^+ influx. It also sets up a sizeable gradient, which has to be overcome by the electromotive force (emf) of the active Na^+ efflux mechanism, i.e. the Na^+ pump.

Chloride distribution across the sarcolemma of skeletal muscle fibers has been generally assumed to be passive and to follow a Donnan-type distribution (Boyle and Conway, 1941). This exclusion of Cl^- by the internal electronegativity of the cell results, on one hand, in the severe depletion of intracellular Cl^- and, on the other, in Cl^- becoming an almost exclusively extracellular anion.

C. Renal Tubular Epithelium

Tissues may be subdivided into two classes: Symmetrical and asymmetrical tissues. Symmetrical tissues include muscle fibers (skeletal, cardiac and smooth), neurons and nerve fibers, red blood cells, etc. The asymmetrical tissues are the epithelia. Epithelia are characterized by an intrinsic asymmetry of their cellular membranes with respect to both structure and function. For over two decades now, Ussing's (Koefoed-Johnsen, V. and Ussing, H.E., 1958) double-membrane model, whose fundamental tenet is the intrinsic asymmetry of the two limiting membranes (apical and basal), has guided investigators in the field of transport.physiology.

The kidney, with its complex and specialized epithelial design, is the homeostatic organ primarily responsible for the overall regulation of the ionic composition of both the extracellular and intracellular fluids. The renal tubular epithelium is essentially a three-compartment system: luminal, intracellular, and interstitial (Fig. 3). The three aqueous phases are separated by two lipid plasma membrane: the apical or luminal and the basal or peritubular cell membrane. The three-compartment approach is an oversimplification since it ignores the lateral intercellular space which is the route for paracellular transepithelial transport. As shown in Fig. 3, the transtubular (transepithelial) approach deals with fluid/plasma transepithelial ratios, thus treating the system as a two-compartment system. The Intracellular Electrochemical Technique, employing double-barreled ion-selective microelectrodes, simultaneously determines the intracellular ionic activity of renal tubular cells and the electrical gradients across the two cell boundaries. It yields simultaneous electrical and chemical trans-cell membrane ratios: cell/fluid and cell/plasma ionic activity ratios. Thus it is basically an intracellular and a transcellular approach capable of directly defining the electrochemical driving forces for the individual ions across the two limiting cellular membranes.

Khuri (1971, 1972) and Khuri et al. (1972b, 1972c) introduced the Intracellular Electrochemical Technique and applied it to map the intensive properties of the trans-cellular route of ion transport across the renal tubular transport. With no intracellular ionic

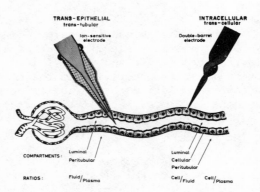

Fig. 3. Transepithelial (transtubular) and intracellular (trans-membrane) activity measurements as applied to renal tubular epithelium.

activity values were available for epithelia, renal physiologists generally assumed that, as in muscle, intracellular K^+ is all free, Na^+ is mostly non-free, and Cl^- is in a state of passive electrochemical equilibrium. As it turns out, these extrapolations with respect to the physical state of intracellular K^+, Na^+ and Cl^- were invalidated by the Intracellular Electrochemical Technique.

METHODS

A. Electrometric Methods

The improved method of construction of double-barreled microelectrodes over that reported by Khuri et al. (1972a) is described below. This improved method is characterized by ease of manufacture and high yield of functional microelectrodes.

Pyrex capillary tubing (Corning Code 7740) with an o.d. 1.2 mm and i.d. 0.6 mm is cleaned with dichromic acid, distilled water, and acetone. The capillaries are dried in the oven. Then a segment of pyrex tubing 10 cm in length is attached to a borosilicate glass capillary with inner filament (WP-Instruments, Cat. No. IB120F), o.d. 1.2 mm and i.d. 0.68 mm, by means of shrinkable tubing (Alpha Wire Corporation, fit 105 3/32"), heated on a microflame. The ends of glass capillaries are fire polished.

The pair of tubing is held over a microflame and when softened rotated 360° and pulled slightly. Then it is mounted on a vertical pipette puller (David Kopf Instrument) and pulled into double-barreled micropipettes with relatively long shanks and tip diameter $<1\mu$. Only the lower micropipette is used. To ensure best electrode performance and maximum yield the sequence in electrode filling is strictly followed. First, the indicator barrel is filled by introducing a column of liquid ion exchanger in the shank of the indicator barrel by means of a filler capillary. Pressure is applied to the column and pushed as far as to the tip of the micropipette. The rest of the shank and the stem of the indicator barrel are then filled with 3 M NaCl as an internal reference solution.

Second, the reference barrel is filled with an appropriate salt bridge electrolyte (3 M NaCl, KCl and Na formate are used for K^+, Na^+ and Cl measurements respectively), by wetting the inner filament of the borosilicate glass capillary. Filling is performed under microscopic inspection to ensure that there is no air bubble trapped in the tip of the reference barrel. However, if an air bubble is trapped in the shank it is removed by applying and releasing pressure by means of a syringe. The rest of the shank and the stem are then filled with a filler capillary. A piece of PE tubing is fitted to the stems of both reference and indicator barrels and are filled with appropriate internal reference solutions, as are mentioned above. Fig. 4 is a diagrammatic representation of the electrode.

The combination electrode was mounted on an Electrode Carrier connected to a hydraulic Micro-Drive (David Kopf, model 1207S). The electrode carrier itself is mounted on a Leitz micromanipulator. An Ag; AgCl wire is inserted into the stem of each barrel as an internal reference element. The indicator barrel is tightly fitted to a lucite chamber, as shown in Fig. 4, filled with internal reference solution. Pressure is applied to the indicator barrel in order to retain the organic ion-exchanger within the confines of the tip. In this manner the aqueous phase is prevented from entering the terminal part of the micropipette shank through the single porous channel at the tip. Leakage of organic exchanger from the tip of the electrode or manifestation of electrical coupling between the two barrels is indicative of broken electrode tips. The leads of the electrode and the external salt bridge reference are connected to the inputs of a differential/dual high impedance electrometer (W-P Instruments, Inc. Model F223A). The readings of the potential measurements were displayed on a Grass Polygraph. Isothermal conditions were maintained at $25 \pm 1^{\circ}C$. All equipment was placed inside a radio frequency shielded room.

Freshly prepared electrodes are immediately tested for any electrical coupling between the two barrels in the region of the tip. This is accomplished by measuring the electrical potential between the reference of the combination electrode and an external reference electrode in solutions with varying ion concentrations. A constant

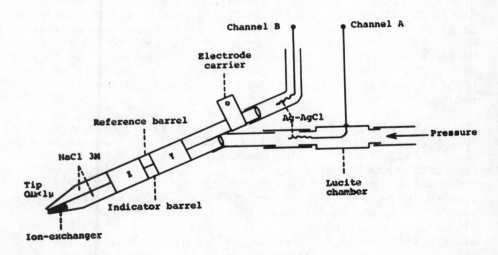

Fig. 4. Improved double-barreled liquid ion-exchanger microelectrode.

negative potential of few millivolts is indicative of no interference. Simultaneously, the sensitivity of the electrode is determined by measuring the potential between the indicator barrel and the external reference electrode. Electrodes exhibiting a response of 55-60 mV/ decade change of ion activity and a response time of less than one second are selected for kinetic studies.

B. Renal Methods

The microperfusion technique described below was developed by Frömter et al. (1971) and Windhager et al. (1970) independently in the rat kidney. This technique was adopted in the Necturus kidney with minor modifications.

Adult Necturus maculosus, weighing 100-130 grams were anesthetized by immersion in tap water containing 0.1% tricaine methanesulfonate. The gills were submerged in water into which air was continuously bubbled. The right kidney was exposed and amphibian Ringer in 2% agar was poured over the kidney. A hole in the center of the agar was filled by a continuous drip with amphibian Ringer solution. All experiments were carried out in situ.

The external reference electrode was made to achieve electrolytic contact with the Ringer solution by means of a fine 3 M NaCl salt bridge. The double-barreled ion-selective microelectrode, mounted on an Electrode Carrier, was introduced into the Ringer solution by means of a Leitz micromanipulator. Opposite to the latter, a double-barreled microinjection pipette with a sharp tip of 20 to 30 μm diameter was immersed in the Ringer solution by means of a manipulator. The tip of the pipette was bevelled and sharpened on a rotating grinding stone. Then it was adequately cleaned and siliconized with trichlorosiloxane. Subsequently, the barrels were respectively filled with the control and test solutions.

Under microscopic control the tips of the combination electrode and the microinjection pipette were advanced very close to the surface of the kidney. An appropriate segment of a proximal tubule was chosen for micropuncture. The choice was limited to tubular segments which were enveloped by the arms of bifurcating peritubular capillaries (Fig. 5). For perfusion, the neck of the bifurcation was punctured. The following sequence was adopted. The combination electrode was made to approach the tubular cell by means of a remotely controled hydraulic Micro-Drive (David Kopf, model 1207S). Upon impalement of the peritubular cell membrane a steep rise in the membrane potential of about 60 to 80 mV (negative) associated with a more gradual change in the ionic potential was recorded (Fig. 2). After reaching a stable value of both potentials a normal Ringer solution was perfused to displace the blood in the peritubular capillaries. Both potentials were recorded. This served as a control (blood perfused tubule) replacement. A colored

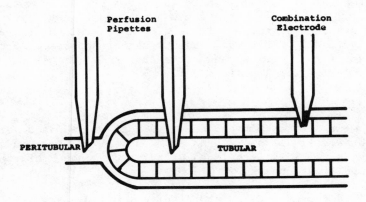

Fig. 5. Model used for monitoring transient changes in electrical
        and chemical potentials of a single cell during tubular
        and peritubular microperfusions.

test solution was perfused and both potentials, electrical and
chemical, were recorded for subsequent comparison with the control
replacement recordings. All perfusions were achieved by pressure
propulsion at high speeds. Occasionally the lumen as well as the
surface of the lumen were perfused either separately or simultaneously with the peritubular capillaries (Fig. 5). The induced
changes are reversible, such that each segment of the lumen serves
as its own control (Fig. 6).

C. Muscle Methods

        The frogs, Rana ridibunda, used for the studies were main-
tained unfed in running tap water at $20^{\circ}C$. The sartorius muscle
of the double pithed frog was exposed. Amphibian Ringer in 2%

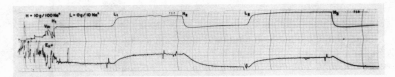

Fig. 6. Use of intracellular electrochemical technique for contin-
        uous monitoring of time course of induced transient changes
        and recoveries of two intracellular events: electrical and
        chemical (ionic) potentials.

agar was poured over the muscle. A hole in the center of the agar was filled with about 2 ml of Ringer solution. All experiments were carried out in situ.

As shown in Fig. 7 a reference electrode is made to achieve electrolytic contact with the Ringer solution by means of a fine 3M NaCl salt bridge. The double-barreled ion-selective micro-electrode is introduced into the Ringer solution by means of a micromanipulator. Opposite to the latter, a microinjection pipette, 5μ in tip diameter and a single chemical electrode are immersed in the Ringer by means of separate micromanipulators. Under micros-copic control the tips of the electrodes and the injection pipette were advanced very close to the surface of a muscle fiber. Subse-quent advances were made for the combination electrode by means of the remote control mechanism. As the electrode impales the sarco-lema, there is a steep rise in the membrane potential of about 80-90 mV (negative) associated with a more gradual change in the ionic potential. After reaching a stable value of both potentials colored test solution is injected from the micropipette at a flow rate of 0.01 μl/sec for 10 sec by means of controlled pressure system. The single electrode next to the tip of the pipette measures the actual concentration of the ion injected, and it is positioned right over the intracellular combination electrode.

The results of these skeletal muscle electrokinetic studies are summarized as follows: With the sudden increase in the external

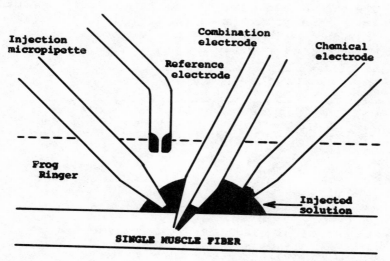

Fig. 7. Model used for monitoring transient changes in electrical and chemical potentials of the frog muscle, in vivo.

potassium which is sensed by the chemical (K^+) electrode, there is an instantaneous triphasic depolarization of the membrane potential. After the cessation of the injection of surface fluid, the concentration of external K^+ and the membrane regain their original levels in 10-12 seconds.

RESULTS

A. Skeletal Muscle
    1. Potassium. Table 1 (Khuri, Kalloghlian, and Agulian, submitted) is a summary of the data obtained in rat muscle during seven different metabolic states. Under control conditions, electrometric intracellular K^+ concentration was 163.2 ± 3.7 mM, a value that is in close agreement with the total apparent K^+ concentration as derived from chemical analyses (Relman et al., 1961; Kendig and Bunker, 1970). This indicates that all the intracellular K^+ is free and evenly distributed within the entire myoplasm of the rat muscle fiber. This has also been shown to be the case for frog skeletal muscle in studies using K^+-selective glass microelectrodes (Lev, 1964; Kostyuk et al., 1969). However, Armstrong and Lee (1971), in studies on frog muscle, and Lee and Fozzard (1975) in studies on rabbit cardiac muscle, using single-barrel K^+-selective glass microelectrodes externally insulated with an inert glass, found that a significant fraction of intracellular K^+ is bound or sequestered.

Table 1.   Rat thigh muscle in-vivo electrometric intracellular and extracellular K^+ concentrations, the concentration ratio, the calculated K^+ equilibrium potential and the simultaneously measured membrane electrical PD under different metabolic conditions. Given values are means ± SEM with the number of measurements in parentheses.

Condition	$[K^+]_{cell}$ mM	$[K^+]_{plasma}^o$ mM	$[K^+]^i/[K^+]^o$	E_K mV	E_m mV
I. Control	163.2±3.7 (70)	4.3±0.1	37.9±0.9 (70)	96.8±0.6 (70)	78.4±0.8 (70)
II. High K^+: chronic	159.8±3.6 (51)	5.4±0.2	29.6±0.7 (51)	90.1±0.6 (51)	70.8±1.0 (51)
III. High K^+: acute	152.7±4.4 (85)	6.8±0.4	22.5±0.7 (85)	82.1±0.8 (85)	68.7±0.9 (85)
IV. Low K^+	123.9±2.3 (54)	2.8±0.1	44.2±0.8 (54)	100.9±0.5 (54)	88.1±0.7 (54)
V. Low Na^+	166.1±3.8 (96)	4.4±0.2	37.8±0.9 (96)	96.2±0.6 (96)	76.3±0.8 (96)
VI. Acidosis: acute	132.7±3.8 (41)	4.8±0.1	27.6±0.8 (41)	88.3±0.8 (41)	76.6±0.7 (41)
VII. Acidosis: chronic	159.4±3.1 (66)	4.6±0.3	34.7±0.7 (66)	94.4±0.5 (66)	91.5±0.9 (66)

They determined an apparent activity coefficient of 0.61 for intracellular K^+ of rabbit cardiac muscle, a value well below that of a simple solution of the same ionic strength. These investigators found close agreement between the calculated K^+ equilibrium potential (-77.0 mV) and the measured resting membrane electrical PD (75.2 ± 1.1 mV) in rabbit cardiac muscle.

With regard to rat muscle (see Table 1) one would predict on the basis of a passive Donnan-type electrochemical equilibrium distribution, an intracellular $[K^+]$ of 83 mM, a value that is about one half of that directly measured for $[K^+]$. Thus the internal electrochemical potential of the K^+ ion is greater than the external one. This is reflected by a K^+ equilibrium potential, E_K, that is 18.4 mV more negative than the simultaneously measured electrical PD (E_m). This disequilibrium can be taken as evidence for active K^+ influx by a coupled Na-K exchange pump. The different metabolic states further demonstrate interesting varying relationships between the magnitude of the transcellular K^+ gradient and the resting membrane PD. Subsequently it was shown (Khuri et al., submitted) that of the major ions that could influence E_m only Cl^- exhibits an electrochemical equilibrium distribution across the skeletal muscle fiber membrane.

Using the bicationic Goldman equation for Na and K, one obtains:

$$E_{(K+Na)} = \frac{RT}{F} \ln \frac{[K^+]_i + P_{Na}/P_K[Na^+]_i}{[K^+]_o + P_{Na}/P_K[Na^+]_o}$$

Using for the permeability ratio, P_{Na}/P_K, a value of 0.01, an electrometric intracellular Na^+ of 5.8 mM (Khuri et al., submitted), and plasma Na of 146.2 ± 1.4 mM, one can calculate the values of the Goldman bicationic potential (E_{K+Na}). This bicationic form of the Goldman equation reduces the difference between E_m and E_K from 14.1 to 7.6 mV.

2. Sodium. Table 2 (Khuri et al., unpublished) summarizes the control steady-state values obtained in rat thigh muscle in vivo by using for a Na^+ sensor a neutral ligand developed by W. Simon. The mean intracellular Na^+ activity of 4.4 ± 0.3 mM and activity coefficient of 0.27 indicate that some 64 percent of cellular Na^+ is bound and/or compartmentalized. The Na^+ may be bound to the muscle protein myosin. The intracellular organelles capable of Na^+ sequestration include the nucleus, the mitochondria, and the sarcoplasmic reticulum.

In the gastrocnemius muscle of the rat (Tables 1 and 2) it is quite apparent that the two major intracellular monovalent cations, K^+ and Na^+, differ markedly in their physical states.

While virtually all the cell K^+ in muscle is in free solution, most of the cell Na^+ is not, suggesting that the intracellular processes

Table 2. Rat thigh muscle (gastrocnemius): in vivo electrical PD(E_m), apparent chemical sodium concentration, electrometric sodium activity $(Na^+)_c$, and the apparent activity coefficient (γ_c).

	E_m	Apparent chemical $[Na^+]_c$	Electrometric $[Na^+]_c$	$(Na^+)_c$	Apparent Na^+ γ_c
	mV	mM	mM	mM	—
Mean	76.2	16.2	5.8	4.4	0.27
±S.E.	1.9	1.2	0.4	0.3	
No.	35	6	35	35	

E_m Resting membrane electrical PD

$[\ ]_c$ Concentration, cellular

$(\ )_c$ Activity, cellular

Apparent chemical$[\ ]_c$ - derived from indirect chemical analysis of total cellular ion content and water content

Apparent $\gamma_c = \dfrac{\text{Electrometric } (\ )_c}{\text{Apparent Chemical}[\ ]_c}$

of sequestration and/or binding have a preferential affinity for the Na^+ over the K^+ ion.

    3. Chloride. Table 3 (Khuri et al., 1980) shows the results of a study in which intracellular Cl^- and the fiber membrane electrical PD (E_m) were measured simultaneously in rat thigh muscle in vivo by means of double-barreled liquid ion-exchanger micro-electrodes. The reference or electrical barrel was filled with 10 mM NaCl in 3M sodium formate to avoid intracellular Cl^- leakage. Sodium formate was chosen as the reference solution for the Cl^- microelectrode because of both the low sensitivity of the Cl^- liquid ion-exchanger to formate anion and the close similarity of the limiting equivalent conductivity of formate and Na^+. Chloride micro-electrodes were selected on the basis of high sensitivity (Nernstian response), high selectivities towards prevalent interfering anions (HCO_3^-, $H_2PO_4^-$, etc.), stability of potential, and fast response (time constant of about 100 ms).

    As summarized in Table 3, the measured electrical PD (E_m) and the transcellular Cl^- equilibrium potential (E_{Cl}) are virtually identical. This shows that, in skeletal muscle, Cl^- is in a state of passive electrochemical equilibrium distribution, at least at physiological concentrations of extracellular chloride. While this result confirms the now classic conclusion of Boyle and Conway (1941), it is at variance with the recent findings of Kernan et al. (1974), though both studies were performed on isolated frog sartorii.

Table 3. Rat thigh muscle: in vivo intracellular chloride concentration, the simultaneously measured electrical PD(E_m), and the calculated transcellular chloride equilibrium potential (E_{Cl}).

	$[Cl]_i$ (mM)	E_m (mV)	E_{Cl^-} (mV)
Mean	7.5	75.9	75.1
± S.E.	0.7	1.3	0.3
Number	42	42	42

Hence, species differences of the preparation (rat vs. frog) are unlikely to account for the observed discrepancies, but comparative electrometric studies based on the same methods have not yet been performed in amphibian and mammalian muscle fibers.

B. Renal Tubular Epithelium
    1. Potassium
        a) Intracellular Potassium. The activity of potassium in the living protoplasm plays a major role in the electrochemistry of cells in general and excitable cells in particular. Studies in skeletal muscle, employing different methods, have generally concluded that all the intracellular K^+ is free and evenly distributed with the entire myoplasm of the muscle fiber.

        b) Proximal Tubule: Necturus. The proximal tubule is the segment of the nephron that reabsorbs the bulk of the filtrate. The Necturus kidney proximal tubule offers a combination of large cells and absence of pulsations, which renders electrometric analysis relatively simple. It is particularly well suited to kinetic analysis where continuous intracellular monitoring is required.

        The first series of electrometric determinations of intracellular K^+ (Khuri et al., 1972c) yielded a mean (K^+) activity of 58.7 ± 2.3mM in Necturus proximal tubule. From this and the apparent total chemical concentration of K^+ of 103 mM, an apparent activity coefficient of 0.57 was obtained. In a subsequent series (Khuri et al., 1978) an even lower apparent K^+ intracellular activity cofficient of 0.46 was obtained. The low intracellular K^+ activity and activity coefficient indicates that some 25-40% of the cell K^+ is either bound or sequestered in some K^+-rich subcellular organelles. Had all the cell K^+ been in free solution in the cytosol, the calculated K^+ equilibrium potential E_K would have been about 95 mV, a value which is well above the mean peritubular PD, that is E_m of 68 mV. The reduction in the intracellular K^+ activity lowered E_K

to 75 mV, a value which is close to but significantly higher than E_m. In effect, K^+ reabsorption by the proximal tubule occurs near electrochemical equilibrium, thus minimizing the work of transport.

In an effort to define the properties of the peritubular membrane, the $[K^+]$ of the peritubular perfusion fluid was raised by the substitution of KCl for NaCl. Figure 8 shows that as the peritubular perfusate $[K^+]$ is increased from the control value of 2.5 mM to 103 mM, the electrometric cell $[K^+]$ rises while the cell $[Na^+]$ falls by almost equivalent amounts. These equivalent but opposing changes in the electrometric cell $[K^+]$ and $[Na^+]$ constitute evidence for a coupled Na^+-K^+ exchange pump in the peritubular membrane.

c) Distal Tubule. Almost all the filtered K^+ is reabsorbed by the proximal tubule, and the variable amount of K^+ that is eliminated in the urine to maintain a state of K^+ balance is derived from distal tubular secretion. The primary determinant of the K^+ secretory and, therefore, excretory rate is the concentration of K^+ within the regulatory distal tubular cells. The other factors that affect distal tubule K^+ secretion are the passive K^+ permeability and the electrical PD across the luminal membrane (Malnic et al., 1966 & Giebisch, 1971).

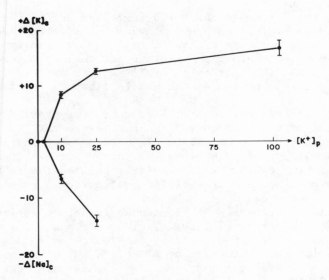

Fig. 8. Changes in cell $(K^+)_c$ and $(Na^+)_c$ activities as peritubular K^+ concentration is elevated from 2.5 to 103 mM. Elevation of $(K^+)_c$ and decline of $(Na^+)_c$ at each new level are equivalent.

In the normal rat, a mean intracellular effective $[K^+]$ of 46.5 ± 1.6 mM was obtained for distal tubule cells, a value which is well below previously (Malnic et al., 1966) assumed values for cell $[K^+]$. Tisher (1976) pointed out that the true distal cells of the rat are columnar and very rich in intracellular organelles (mitochondria and vesicles). These organelles could sequester K^+, thus contributing to the low cytoplasmic K^+ values. In kaliuretic states resulting from high K^+ diet or metabolic alkalosis, distal cell $[K^+]$ increased; whereas in the kaliupenic states resulting from low K^+ diet, metabolic acidosis and adrenalectomy cell $[K^+]$ decreased. This adaptive response of renal cell $[K^+]$ resulting in labile changes in cell $[K^+]$ is more suggestive of intracellular compartmentalization than binding.

While the Necturus kidney is the ideal preparation for the proximal tubular system, the Amphiuma kidney (Sullivan, 1968) is the preparation most suitable for the study of the distal tubule. The ventral surface of the Amphiuma kidney is composed almost exclusively of distal tubules. As shown in Table 4 the intracellular K^+ activity of control, blood-perfused distal tubule cells of Amphiuma is 47.0 ± 2.0 mM, a mean value which when taken in conjunction with an apparent chemical K^+ concentration of 103.2 mM yields an apparent activity coefficient for cell K^+ of 0.46. This suggests that only 60% of total cell K^+ is accessible to the impaling microelectrode within the aqueous cytosol, whereas some 40% of the cell K^+ is sequestered and/or bound. Kimura et al. (1977), using single-barreled K^+ microeletrodes found an intracellular K^+ activity of 41.2 ± 0.5 mM and an apparent activity coefficient of 0.32 in the toad bladder, a tissue often considered a good functional model for the

Table 4. Cellular Na^+ and K^+ activities in Amphiuma distal tubule.

| Activity | Luminal perfusions | | Blood-perfused controls | |
	$[Na^+]l=10$	$[Na^+]l=100$	Activities	Apparent γ_c
mM	mM	mM	mM	–
$(Na^+)_c$	8.6	21.3	16.3	0.45
	±1.3	±2.8	±1.5	
	(12)	(12)	(12)	
$(K^+)_c$	43.5	53.8	47.0	0.46
	±3.0	±3.8	±2.0	
	(17)	(12)	(28)	

Right panel: The cellular activities of $(Na^+)_c$ and $(K^+)_c$ and the apparent activity coefficients of blood-perfused intact Amphiuma distal tubular cells.

Left panel: The effect of changing the concentration of Na^+ in the luminal perfusion fluid $[Na^+]_1$ on the cellular $(Na^+)_c$ and $(K^+)_c$ ionic activities. Values given are those of the mean ± SE (Number).

distal nephron. White (1976) obtained an intracellular K^+ activity of 41.6 ± 1.5 mM in absorptive cells lining the small intestine of Amphiuma; the apparent activity coefficient was 0.28.

2. Sodium
            a) Intracellular Sodium. Several studies of intracellular Na^+ of muscle have been carried out with Na^+-sensitive glass microelectrodes in large fibers. Hinke (1959) obtained an apparent activity coefficient of 0.3 in crab muscle and later by McLaughlin and Hinke, 1966 an activity coefficient of 0.2 in squid axon. Lev in 1964 and Kostyuk et al. in 1969 obtained an apparent Na^+ activity coefficient of 0.3 in frog sartorius muscle.

In the first use of liquid ion-exchanger microelectrodes to determine cell Na^+, Khuri et al. (1978) used a neutral Na^+ ligand developed by Simon. In rat gastrocnemius muscle a mean intracellular activity of 4.4 ± 0.3 mM and activity coefficient of 0.27 indicate that some 64% of cell Na^+ is bound and/or compartmentalized. The Na^+ ion may be bound to the muscle protein myosin. The sarcoplasmic reticulum can accumulate Na^+. In the gastrocnemius of the rat it is quite apparent that the two major intracellular monovalent cations, K^+ and Na^+, differ markedly in their physical states. While virtually all the cell K^+ in muscle is in free solution, most of the cell Na^+ is not, suggesting that the intracellular processes of sequestration and/or binding have a preference for the Na^+ over the K^+ ion.

b) Proximal Tubule: Necturus. The proximal tubule performs the bulk of the operation of Na^+ reabsorption from the filtrate. Table 5 (Khuri et al., 1978) represents the first direct electrometric determinations of intracellular Na^+ activity in the renal epithelium. Against the background of estimates of the Na transport pool of about 1 mM by radiokinetic methods, much to our surprise we found that some 60% of renal cell Na^+ is free. In addition, the intracellular Na^+ and K^+ activity coefficients in cells of the proximal tubule of Necturus are quite similar, indicating no preferential binding and/or sequestration of the sodium ion. In contrast, a marked difference between the intracellular activity coefficient of K^+ (γ^k=0.75) and Na^+ (γ^{Na}=0.27) exists in muscle, which suggests that the intracellular binding process is highly selective for Na^+.

With a double-barreled ion-selective microelectrode continuously recording cell Na^+ and the electrical PD, two luminal perfusion solutions were injected alternatively via a double-barreled luminal pipet into single proximal tubules of Necturus, each cell serving as its own control. Increasing luminal $[Na^+]$ and the addition of glucose to luminal fluid resulted in increases in cell $[Na^+]$. The increases in cell $[Na^+]$ were accompanied by parallel and equivalent changes in cell $[K^+]$.

Table 5. Intracellular sodium activity $(Na)_c$ and the peritubular membrane electrical $PD(V_m)$ as measured simultaneously with Na^+-selective double-barreled liquid ion-exchange microelectrodes in the proximal tubule of normal blood-perfused Necturus.

	V_m	Apparent Chemical $[Na^+]_c$	Electrometric $[Na^+]_c$	$(Na^+)_c$	Apparent Na^+ γ_c
	mV	mM	mM	mM	−
Mean	68.2	42.0	25.2	20.0	
±S.E.	2.6	±2.2	±1.6	±1.3	0.48
#	37	8	37	37	

V_m Peritubular membrane electrical PD

Rest of symbols as in Table 2.

The parallel changes in cell Na^+ and K^+ activities induced by luminal perfusions (Fig. 6) and the reciprocal changes (Fig. 8) induced by peritubular perfusions represent strong and direct evidence for coupled Na^+-K^+ active exchange in the basal membrane. The following sequence of events is proposed: increasing luminal $[Na^+]$ increases Na^+ influx, followed by a rise in cytoplasmic $[Na^+]_c$, which by mass action drives an augmented Na^+ efflux and coupled K^+ influx across the basal membrane. As a consequence, cell $[K^+]$ rises. The direct confirmation of this sequence of predictions lends strong support to Ussing's double-membrane epithelial transport model.

The dependence of intracellular $[Na^+]_c$ on the lumen/cell Cl^- gradient was evaluated using paired luminal perfusions in which Isethionate was substituted for Cl^-. Switching from a luminal $[Cl^-]$ of 5.6 mM to 98.1 mM was accompanied by a rise in cell $[Na^+]$ from 20.5 to 30.5 mM. This supports cotransport of Na and Cl (Spring and Kimura, 1977).

The concept of the sodium transport pool was formulated to relate transcellular transport to intracellular ion levels. The intracellular Na transport pool is that fraction of intracellular Na^+ that exchanges readily with external Na^+ during its reabsorptive transit through the cell interior. Estimates of the size of the Na^+ pool by radiokinetic methods generally suggest that in epithelia the pool is only a small fraction of total cellular Na^+ content. The marked sensitivity of changes in cell $[Na^+]$ to maneuvers that stimulate or inhibit Na^+ transport suggests that the cytoplasmic $[Na^+]$ as measured electrometrically (60% of total cell Na^+) represents the Na^+ transport pool.

c) Distal Tubule. The distal tubular Na^+ reabsorptive system is responsible for the fine adjustment of renal Na^+ regulation. Table 4 (Khuri et al., submitted) gives the mean values obtained from an electrometric study of Amphiuma distal tubules. The mean intracellular Na^+ activity of 16.3 mM corresponds to an apparent Na^+ activity coefficient of 0.45; about 60% of cell Na^+ is free in the Amphiuma distal tubule, a value which is identical with cell Na^+ in Necturus proximal tubule. Table 4 also shows that the activity coefficients of Na^+ and K^+ are equally reduced in distal tubular cells of Amphiuma.

As luminal $[Na^+]$ was increased (Table 4), electrometric cell $[Na^+]$ and cell $[K^+]$ increased by equivalent amounts. The magnitude of these increases in Amphiuma distal tubule are comparable to the change in Necturus proximal tubule when the same luminal maneuver was performed. In both cases these increases are mediated by the stimulation of a Na^+-K^+ active exchange pump mechanism in the peritubular cell membrane. The mean intracellular Na^+ activity of 16.4 $\pm$ 1.9 mM (Khuri et al., submitted) obtained in the rat distal tubule is in close agreement with the value obtained in Amphiuma.

3. Chloride

a) Intracellular Chloride. The passive distribution of Cl^- ions between the extracellular and intracellular water is uneven (ratio of about 20:1). A small error in the chemical estimation of extracellular space would result in a large error in the estimation of intracellular $[Cl^-]$ by indirect chemical methods. Kernan et al. (1974) challenged the passive distribution theory of Cl^- in muscle. They used chlorided silver wires mounted inside glass micropipettes. However, using Cl^--selective liquid ion-exchanger microelectrodes, Khuri et al. (submitted) found that in the gastrocnemius muscle of the rat in vivo the measured electrical PD (E_m) and the transcellular Cl^- equilibrium potential (E_{Cl}) are virtually identical. This means that in skeletal muscle Cl^- is in a state of passive electrochemical equilibrium distribution.

b) Proximal Tubule: Necturus. Considering the transepithelial distribution of Cl^-, it is generally assumed that proximal tubular Cl^- transport is passive (Danielson et al., 1970; Giebisch and Windhager, 1964). However, intracellular Cl^- electrochemical analysis in the proximal tubule of Necturus (Khuri et al., 1975) yielded a mean cell $[Cl^-]$ of 18.7 $\pm$ 1.3 mM a value which places intracellular Cl^- at a higher electrochemical potential than either luminal or peritubular fluid. This will drive passive efflux of Cl^- across the luminal and peritubular cell membranes. However, to maintain the high intracellular Cl^- level in the steady state, the cell must possess a mechanism for active Cl^- influx in the luminal membrane or, alternatively, a mechanism that coupled uphill chloride entry to the downhill movement of another ion species.

Spring and Kimura (1978) have suggested that transluminal chloride movement could be coupled to sodium entry and that it proceeds by neutral NaCl translocation.

c) Distal Tubule. This segment of the nephron reabsorbs both Na^+ and Cl^- against sizable transepithelial gradients and is mostly responsible for the fine regulation of renal NaCl excretion. Controversy about the mechanism of chloride transport across the distal tubule epithelium persists. Most investigators (Danielson, 1970b; Kashgarian et al., 1963) have not found it necessary to assume the existence of active Cl^- reabsorption in the distal tubule.

Using Cl^--selective liquid ion-exchange microelectrodes, Khuri et al. (1974c) found a cell $[Cl^-]$ of 42.3 mM in cells of the distal tubule of the rat. Thus intracellular Cl^- ion is at a higher electrochemical potential than either the luminal or peritubular fluid Cl^-. A net force would drive the passive efflux of Cl^- across both cell membranes. These passive effluxes must, in the steady state, be balanced by equal and opposite active Cl^- influx from lumen to cell. This active mechanism in the luminal cell membrane could be either a Cl^- anionic pump or an electrically neutral NaCl cotransport pump.

Thus in the distal tubule, like in the proximal tubule, Cl^- reabsorptive process consists of two steps in series: primary (Cl^- anionic pump) or secondary (cotransport of NaCl) active Cl^- transport from lumen to cell, and passive diffusion of Cl^- from cell to interstitium. In contrast, Na transport is passive across the apical membrane and active across the basal membrane.

CONCLUSION

Figure 9 is a schema of the Necturus proximal tubule cell based on the total direct evidence obtained from electrochemical studies. The primary active event is the operation of the peritubular active Na^+-K^+ exchange pump. This Na^+ extrusion generates a favorable driving force for passive luminal Na^+ influx. This transluminal Na^+ electrochemical gradient (93 mV) may provide a sufficient driving force to drive several ionic species uphill into the cell. These include cotransport of Na^+ with Cl^- and HCO_3^-. The latter is indistinguishable from the countertransport of Na^+ and H^+. They also include the cotransport of Na^+ with glucose and amino acids, which represents electrogenic transport that depolarizes the luminal membrane.

The intracellular electrochemical technique is a new methodological development that has improved our definition of individual transport mechanisms at the cellular level, since the simultaneous determination of the electrical and chemical potentials results in more accurate measurement of each parameter alone.

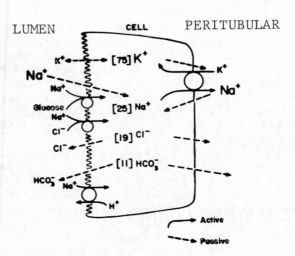

Fig. 9. Scheme of Necturus proximal tubule cell, incorporating all
        electrometric evidence obtained for different ions both
        under steady-state conditions and from kinetics of induced
        transient changes.

Thus, the study of the electrochemistry of the nephron has
demonstrated some clear distinction between skeletal muscle and
renal tubular epithelium. Some additional conclusions can be
drawn. First, as stated above, the discrepancy between the intracellular activity coefficients of K^+ and Na^+, suggesting differences
in the cytoplasmic states of these two ions, while true for skeletal
muscle, does not seem to hold for renal tubular epithelium. Second,
no major electrochemical distinction could be observed between the
two major segments of the nephron, that is, the proximal tubule and
distal tubule cells. Third, since the Na^+ transport pool is so
substantial, it can tentatively be assumed that it is unlikely that
there are two or more functionally important Na^+ pools in kidney
cells. Thus, the study of the electrochemistry of the nephron has
provided direct evidence in support of Ussing's "Double membrane"
theory for epithelia and in support of the general membrane theory.

REFERENCES

Armstrong, W. McD., Lee, C. O., 1971, Sodium and potassium activities
        in normal and "sodium-rich" skeletal muscle, Science, 171:413.
Boyle, P. J., Conway, E. J., 1941, Potassium accumulation in muscle
        and associated changes, J. Physiol., 100:1.
Caldwell, P. C., 1954, An investigation of the intracellular pH of
        crab muscle fibers by means of microglass and micro-tungsten
        electrodes, J. Physiol., 126:169.

Danielson, B. G., Persson, E., Ulfendahl, H. R., 1970a, Transmembrane transport of chloride and iodide in proximal rat tubules, Acta Physiol. Scand., 78:339.

Danielson, B. G., Persson, E., Ulfendahl, H. R., 1970b, The transport of halide ions across the membrane of distal rat tubules, Acta Physiol. Scand., 78:347.

Frömter, E., Muller, C. W., Wick, T., 1971, Permeability properties of the proximal tubular epithelium of the rat kidney studied with electrophysiological methods. In "Electrophysiology of Epithelial Cells" (Symp. Med. Hoechst). Stuttgart, Schatteauer, p. 119.

Giebisch, G., Windhager, E. E., 1964, Renal tubular transfer of sodium, chloride and potassium, Am. J. Med., 36:643-669.

Giebisch, G., 1971, Renal potassium excretion. In "The Kidney: Morphology, Biochemistry, Physiology" (C. Rouiller and C.W. Mueller, eds.), 3:329-382, Academic Press, New York.

Hinke, J. A. M., 1959, Glass microelectrodes for measuring intracellular activities of sodium and potassium, Nature (Lond.), 184:257.

Kashgarian, M. H., Stöckle, H., Gottschalk, C. W., Ullrich, J. J., 1963, Transtubular electrochemical potentials of sodium and chloride in proximal and distal renal tubule during antidiuresis and water diuresis (diabetes insipidus), Pflügers Arch., 277:89.

Kendig, J. J., Bunker, J. P., 1970, Extracellular space, electrolyte distribution and resting potential in K depletion, Am. J. Physiol., 218:1737.

Kernan, R. P., MacDermott, M., Wesphal, W., 1974, Measurement of chloride activity within frog sartorius muscle fibers by means of chloride-sensitive microelectrodes, J. Physiol., 241:60P.

Khuri, R. N., 1971, Intracellular potassium and the electrochemical propertie of striated muscle fibers, Proc. IUPS 9:301.

Khuri, R. N., 1972, Intracellular potassium in cells of the distal tubule, Yale J. Biol. Med., 45:384.

Khuri, R. N., Hajar, J. J., Agulian, S. K., 1972a, Measurement of intracellular potassium with liquid ion-exchange microelectrodes, J. Appl. Physiol., 32:419.

Khuri, R. N., Agulian, S. K., Kalloghlian, A., 1972b, Intracellular potassium in cells of the distal tubule, Pfluegers Arch., 335:297.

Khuri, R. N., Hajjar, J. J., Agulian, S. K., Bogharian, K., Kalloghlian, A., Aklanjian, D., Bizri, H., 1972c, Intracellular potassium in cells of the proximal tubule of Necturus, Pfluegers Arch., 338:73.

Khuri, R. N., Agulian, S. K., Bogharian, K., 1974c, Electrochemical potentials of chloride in distal renal tubule of the rat, Am. J. Physiol., 227:1352.

Khuri, R. N., Agulian, S. K., Bogharian, K., Aklanjian, D., 1975, Electrochemical potentials of chloride in proximal renal tubule of Necturus maculosus, Comp. Biochem. Physiol., A50:695.

Khuri, R. N., Agulian, S. K., Boulpaep, E. L., Simon, W., Giebisch, G. H., 1978, Changes in the intracellular electrochemical potentials of Na^+, K^+ and Cl^- in single cells of the proximal tubules of the Necturus kidney induced by rapid changes in the extracellular perfusion fluids, Drug Res., 28:879.

Khuri, R. N., Agulian, S. K., AbdelNour, S., (submitted), Intracellular activity of sodium in the distal tubule of the rat, Pfluegers Arch.

Khuri, R. N., Agulian, S. K., Giebisch, G., (submitted), Electrochemical potentials of Na^+ and K^+ in the distal tubule of Amphiuma, Am. J.Physiol.

Khuri, R. N., Kalloghlian, A., Agulian, S. K., (submitted), Intracellular potassium in rat muscle under different metabolic states, Pfluegers Arch.

Koefoed-Johnsen, V., Ussing, H. E., 1958, The nature of the frog skin potential, Acta Physiol. Scand., 42:298.

Kimura, T., Urakabe, S., Yuasa, S., Miki, S., Takamitsu, Y., 1977, Potassium activity and plasma membrane potentials in epithelial cells of toad bladder, Am. J. Physiol., 232:F196.

Kostyuk, P. G., Sorokina, Z. A., Kholodova, Yu. D., 1969, Measurement of activity of hydrogen, potassium and sodium ions in striated muscle fibers and nerve cells. In: Lavallee M, Schanne, O. F., Hebert, N. C. (eds), Glass Microelectrodes. Wiley, New York pp. 322-348.

Lev, A. A., 1964, Determination of activity coefficients of potassium and sodium ions in frog muscle fibers, Nature (Lond.) 201:1132.

Lee, C. O., Fozzard, H. A., 1975, Activities of potassium and sodium ions in rabbit heart muscle, J. Gen. Physiol., 65:695.

Ling, G., Gerard, R. W., 1949, Measurement of the transmembrane electrical potential of frog sartorius muscle fibers, J. Cell Comp. Physiol., 34:383-395.

Malnic, G., Klose, R. M., Giebisch, G., 1966, Microperfusion study of distal tubular potassium and sodium transfer in rat kidney, Am. J. Physiol., 211:548-559.

McLaughlin, S. G. A., Hinke, J. A. M., 1966, Sodium and water binding in single striated muscle fibers of the giant barnacle, Can. J. Physiol. Pharmacol., 44:837.

Relman, A. S., Gorham, G. W., Levinsky, N. G., 1961, The relation between external potassium concentration and the electrolyte content of isolated rat muscle in the steady state, J. Clin. Invest., 40:386.

Spring, K. R., Kimura, G., 1978, Chloride reabsorption by renal proximal tubules of Necturus, J. Membr. Biol., 38:233-254.

Sullivan, W. J., 1968, Electrical potential differences across distal renal tubules of Amphiuma, Am. J. Physiol., 214:1096.

White, J. E., 1976, Intracellular potassium activities in Amphiuma small intestine, Am. J. Physiol., 231:1214.
Windhager, E., Spitzer, A., 1970, Effect of peritubular oncotic pressure changes on proximal fluid reabsorption, Am. J. Physiol., 218_1188.

MEASUREMENT OF INTRACELLULAR CALCIUM ACTIVITIES

Josephine O'Doherty and Robert J. Stark*

Department of Physiology
Indiana University School of Medicine
*Department of Biology
Purdue University School of Science
Indianapolis, Indiana, USA

Accurate measurement of intracellular calcium activities has become possible with the development of the neutral lipophilic carrier molecule N,N'-di(11-ethoxycarbonyl)undecyl N,N' 4,5 tetramethyl-3,6 -dioxaoctane diacid diamide designed and synthetized by Simon (Simon et al., 1978). We have developed a liquid ion-exchanger microelectrode using this neutral carrier as the calcium selective component to measure intracellular Ca^{++} activities in rat soleus muscle fibers and adipose tissue. The advantage of using liquid ion-exchangers as the sensing element is the degree of miniaturization that can be obtained, making possible electrophysiological measurements of intracellular ionic activities. The microelectrodes used in our experiments had tip diameters of approximately 0.4 μm. In order for these carrier molecules to behave as liquid ion-exchangers, the carrier and the ion complexed carrier must be soluble in the membrane phase, have adequate mobility, and the uncomplexed carrier must be present in excess to get a cation response. 10% (w/v) of the above neutral carrier molecule dissolved in 3-nitro-o-xylene satisfied all of these conditions. It formed a liquid ion-exchange membrane which was permeable only to calcium. In order that the ion-exchange kinetics be compaible with a sufficiently fast microelectrode response, the lipophilic salt calcium 3,5 dibromosalicylate (1 percent, w/v) was incorporated into the system. This addition to the liquid membrane provided a charged "site" ion of opposite sign and dramatically improved the response time of these electrodes. The apparent response time was of the order of one second. Since the response of liquid ion-exchanger microelectrodes is affected by internal capacitances in the recording systems, the intrinsic response time of the microelectrode is probably much less than one second.

Since the response of liquid ion-exchanger microelectrodes is affected by internal capacitances in the recording systems, the intrinsic response time of the microelectrode is probably much less than one second.

The cytoplasmic concentrations of free Ca^{++} are very low, therefore the electrical potential of the microelectrode (E_{Ca}), must adequately respond to changes in calcium activities in the range 10^{-6} to 10^{-7} mol/l. To obtain maximum calcium sensitivity, we attempted to eliminate the conductance that exists between the inner surface of the pipette and the membrane phase. This conductance tends to short circuit the sensing membrane potential, especially when the tip diameter is small, and as a result, drastically lowers the slope of the electrode. To reduce this conductance, the micropipettes were equilibrated for four hours under carefully controlled temperature and humidity conditions (60 °C, R.H. 30%) and then were rendered hydrophobic with the vapor of chlorotrimethylsilane. The inner glass surface of the pipette must be coated with the right number of adsorbed water molecules to be properly coated. The correct relative humidity was established empirically and was applicable to the type of glass used *. This is one of the most painstaking, but probably the most important step in the preparation of a good calcium microelectrode. The most specific ionophore will not function properly in poorly siliconized glass. Careful pretreatment of the micropipettes in this way increased the slope of the electrode, particularly in the critical range of 10^{-5} to 10^{-7} mol/l. Most significantly, the actual difference in potential measured between these two concentrations was 53.5 ± 2.6 mV.

We calibrated the microelectrodes in solutions that were adjusted to approximate the ionic strength of the cell interior (Stark et al., 1980), so that the calcium present in the calibration standards, the mammalian Ringer's solution, and the cytosol, all had the same ionic activity coefficient. In addition, two solutions were used in which Ca^{++} was buffered to a calculated P_{Ca} of 6 and 7 respectively with calcium disodium and disodium salts of EDTA. KCl was added to these solutions to bring them to virtually the same ionic strength (0.150 mol/l) as the other calibrating solutions. Mg^{++} complexes with EDTA and therefore was not added to these solutions as it would complicate the calculation of P_{Ca}.

A representative calibration is shown in Fig. 1. It is apparent from this calibration that the microelectrode response to Ca^{++} was a linear function of $\log a_{Ca}$ between 10^{-3} and 10^{-7} mol/l and that E_{Ca} is not affected by physiological concentrations of K^+, Na^+ and Mg^{++} usually present in either the cytosol or extracellular fluid.

---

*Kwik-Fil borosilicate glass tubing (O.D., 1.2 mm, I.D. 0.68 mm; W.P. Instruments, New Haven, Conn.)

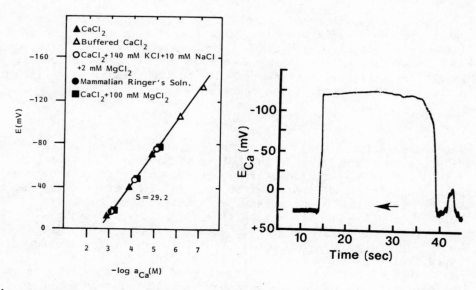

Fig. 1. Steady state electrical potentials registered by a Ca^{++}-selective microelectrode plotted as a function of log a_{Ca}. Lines were fitted to the data by least-squares analysis.

Fig. 2. Impalement of a rat adipocyte with a Ca^{++}-selective microelectrode.

Despite the difference in composition of the mammalian Ringer's solution used to bathe the tissue, E_{Ca} in this solution corresponds exactly with that registered in the calibrating solution containing the same amount of Ca^{++} and having the same ionic strength. The fact that Mg^{++} does not interfere with E_{Ca} can also be determined from Fig. 1. E_{Ca} was measured in solutions containing 2×10^{-3} mol/l, 2×10^{-4} mol/l, 2×10^{-5} mol/l $CaCl_2$ either alone or together with 100 mmol/l $MgCl_2$. Activity coefficients for Ca^{++} under these conditions were either directly taken or estimated from Butler's analysis (Butler, 1968). When the difference in activity coefficients was taken into account, E_{Ca} both in pure $CaCl_2$ solution and the 100 mmol/l $MgCl_2$ mixture fell on the regression line calculated for mixtures containing K^+, Na^+ and Mg^+ indicating that, aside from their effect on ionic strength, these ions did not affect E_{Ca}. The average slope of twenty electrodes calibrated in this way was 26.9 ± 0.8 mV.

Either isolated soleus muscle fibers or adipose tissue of the rat were mounted in a simple organ chamber, under open circuit conditions at 37 °C and bathed with an oxygenated mammalian Ringer's solution containing 145 mmol/l Na^+ and 4.7. mmol/l K^+, 2 mmol/l Ca^{++} 1.5 mmol/l Mg^{++}, and 154 mmol/l Cl^- (pH 7.4). The muscle fibers or adipocytes were impaled with conventional and Ca^{++}-selective microelectrodes. Fig. 2 is an oscilloscope tracing of a cell impalement

in adipose tissue recorded in one of these experiments. After impalement there was a rapid downward (negative) deflection of the microelectrode potential, which reached a minimum (-127 mV). The potential
remained steady until the microelectrode was withdawn. After with-
drawal, the potential returned rapidly to its initial value (+25 mV)
in the Ringer's solution. The equation

$$a^i_{Ca}/a^o_{Ca} = 2.303 \ exp[(\Delta E - \overline{Em})/s_{Ca}]$$

was used to calculate a^i_{Ca} from 20 recordings, similar to Fig. 2, in
adipose tissue and 21 recordings of impalements in muscle fibers.
Here ΔE is the potential difference of the Ca^{++} electrode between
the steady-state potentials in the cell interior and the bathing medium. $\overline{Em}$ is the average membrane potential for the adipocytes (-46.1
$\pm$ 0.9 mV, n = 35) and the muscle fibers (-77.8 $\pm$ 1.3 mV; n = 51) and
s_{Ca} is the slope of the electrode used to measure each value of ΔE.
The a^i_{Ca} for adipocytes and muscle fibers in these experiments were
respectively 4.1 $\pm$ 1.2 x 10^{-7} mol/1, (n = 20), and 4.9 + 1.1 x 10^{-7}
mol/1, (n = 21). These results are in good agreement with those found
previously in the epithelium cells of the fly salivary gland (8.7
x 10^{-7}) (O'Doherty et al., 1980).

ACKNOWLEDGEMENTS

This work was supported by USPHS grant AM 26246 and the American
Diabes Association. R.J. Stark was the recipient of a XL Faculty Grant
from the Purdue Research Foundation and an Indiana University UROC
grant.

REFERENCES

Butler, J.N., 1968, The thermodynamic activity of calcium ion in
    chloride-calcium chloride electrolytes, Biophysical. J., 8:1426.
O'Doherty, J., Stark, R.J., and Armstrong, W.,McD. 1980,Calcium re-
    gulation during stimulus-secretion coupling: Continuous measur-
    ement of intracellular calcium activities, Science, (In Press).
Simon, W., Amenesu, D., Oehme, M., and Morf, W.E., 1978, Calcium-
    selective electrodes, Ann. N. Y. Acad. Sci., 307:52.
Stark, R.J., Read, P.D., and O'Doherty, J., 1980,Measurements of
    intracellular Na^+ and K^+ during insulin stimulation of skeletal
    muscle, The Physiologist, (In Press).

pH RELATED POTASSIUM MOVEMENTS IN RABBIT ATRIUM

Diana L. Kunze and John M. Russell

Department of Physiology and Biophysics
University of Texas Medical Branch
Galveston, Texas 77550

INTRODUCTION

A relationship between the distribution of hydrogen and potassium ions across cell membranes has been documented by numerous studies using both in vivo and in vitro preparations (Adler and Fray, 1977). Potassium appears to leave the cells of both skeletal and cardiac muscle when extracellular acidosis is produced and to enter the cells under conditions of extracellular alkalosis. There has as yet been no explanation for the mechanism of the exchange. We were particularly interested in this problem because a period of myocardial ischemia results in both an extracellular acidosis and a movement of potassium from the myocardial cells (Case et al., 1969). The specific question we asked was whether the decrease in extracellular pH could be the initiating factor in potassium loss. To investigate this, we chose an isolated rabbit atrial preparation which could be superfused with solutions of various composition while recording both intracellular and extracellular potassium activity.

METHODS AND RESULTS

Rabbits were killed by cervical dislocation. The heart was excised and the atria quickly removed. Either the left or right atrium was pinned endocardial surface up. When the right atrium was used, the pacemaker tissue was cut away. All studies were done with quiescent tissue. The tissue was superfused with Krebs Henseleit solution gassed with 95% O_2/5% CO_2 and maintained at 37 °C. Both intracellular and extracellular potassium were measured using double barrel potassium liquid ion sensitive microelectrodes inserted into either the intracellular or in the extracellular space within one or two cell layers of the surface. An acidosis was produced when the pH of the extra-

95

cellular perfusate was reduced from 7.45 to 6.8, or 6.1, by decreasing the bicarbonate concentration from 25 mmol/l to 5 mmol/l or 1 mmol/l at constant pCO_2. When extracellular pH was reduced to 6.8, extracellular potassium activity increased from 3.6 mmol/l to 3.9 mmol/l within thirty minutes at which time the value stabilized. The effect was fully reversible over a 20-30 minute period when the bathing solution was returned to a normal pH of 7.45. Intracellular measurements of potassium activity while pH_o was maintained at 6.8 showed that the potassium activity value of 91 $\pm$ 0.2 mmol/l at pH 7.45 fell to 86 $\pm$ 0.2 mmol/l after one hour. The changes were greater when pH was reduced to 6.1 (Table 1). These studies showed a net movement of potassium from the intracellular to extracellular space occurring when the pH was reduced by lowering extracellular HCO_3^-. Was this an effect of extracellular H+ activity? If so, a decrease in pH_o produced by a means other than reducing HCO_3^- should also produce a K^+ loss. This was tested by the following experiment. Potassium in the extracellular space was measured when the pH_o was reduced from 7.45 to 7.2 or 6.85 by increasing the CO_2 content from 5% to 10% or 20% while maintaining the bicarbonate constant. When the CO_2 of the superfusate was increased from 5% to 10% or 20%, there was no change in the extracellular potassium. Measurements of intracellular potassium over a one hour period at pH 6.86 showed no change from control (92 $\pm$ 0.3). Thus, the redistribution of potassium was not dependent solely upon the extracellular pH. An obvious difference between the two methods of reducing the pH is that a rapid development of an intracellular acidosis is expected when the extracellular pH_o is reduced by increasing CO_2 while a more slowly developing intracellular acidosis is expected when the extracellular pH is reduced by decreasing bicarbonate (Ellis and Thomas, 1977; Aickin and Thomas, 1977). To determine whether the time course of the development of the intracellular acidosis could explain the results we measured intracellular pH using the Thomas type recessed tip glass pH microelectrodes. A single barrel electrode of the same shape and tip as the insulating barrel of the pH electrode was filled with 3 mol/l KCl and served as the intracellular potential measuring electrode. This electrode was placed in the tissue adjacent to the pH electrode. The intracellular pH was measured when the pH_o was reduced to 6.8 by reducing bicarbonate from 25 mmol/l to 5 mmol/l. The pH fell from a value of 7.01 $\pm$ 01 to 6.81 $\pm$ 0.4 (n = 6) within the thirty minute time period during which extracellular potassium would have been increasing. In another series of experiments, the CO_2 was increased to 20%, and the intracellular pH fell rapidly from 7.00 $\pm$ .01 to 6.76 $\pm$ .05 (n = 6). pH_i was reduced in the two cases but the tissue in which pH_o was reduced by lowering bicarbonate was losing potassium while the other was not. Thus, neither intracellular nor extracellular pH alone is responsible for the potassium loss during the acidosis produced by lowering HCO_3^-.

Alternate explanations include the dependence of potassium movements on the hydrogen or bicarbonate ion gradients. Data confirming

Table 1. Effects of pH on intracellular and
extracellular potassium

pH	CO_2	HCO_3^-	K_i(one hour)	K_o(30 min)
7.40	5%	25 mmol/l	91±0.2 mmol/l	3.6 mmol/l
6.80	5%	5 mmol/l	86±0.2 mmol/l	3.9±0.01 mmol/l
6.10	5%	1 mmol/l	80±0.3 mmol/l	5.0±0.02 mmol/l
7.45	5%	25 mmol/l	92±0.3 mmol/l	3.6 mmol/l
7.20	10%	25 mmol/l	92±0.3 mmol/l	3.6±0.01 mmol/l
6.85	20%	25 mmol/l	92±0.3 mmol/l	3.6±0.01 mmol/l

+p≤ .05
*p≤ .01

either of these will come from studies examining the gradients over
a wide range of combinations of pH, CO_2 and HCO_3^-.

REFERENCES

Adler, S., and Fray, D.S., 1977, Potassium and intracellular pH,
Kidney Int., 11:433.

Aickin, C., and Thomas, R.C., 1977, Micro-electrode measurement of
the intracellular pH and buffering power of mouse soleus muscle
fibres, J. Physiol., 267:791.

Case, R.B., Nasser, M.G., and Crampton, R.S., 1969, Biochemical
aspects of early myocardial ischemia, Am. J. Card., 24:766.

Ellis, D., and Thomas, R.C., 1976, Direct Measurement of the intracellular pH of mammalian cardiac muscle, J. Physiol., 262:755.

INTRACELLULAR FREE CALCIUM AFFECTS ELECTRIC MEMBRANE PROPERTIES.

A STUDY WITH CALCIUM-SELECTIVE MICROELECTRODES AND WITH

ARSENAZO III IN HELIX NEURONS

H.D. Lux, G. Hofmeier and J.B. Aldenhoff

Max-Planck-Institute of Psychiatry
Kraepelinstrasse 2, D-8000 Muenchen 40, F.R.G.

INTRODUCTION

Calcium activated membrane permeabilities appear usually as a consequence of calcium currents. To correlate the dynamics of Ca-entry with its effects one would wish to have a measure of steady state and transient changes of intracellular free Ca ($[Ca]_i$). Estimates by various methods suggest that the resting level of $[Ca]_i$ is at least 5 orders of magnitude lower than the value expected from a passive distribution (for review see Ashley and Campbell, 1979). Even if the increase in $[Ca]_i$ during excitation is small in absolute terms, it may be a large relative change compared to the low background level and may have an important messenger function.

Determination of intracellular free Ca-activity requires sensitive methods of detection. An indicator should possess low toxicity and little interference with the regulation of $[Ca]_i$. Ideal in all these respects are ion-selective microelectrodes (ISMs) for calcium (Brown et al., 1976; Christoffersen and Simonsen, 1977; Heinemann et al., 1977) which can now be constructed on the basis of neutral Ca-carriers (Ammann et al., 1975; see also Simon et al., 1978) to allow detection of very small steady-state changes of $[Ca]_i$. The specific advantage of these electrodes is that they give a most direct and nearly undisturbed account of changes in ionic activity. This compares favorably with the mode of action of dye indicators such as arsenazo III (Budesinsky, 1969) which bind Ca to a considerable degree in competition with intracellular Ca-buffers. However, dye indicators appear to be indispensable for recording transient changes in $[Ca]_i$ in larger nerve cells (Brown et al., 1975, 1977; Thomas and Gorman, 1977; Ahmed and Connor, 1979) since the Ca-electrode cannot be systematically positioned at the very place where these changes occur. This applies especially to the situation in which large but localized changes in Ca-activity are produced by inward Ca-currents through the neuronal membrane. Furthermore, the electrical properties of the ISMs limit the resolution of Ca-signals during membrane currents which are activated by step changes of the membrane potential. In many applications the results obtained with the indicator dye method are complementary to those from experiments with ISMs. This will be demonstrated in some examples.

METHODS

Fabrication and Calibration of Electrodes

Ca-selective microelectrodes were made following basically the techniques described by Lux and Neher (1973). The ion-selective element of these electrodes is the liquid neutral-carrier compound ETH 1001 (Ammann et al., 1975; Simon et al., 1978). The electrodes were calibrated at a range of $[Ca]$ from 10 mM down to 7 nM. Since the electrodes were meant to be used intracellularly all calibration solutions contained 100 mM KCl. Values of $[Ca]$ of less than 1 mM were adjusted by the addition of 10 mM of Ca-buffers plus the appropriate amounts of $CaCl_2$ (between 1 and 9 mM). The necessary range of $[Ca]$ is covered by three buffers with different stability constants: NTA (Merck), HEDTA (Sigma) and EGTA (Merck). The pH of the solutions was kept constant at 7.25 with 10 mM of Tris/HCl buffer. Apparent stability constants were calculated from tabulated data (Bjerrum et al., 1957) by the equations given by Portzehl et al. (1964). Numerical values obtained were 1.18×10^{-4} (NTA), 2.17×10^{-6} (HEDTA) and 6.6×10^{-8} (EGTA). The responses of the electrodes were fitted to the modified Nernst equation (IUPAC, 1976) by a nonlinear least-square computer fitting program. Amplifiers with an input resistance of more than 10^{15} Ohms and with compensation of the input capacitance were used for all measurements.

For the injection experiments (see RESULTS) we used electrodes made from the same sample of ion-exchanger which had already been used by Heinemann et al. (1977) for extracellular work. The limit of detection (IUPAC, 1976) of these electrodes was at 3.8 µM, and the slope was 29 mV per decade in Ca-concentration. These characteristics were found to be sufficient to measure the time-course of rise and fall of $[Ca]_i$ after intracellular microinjection of $CaCl_2$ solution.

The response time of these electrodes to changes in [Ca] in the same range as those induced intracellularly by the injections was tested by a fast exchange methode. The test 'chamber' was a 4µl drop hanging in a small coil of a grounded chlorided silver wire. Changes in [Ca] were performed by exchanging HEDTA-buffered solutions through a 1.5 mm capillary with its tip about 5 mm away and directed onto the drop. New readings of the potential of the Ca-ISM (Vca) were immediately stable after a period of artifacts from the exchange procedure lasting for about 200 ms.

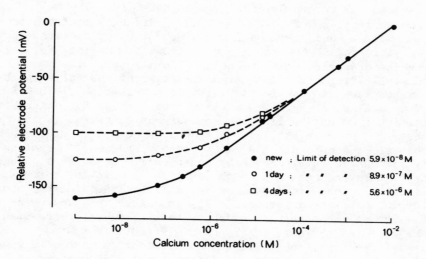

Fig.1: Calibration curves of a single-barrelled Ca-selective microelectrode for the determination of resting $[Ca]_i$ at different times after its preparation.

For the determination of the resting level of $[Ca]_i$ we prepared single-barrelled electrodes from a new sample of ETH 1001 ion-exchanger. When measured shortly after filling they displayed a limit of detection of 30 nM, corresponding to a maximal difference in Vca between 10 mM Ca (the amount of calcium in normal snail ringer) and zero Ca (in a solution with 10 mM EGTA without additional calcium) of 160 mV. As shown in Fig.1 this limit of detection increases with time, and after between one and four days the calibration curves of these electrodes were very similar to those of the electrodes made from the older sample of ion-exchanger. The original detection limit of the electrodes could be restored by freshly silanizing and then refilling them. It thus seems probable that the increase in detection limit is due to the development of a leakage conductance along the ion-exchanger/glass interface, which partly shorts Vca. Interference by Mg is not considered to be substantial, since Simon et al. (1978) give a

Mg-selectivity factor log K(CaMg) of -5.10. It is improbable that $[Mg]_i$ in snail neurons is higher than the value of about 4 mM reported for marine preparations (Brinley and Scarpa, 1975; Brinley et al., 1977), and thus the Mg-contribution in the intracellular measurements would not be more than the 30 nM detection limit without any Mg.

Measurements with Arsenazo III

Arsenazo III (Sigma Grade I) was injected into the cells to a final concentration of 0.2 to 1 mM by directly controlling the injection volume (Hofmeier and Lux, 1980). Light of a quartz-iodide lamp was filtered at 660 and 685 nm (bandwidth 5 nm) and focused by a microscope objective onto the cell to form a spot with the size of the cell diameter. The transmitted light was collected by a small fibre glass rod coupled to a photomultiplier (EMI-GENCOM QL 30). The dual-wavelength measurement was made by alternating illumination (500 Hz) by the two monochromatic beams, using the time-sharing spectrophotometer of Chance et al. (1975). The differential readout at the two closely adjacent wavelengths greatly decreased interference by non-specific absorbance changes, such as transparency changes of the cell due to flow of current, to the inserted micro-electrodes or to cell swelling. Another source of error in correlating arsenazo III signals to $[Ca]_i$ is its sensitivity to magnesium and hydrogen ions. The difference spectra for changes in pH and $[Mg]$ are distinct from the calcium difference spectrum, but if the measurement is done at a single wavelength mistakes are possible. Although the absolute size of the Ca-signal is higher at other wavelengths or wavelength pairs, the rejection of contributions by $[Mg]$ and pH is near optimum, by about 3 orders of magnitude (see also Scarpa, 1979), at 660/685 nm, but is much lower at the invidual wavelengths. Mg-signals may possibly become important with strong depolarization to near the Ca-equilibrium potential with the result of a near zero Ca-entry, but with the possibility to produce some outward Mg-current. This suggestion is supported by the occasional finding of a transient decrease of absorbance at 660 nm during such depolarizations without a signal in the difference measurement.

At low values of $[Ca]$ the absorbance changes of arsenazo III vary linearly with $[Ca]$ (Michaylova and Kouleva, 1973; Kendrick et al., 1977) which probably holds also for variations of low dye concentrations at constant $[Ca]$. For dye concentrations far exceeding the calcium concentrations a second order complex formation between Ca and arsenazo III has been proposed (Thomas and Gorman, 1978). Absorbance signals can be expressed in terms of free Ca from 'in vitro' determinations by assuming identity of optical paths with and without the cell. Alternatively, with the knowledge of the specific extinction coefficients, the dissociation constant, and the intracellular dye concentration it is possible to calculate the 'in vivo' Ca-concentration, since the ratio of the absorbance of the arsenazo III- Ca complex to that of the uncomplexed dye is proportional to $[Ca]_i$. Although this formulation has the advantage of being free of optical parameters its application to the experimental situation is limited. The most important error arises from the determination of the dye concentration by measuring absorbance, which in the cell does not properly represent the 'in vitro' value. It is also not known whether the absorbance coefficients remain unaltered in the presence of cytoplasmic Ca-buffers. Since an error in the determination of resting $[Ca]_i$ by one order of magnitude is entirely possible, controlled injection of arsenazo III and determination of resting $[Ca]_i$ by Ca-ISMs is preferable. Other details of the experimental procedure are similar to those found in Gorman and Thomas (1978) and Ahmed and Connor (1979).

Experimental Preparation

Two types of cells were used, the fast burster cell (Heyer and Lux, 1976) in the right parietal ganglion of the subesophageal mass of Helix pomatia, and cells in the group D cluster (Sakharov and Salanki, 1969) of this ganglion which are characterized by predominant inward Ca-currents. Almost all of the outward currents of the latter cells are activated during depolarization under the additional condition that extracellular Ca is present. All experiments were performed at 18°C and pH 7.6 in saline containing (in mM) 80 NaCl, 4 KCl, 10 $CaCl_2$, 5 $MgCl_2$, and 10 HEPES buffer. In Ni or Mg saline all $CaCl_2$ was substituted by $NiCl_2$ or $MgCl_2$. The voltage clamp arrangement was similar to that used by Heyer and Lux(1976).

RESULTS

Resting Intracellular $[Ca]$

With freshly made ISMs which had a calibration curve as shown in Fig.1 the potential drop on penetration of the membrane measured differentially against the normal intracellular electrode amounted to values of about -150 mV in neurones clamped to a constant holding potential of -50 mV. From the calibration curve and with the single-ion activity coefficient for extracellular Ca of 0.25 at the ionic strength of the Ringer solution (Bates et al., 1970) an intracellular Ca-activity of about 10 nM is calculated. This is considerably lower than values reported before from measurements with electrodes employing different types of ion-exchangers (Owen et al., 1977, Christoffersen and Simonsen, 1977).

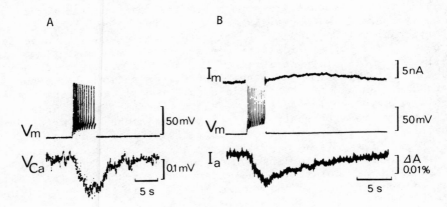

Fig.2: Response of the external Ca-selective microelectrode (A) and of the intracellular arsenazo III absorbance change (B) accompanying trains of action potentials in two pacemaker cells. The cells were kept at -60 mV holding potential (Vm) and action potentials were elicited by step changes into current clamp mode. A) The ISM recording (Vca) of the decrease in $[Ca]_o$ was made close to the apparent (glia covered) surface of the cell body. B) Upper trace (Im) membrane current; note the delayed appearence of a small outward current after the spikes. Middle trace (Vm) membrane voltage with action potentials. Lower trace (anode current Ia) records the arsenazo III absorbance changes during and after the spikes.

Signals Recorded During Discharge Activity

It was not yet possible to detect significant signals of the intracellular Ca-ISM during action potentials, either spontaneous or evoked by depolarizing current. However, decreases of extracellular Ca-activity ($[Ca]_o$) are well detectable by the ISM during bursts of spikes (Fig.2A). The recording was made close to the glial cover of the cell and was repeated at varied distances from the cell surface to achieve an approximation of the total amount of Ca which was lost from the surround (Neher and Lux, 1973). The resulting gain of intracellular Ca can be estimated by assuming a cytoplasmic diffusion coefficient of $6 \times 10^2 \ \mu m^2/s$ (Hodgkin and Keynes, 1957) and using the expression for diffusion of Ca during constant flux through the membrane (Carslaw and Jaeger, 1959). At distance zero under the membrane a value near 50μM is obtained for the local Ca-concentration. The estimate of the Ca-gain from the absorbance signal in Fig.2B from a similar cell suggests an average increase of $[Ca]_i$ by only about 50 nM, near to the values found in comparable cells of other species during similar trains of spikes (Gorman and Thomas, 1978).

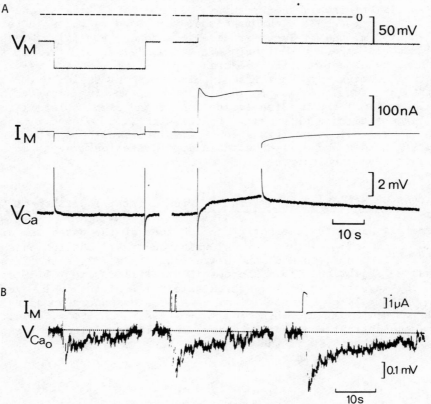

Fig.3: Intracellular and extracellular responses of Ca-selective microelectrodes during depolarizing voltage clamp pulses. A) The electrode was inserted into a voltage clamped burster neuron (holding potential -50 mV) and longlasting step changes of voltage were applied (Vm). The Im trace shows membrane currents during the voltage steps. No signal of the Ca-ISM (Vca) with the hyperpolarizing pulse. A small, slowly rising signal appears throughout the depolarizing step which produces outward K-currents after a relatively short inward Ca-current transient. B) The external ISM recording (Vca) was made close (about 10 μm) to the cell body of another burster cell which was depolarized to +35 mV by voltage steps from a holding potential of -50 mV. Note the large increase of the signal with double step application (middle) and with pulse prolongation (right).

The comparison of the observations in Fig.2A and B is limited by the inherent approximations but may be useful to illustrate the probably extreme differences between average and local Ca-concentrations due to steep gradients within the cytoplasm.

Weak intracellular Ca-signals were observed with ISMs during depolarizing voltage clamp steps to membrane potentials at which the persistent inward Ca-current is turned on (Eckert and Lux, 1976). To produce a clear response, the steps to voltages between -20 and +30 mV had to last for several seconds (Fig.3A). Rises in $[Ca]_i$ could then be clearly distinguished from the artifacts produced by stepping the membrane potential, which were also observed during hyperpolarizing pulses without Ca-influx. Because of the low sensitivity of the electrode at the intracellular baseline level the precise evaluation of the signals is difficult. The largest signals obtained with ISMs with 4 µM detection limit were 2 mV, indicating that a considerable elevation of $[Ca]_i$ up to about 1 µM does occur with suitable depolarizations even at some distance from the membrane.

Time Course of $[Ca]_i$ and Membrane Currents after Injection of $CaCl_2$

Fig.4 shows the characteristic changes of the potential of the Ca-ISM and of membrane current which occur at constant potential (-50 mV) in consequence of the elevation of $[Ca]_i$ by a shortlasting pressure injection with a microcapillary filled with 100 mM $CaCl_2$. With the injected quantity, approximately 1 % of the cell volume, peak Vca values of about 30 mV were attained, corresponding to a Ca-level of 50 µM. The mean time to peak was about 11 s, and it can be assumed that Ca has then largely equilibrated inside the cell. Thus, only about 5 % of the injected ions appeared to be left unsequestered after this time.

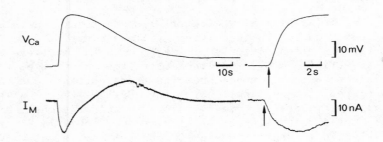

Fig.4: Intracellular response of a Ca-ISM (Vca) and membrane current (Im) at a holding potential of -50 mV after a short intracellular injection (arrow) of 100 mM $CaCl_2$ solution (ca. 1% of cell volume). Left, slower speed recording; right, recording with faster speed to show the initial phase of the response.

It should be noted that the peak $[Ca]_i$ achieved by the injection is entirely comparable to concentrations under the membrane which are expected to occur in the course of several

Ca-injecting action potentials or during maximum inward Ca-currents with step depolarizations of about 100 ms duration. This can be inferred from the density of peak inward Ca-current (of the order of $10-12$ A/μm^2) at zero potential of these neurons.

The earliest effect of a micromolar increase in $[Ca]_i$ was always the development of an inward current, while the Vca signal rose with some delay. This delay was caused by the diffusion of the injected Ca across the cell towards the ISM which was opposite to the injection pipette to ensure an earlier arrival of Ca at the membrane. The inward current was transient and the current turned outward after the peak of Vca and reached a maximum about four times slower than Vca. The relative sizes of the two phases of injection-induced currents as well as their timing were variable in different experiments, but the sequence of currents was constant and the outward current was always observed to peak during the decay of Vca.

The similarity between the time course of the rise of the inward current with that of the Vca signal suggests that it is due to direct action of the injected Ca-ions, as they spread throughout the cell and reach an increasingly larger part of the internal membrane surface. The peak of the inward transient always occurred somewhat earlier than that of Vca. This may be due to the subsequent activation of the oppositely directed outward current, produced by the K-conductance originally observed by Meech (1972,1979). The peak of this secondary effect of calcium-injection on membrane current occurs clearly rather late during the phase of declining Vca. By pulsing the membrane to different potentials during the two phases of current activation, the equilibrium potentials of the two currents can be calculated and it becomes possible to separate the two conductances carrying the initial unspecific inward current and the later outward K-current.

Control injections of 100 mM KCl, pure water or the ion-exchanger in the injection pipette were without any effect on membrane current, excluding artifactual origin of the observed inward-outward current sequence from our injection technique. If sufficient time was allowed for the neurons to recover from each injection - and if the injection pipette did not block in the course of the experiment - the sequence of inward-outward current responses can be elicited by repeated injections for an arbitrary number of times. In one such experiment lasting for several hours calcium was injected 42 times with qualitatively identical effects, but some slowing of the time courses at later times.

These findings can give a satisfactory account for the origin of the spontaneous activity pattern of bursting pacemaker neurons. One of the most prominent features of this activity is the biphasic time course of the discharge frequency during each burst. The initial increase in the rate of action potentials is in line with a production of inward currents as a consequence of the considerable elevation of the submembrane Ca-level produced by first spikes. This phenomenon is difficult to understand on the basis of a K conductance as a primary result of the increase in $[Ca]_i$. The observations of the delayed appearence of the K-current also explains the fact that the maximum of the post-burst-hyperpolarization is delayed by several seconds in respect to the last action potential of the burst, and thus from the absolute peak in internal Ca-activity. With sporadic low frequency activity on the basis of a higher resting membrane conductance, both Ca mediated effects could overlap with the result of a less pronounced biphasic discharge activity.

Aftereffects of Elevated $[Ca]_i$ by Membrane Currents

An overlasting inward current component that appears after a series of action potentials in related bursting pacemaker neurons has already been observed by observed by Gola (1974) and Smith et al.(1975). Amplitude and time course of this phenomenon is well comparable to that after intracellular Ca-injection. It is more difficult to study the aftereffects of the Ca-entry by Ca-currents during depolarizing voltage clamp pulses. These pulses produce outward K-currents of considerable amplitude shortly after the initial Ca-current. Although the tail currents after the pulse show reversal potentials that are distinctly positive from the K equilibrium potential, it is not possible to simply attribute this finding to an overlasting inward current. This cannot always be separated from the shift of the K-potential which is produced by the external K-accumulation during the outward current. However, indirect evidence supports the suggestion of increased inward, fast as well as slow, tail current components in the course of repetitive Ca-injecting clamp pulses in bursting pacemaker neurons (Heyer and Lux, 1976).

As suggested by the results of intracellular Ca-injection, aftereffects of Ca-currents during a clamp pulse can be longlasting and a typical example of this is shown in Fig.4. The results are principally similar to observations of Tillotson and Horn (1978) and Tillotson (1979) with similar clamp pulse paradigms in preparations with reduced K-currents. The pulse presented with an interval to an identical pulse showed a considerably depressed net peak inward current which was largely carried by Ca since it disappeared reversibly when external Ca was substituted by Ni. The depression of the peak inward Ca-current was previously taken to indicate significant inactivation of Ca-currents by $[Ca]_i$ that was elevated by the first pulse. This conclusion was strengthened by the additional observation that varied first pulse amplitudes produced a depression of the net inward current of the second pulse

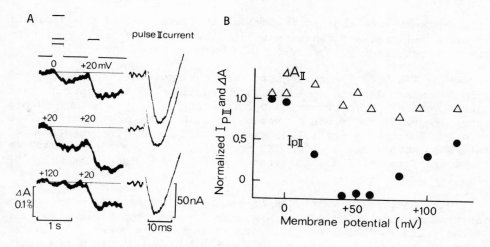

Fig.5: Effects of varying the voltage of a prepulse on the transient net inward current of a subsequent pulse. A) Arsenazo III absorbance signals of the pulses (left) and the initial net inward current (right) of the subsequent test pulse. Three examples of the conditioning pulse - testpulse paradigm (see top trace) are given. Note the variation in the arsenazo III signal during the leading pulse and the constancy of the absorbance signal of the test pulse. B) Peak amplitudes of the net inward currents and maximum ansorbance changes during the second pulse are plotted against membrane potential of the first pulse (abscissa). The data are normalized in respect to those of a pulse to +20 mV in the absence of a preceding pulse. Holding potential was -50 mV.

in close correlation to the Ca-current of the first pulse (Tillotson, 1979). Again, this applies to the net peak inward current of the cells in our study but not to the Ca-entry which was simultaneously recorded with the arsenazo III absorbance (compare Fig.5A and B). In fact, the absorbance signal of the second pulse is not much affected by the leading pulse and often an even slightly larger second signal was obvious if the first signal was near maximum. The considerable divergence between the behaviour of net inward current and Ca-entry has probably a simple explanation. The depression of the peak inward current is merely the result of overlasting membrane conductances due to the Ca-entry of the first pulse which at positive membrane potentials produces an instantaneous outward current that obscures the true inward Ca-current of the second pulse. In addition, voltage dependent activation of the Ca-mediated outward K-current (see below) may occur during the second pulse which could assist to reduce the inward current transient. Such effects do not seem to be excluded in the experiments of Tillotson (1979). The strenghth of the aftereffects of preceding Ca-entry may vary amongst different cells and preparations, but it is obvious that net current measurements without independent assessment of the Ca-entry can lead to misinterpretations of specific ionic current flow.

Also ISM recordings suggested an unchanged Ca-entry during the second pulse despite the drastic reduction of its apparent peak inward current. With intervals below about 300 ms preceding pulses were observed to produce probably voltage dependent inactivation effects. These were partial, however, and even prolongation of pulses up to several seconds did not fully suppress the Ca-entry as concluded from both, the absorbance signals and the external ISM signals.

With interpulse intervals of one second a particularly large increase by about 60 % of the arsenazo III absorbance signal of the second pulse was observed in several bursting pacemaker cells at membrane potentials between +10 and +30 mV. These observations are in line with earlier results by another method of an increased inward current component during subsequent pulses (Heyer and Lux, 1976). The observation that the amplitudes of the arsenazo III absorbance signals are maintained or increased during second or third pulses of pulse series with suitable intervals deserves some comment. There is the definite property of the arsenazo III - Ca reaction in the intracellular situation to increase less than linearly with increasing availability of free Ca. This is due to the fact that experimentally useful dye concentrations are restricted to the millimolar range (2 mM) to avoid significant disturbances of the intracellular Ca-equilibration by the arsenazo III - Ca complex (Brown et al., 1977). In this situation and since the dissociation constant of the arsenazo III - Ca reaction of 50μM (Scarpa, 1979) is in the range of expected submembrane Ca-concentrations it appears to be entirely possible that the reaction becomes locally depressed since it approaches saturation. From this argument a less than proportional increase of the arsenazo III absorbance for an increment in Ca-entry should be expected in line with results of Ahmed and Connor (1979). An increase of the arsenazo III absorbance change during a subsequent pulse in a series should be more significant for an increased Ca-entry in comparison with that of the first pulse. However, there is an alternative explanation based on the hypothesis of specific localized cytoplasm Ca-buffers that make less free Ca available for reaction with dye unless the capacity of the system becomes exhausted. Some of the early entering Ca may be lost into the Ca-sequestering buffer system of high affinity (Baker and Schlaepfer, 1978) but it cannot be decided wether such a possible loss of resolution of the true Ca-entry applies to the double pulses as well as to the single pulse situation. A systematic study of this problem with the extracellular Ca-ISM could be ideal but the ISMs are very sensitive to the large voltage change of the adjacent current injecting electrodes in the voltage clamp situation. Thus, large transient artifacts must usually be separated from a small ΔVca ($<$ 1 mV) and the measurement of Vca is necessarily confined to times several seconds after the pulses. This obstacle limits the systematic use of ISMs in such studies.

External Ca-Measurements and Arsenazo III Signals in Current-Voltage Determinations

Estimates of the actual Ca-entry by inward Ca-currents are difficult to obtain from the arsenazo III absorbance changes. These represent an undefined average of the reaction with internal free Ca over the cell volume. This average is certainly time dependent and conclusions towards amounts of Ca that entered the cells or towards submembrane Ca-levels are possible only with detailed knowledge of the equilibration kinetics of free intracellular Ca. It is also not known wether intracellular Ca buffering systems are uniform inside the cell. This difficulty adds to uncertainties of calibrating the absorbance changes in terms of absolute levels of free Ca.

Theoretically it is more simple to gather an estimate of the Ca-entry from the loss of external Ca-activity as the result of inward Ca-currents. The external ISM signals can be anticipated to follow diffusion kinetics with relatively small distortion by secondary processes such as Ca-pumping. One method of a direct determination of absolute sizes of ion fluxes by external ISM recordings at varied distances from the cell surface has already been described (Neher and Lux, 1973). In cases where the peak and the decay times of the external Ca-signal are well determined, the significant parameters diffusional distance and diffusion coefficient can be received from the mathematical analysis of the slope characteristics of the ISM signal (Lux and Hofmeier, 1979). It turned out that the diffusion coefficient at distances near the cell surface is smaller than in the bathing medium, which is attributable to the glial layer which restricts the access to the neuronal membrane. A best fit procedure to describe the time course of the external Ca-changes resulted in values of about 1/4 of that in free solution. In practice, due to the radial geometry, the calculated flux values were less than linearly dependent on the choice of the effective diffusion coefficient. An error of a factor of 2 in its estimation or in that of decay times would result in about the same error in flux values. The average current for a pulse of 300 ms duration producing maximum Ca-entry, i.e. Ca-loss from the outside, at membrane potentials near + 50 mV was calculated to be between 50 - 300 nA and thus in the 10 % range of the outward current. The resulting increase in intracellular Ca was found to be considerably higher, by two orders of magnitude, than the changes in free Ca calculated from the arsenazo III measurements.

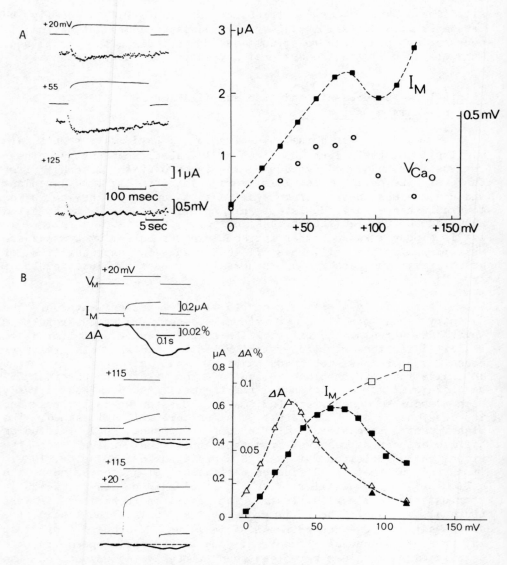

Fig.6: A) Current-voltage (■) and [Ca]$_o$-voltage (○) relationships of a fast burster neuron (each measurement averaged from 8 trials). Left: Examples of membrane currents and of external Ca-loss.
B) Current-voltage (■) and absorbance-voltage (△) relationships of a cell with predominant inward Ca-currents and Ca-dependent outward currents. Left: Examples of clamp pulses (Vm) with membrane currents (Im) and arsenazo III absorbance changes (△A) (each trace averaged from 4 trials). The lowermost traces were obtained with a prepulse to +20 mV of 6 ms duration. Open symbols in the I/V -plot on the right denote signals with prepulse activation.

The peak Ca-loss which is estimated from the external ISM signals appears to occur at somewhat higher depolarizations than in the measurements with arsenazo III. This is probably due to residual voltage artifacts which produce increased distortions of Vca with increasing amplitudes of currents in the voltage clamp situation. The signal at + 125 mV membrane potential in Fig.6A was probably of artifactual nature, and if proportionally sized distortions are subtracted the probable peak Ca-loss would be near or below + 50 mV. Determinations by the indicator dye method are more reliable in this situation and fewer repetitions are necessary to achieve a sufficient signal to noise ratio. The peak entry suggested by these recordings was at between +20 and +40mV for pulse durations of 100 to 300 ms (Fig.6B). With stronger depolarization beyond +120 mV the absorbance signal decreased towards zero. An inversion of the signal was never observed with the differential absorbance method.

The experiment of Fig.6B presents also a characteristic example of the strong activation of the Ca-dependent K-current ($I(K,Ca)$) by a shortlasting preceding pulse. The Ca-injecting prepulse plus the subsequent pulse to + 115 mV produced a rather small absorbance signal. This signal was not significantly different from that without the prepulse. Thus a large activation of the Ca-dependent outward current can occur in the absence of a significant Ca-entry as indicated by the unchanged arsenazo III-absorbance signal. Ca-entry and activation of the Ca-dependent outward current are obviously not proportional. Prepulses to +20 mV of 10ms duration were maximally effective in activating the outward current, but produced hardly detectable absorbance changes. These were in any case smaller than the absorbance signals of longlasting (> 200 ms) depolarizations to membrane potentials between +80 and +110 mV, at which $I(K,Ca)$ was poorly activated. Thus, activation of $I(K,Ca)$ appears to require relatively little inward Ca-movement.

It has already been noted that activation of the Ca-mediated K-current $I(K,Ca)$ (Lux and Hofmeier, 1979a,b) is voltage dependent and thus different from the non-rectifying outward K-current which appears late after elevation of $[Ca]_i$ by injection of Ca-salts (Hofmeier and Lux, 1980). In fact, increased $[Ca]_i$ has an early depressing action on $I(K,Ca)$ (Heyer and Lux, 1976) particularly in the bursting pacemaker cells.

CONCLUSIONS

Ca-dependent functions in nerve cells are manifold and important electrogenic changes in membrane properties are coupled to intracellular changes in free Ca or directly to Ca-movement through the membranes. In many instances net Ca-currents through the membrane cannot be separated from other currents, including those activated by Ca. Independent measurements of the Ca-entry with the help of ISMs and dye indicators are necessary in this situation to identify Ca-coupled processes. Although the true time course of Ca-currents and the exact intracellular, particularly submembrane Ca-activity is not determinable by either method, ISM and dye methods are useful for achieving a quantitative account for the relationship between inward Ca-currents and changes in intracellular free Ca with subsequent alterations in electric membrane properties, as has been shown in some examples. Quantitative estimates of Ca-fluxes are difficult and probably more reliable with ISM methods than with the arsenazo III-Ca reaction, since the latter competes with intracellular Ca-buffering and is subject to large gradients of intracellular Ca-activity. In addition, there is the possibility of saturation of the dye-Ca reaction due to a considerable submembrane Ca-concentration in the case of inward Ca-current. Use of ISMs could be preferable for this purpose, but it is impeded by the enormous difficulties of a sufficiently precise intracellular localisation of the ISM. Measurements of steady state $[Ca]_i$ with ISMs can be important to ascertain the true intracellular Ca-activity in experiments recording transient changes by the indicator dye method.

REFERENCES

Ahmed, Z., and Connor, J.A., 1979, Measurement of calcium influx under voltage clamp in molluscan neurones using the metallo-chromic dye arsenazo III, J. Physiol. (Lond.), 286:61.

Ammann, D., Güggi, M., Pretsch, E., and Simon, W., 1975, Improved calcium selective electrode based on a neutral carrier, Analyt. Lett., 8:709.

Ashley, C.C., and Campbell, A.K., eds., 1979, Detection and measurement of free Ca^{++} in cells, Elsevier, Amsterdam.

Baker, P.F., and Schlaepfer, W.W., 1978, Uptake and binding of calcium by axoplasm isolated from giant axons of Loligo and Myxicola, J. Physiol. (Lond.), 276:103.

Bates, R.G., Staples, B.R., and Robinson, R.A., 1970, Ionic hydration and single ion activities in unassociated chlorides at high ionic strengths, Anal. Chem., 42:867.

Bjerrum, I., Schwarzenbach, G., and Sillen, L.G., 1957, Stability constants, Part I: Organic ligands, The Chemical Society, London.

Brinley, F.J., and Scarpa, A., 1975, Ionized magnesium concentration in axoplasm of dialyzed squid axons, FEBS Lett., 50:82.

Brinley, F.J., Scarpa, A., and Tiffert, T., 1977, The concentration of ionized magnesium in barnacle muscle fibres, J. Physiol. (Lond.), 266:545.

Brown, H.M., Pemberton, J.P., and Owen, J.D., 1976, A calcium-sensitive microelectrode suitable for intracellular measurement of calcium(II) activity, Anal. Chim. Acta, 85:261.

Brown, J.E., Cohen, L.B., DeWeer, P., Pinto, L.H., Ross, W.N., and Salzberg, B.M., 1975, Rapid changes of intracellular free calcium concentration: Detection by metallochromic indicator dyes in squid giant axon, Biophys. J., 15:1155.

Brown, J.E., Brown, P.K., and Pinto, L.H., 1977, Detection of light-induced change of intracellular ionized calcium concentration in Limulus neural photoreceptors using arsenazo III, J. Physiol. (Lond.), 267:299.

Budesinsky, B., 1969, Monoarylazo and bis(arylazo) derivations of chromotropic acid as photometric reagents, in:'Chelates in Analytical Chemistry, vol. 2:1', Flaschka, H.A., and Bamard, A.S., eds., M. Dekker, New York.

Carslaw, H.S., and Jaeger, J.C., 1959, Conduction of heat in soldis, Clarendon Press, Oxford.

Chance, B., Legallais, V., Sorge, J., and Graham, N., 1975, A versatile time-sharing multi-channel spectrophotometer, reflecto-meter, and fluorometer, Analyt. Biochem., 66:498.

Christoffersen, G.R.J., and Simonsen, L., 1977, Ca^{2+}-sensitive microelectrode: Intracellular steady state measurement in nerve cell, Acta Physiol. Scand., 101:492.

Eckert, R., Lux, H.D., 1976, A voltage-sensitive persistent calcium conductance in neuronal somata of Helix, J. Physiol. (Lond.), 254:129.

Gola, M., 1974, Neurones a ondes-salves des mollusques, Pflüger's Arch., 352:17.

Gorman, A.L.F., and Thomas, M.V., 1978, Changes in the intracellular concentration of free calcium ions in a pacemaker neurone, measured with the metallochromic indicator dye arsenazo III, J. Physiol. (Lond.), 275:357

Heinemann, U., Lux, H.D., and Gutnick, M.J., 1977, Extracellular free calcium and potassium during paroxysmal activity in the cerebral cortex of the cat, Expl. Brain Res., 27:237.

Heyer, C.B., and Lux, H.D., 1976, Properties of a facilitating calcium current in pacemaker neurones of the snail, Helix pomatia, J. Physiol. (Lond.), 262:349.

Hodgkin, A.L., and Keynes, R.D., 1957, Movements of labelled calcium in squid giant axons, J. Physiol. (Lond.), 138:253.

Hofmeier, G., and Lux, H.D., 1980, Intracellular applications of Ca-selective microelectrodes in voltage-clamped snail neurons, in: 'Ion-selective electrodes in physiology and medicine II', Lübbers, D.W., ed., Springer, Heidelberg (in press).

International Union of pure and applied chemistry, 1976, Recommen-dations for nomenclature of ion-selective electrodes, Pure and Appl. Chem., 48:127.

Kendrick, N.C., Ratzlaff, R.W., and Blaustein, M.P., 1977, Arsenazo III as an indicator for ionized calcium in physiological salt solutions: its use for determination of the Ca-ATP disso-ciation constant, Analyt. Biochem., 48:433.

Lux, H.D., and Hofmeier, G., 1979a, Effects of calcium currents and intracellular free calcium in Helix neurons, in: 'Detection and measurement of free Ca^{++} in cells', Ashley C.C., and Campbell, A.K., eds., Elsevier, Amsterdam.

Lux, H.D., and Hofmeier, G., 1979b, The voltage dependence of the calcium mediated K current $(I(K,Ca))$ in Helix neurons, Neurosc. Lett., Suppl.3:582.

Lux. H.D., and Neher, E., 1973, The equilibration time course of $[K^+]_o$ in cat cortex, Expl. Brain Res., 17:190.

Meech, R.W., 1972, Intracellular calcium injection causes increased potassium conductance in Aplysia nerve cells, Comp. Biochem. Physiol., 42A:493.

Meech, R.W., 1979, Membrane potential oscillations in molluscan "burster" neurones, J. Exp. Biol., 81:93.

Michaylova, V., and Kouleva, N., 1973, Arsenazo III as metallo-chromic indicator for complexometric determination of calcium in slightly alkaline medium, Talanta, 20:453.

Neher, E., and Lux, H.D., 1973, Rapid changes of potassium concentration at the outer surface of exposed single neurons during membrane current flow, J. Gen. Physiol., 61:385.

Owen, J.D., Brown, H.M., and Pemberton, J.P., 1977, Neurophysiological application of a calcium-selective micrelectrode, Anal. Chim. Acta, 90:241.

Portzehl, H., Caldwell, P.C., and Ruegg, J.C., 1964, The dependence of contraction and relaxation of muscle fibres from the crab Maia squinado on the internal concentration of free calcium ions, Biochim. Biophys. Acta, 79:581.

Sakharov, D.A., and Salanki, J., 1969, Physiological and pharmacological identification of neurons in the central nervous system of Helix pomatia L., Acta Physiol. Acad. Sci. Hung., 35:19.

Scarpa, A., 1979, Measurement of calcium ion concentrations with metallochromic indicators, in:'Detection and measurement of free Ca^{++} in cells', Ashley, C.C., and Campbell, A.K., eds., Elsevier, Amsterdam.

Simon, W., Ammann, D., Oehme, M., and Morf, W.E., 1978, Calcium-selective electrodes, in:'Calcium Transport and Cell Function', Scarpa, A., and Carafoli, E., eds., Ann. N. Y. Acad. Sci., 307:52.

Smith, T.G., Barker, J.L., and Gainer, H., 1975, Requirements for bursting pacemaker potential activity in molluscan neurones, Nature, 253:450.

Thomas, M.V., and Gorman, A.L.F., 1977, Internal calcium changes in a bursting pacemaker neuron measured with arsenazo III, Science, 196:531.

Thomas, M.V., and Gorman, A.L.F., 1978, Arsenazo III forms a 2:1 complex with Ca under physiological conditions, Biophys. J., 21:53a.

Tillotson, D., and Horn, R., 1978, Interaction without facilitation of calcium conductances in caesium-loaded neurons of Aplysia, Nature, 273:312.

Tillotson, D., 1979, Inactivation of Ca conductance dependent on entry of Ca ions in molluscan neurons, Proc. Natl. Acad. Sci. USA, 76:1497.

MEASUREMENT OF FREE Ca^{2+} IN NERVE CELL BODIES

F.J. Alvarez-Leefmans*, T.J. Rink and R.Y. Tsien

Physiological Laboratory, Downing Street,
Cambridge CB 2 3EG, U.K. and *Departamento
de Neurociencias, Centro de Investigacion del
I.P.N., Apartado Postal 14-740, Mexico 14, D.F.

INTRODUCTION

In principle it is simple to insert an ion-selective micro-electrode into a cell, measure the drop in potential, subtract from it the membrane potential to give the differential signal, and calculate from that the free ion concentration. In practice, particularly with Ca^{2+}, it is not so straightforward and here we outline some of the problems to be overcome and precautions needed in obtaining believable data, and summarize some of the results we have obtained in giant neurones of Helix aspersa (Alvarez-Leefmans et al., submitted for publication).

ELECTRODES

It has proved difficult to produce calcium-selective microelectrodes with tips ≤ 1 μm that have adequate performance for measuring the very low levels of Ca^{2+} in cytoplasm. The organophosphate based sensors appear to have inadequate Mg^{2+} rejection (Owen and Brown, 1979) and their use with tips ≤ 1 μm has not been reported. The neutral carrier, liquid sensor formulation of Oehme, Kessler and Simon (Oehme et al., 1976) has been quite widely used in microelectrodes and has excellent Mg rejection. But in submicron electrodes this sensor usually gives little response below 1 μM Ca^{2+} in the presence of intracellular K^+ concentrations (Tsien and Rink, 1980; Coray et al., 1980; Berridge, 1980) non-Nernstian responses from 1 to 100 μM Ca^{2+} (Tsien and Rink, 1980; Coray et al., 1980; Berridge, 1980) and frequently, hysteresis where a given $[Ca^{2+}]$ gives a different electrode potential depending on whether the preceding level was higher or lower (Oehme et al., 1976). The lifetime of these electrodes is often very short, the performance deteriorating within an hour or two of fabrication. We have used electrodes with a novel PVC-gelled neutral carrier sensor, as described by Rink and Tsien (1980), which gives a performance in fine electrodes, much superior to that of the liquid sensor. The sensor contains 10% w/w of the neutral carrier (Oehme et al., 1976), 8% w/w of the intensely hydrophobic salt tetraphenyl arsonium tetrakis (p-biphenylyl)borate, 13% PVC and 69% (o-nitrophenyl)ocyl ether. (The exact proportions are not critical.) Submicron, bevelled electrodes of this type have been used successfully to measure intracellular free calcium concentration, $[Ca^{2+}]_i$, in ferret ventricular myocardium where the cells are only about 15 μm across (Harban et al., 1980). For use in snail neurones the electrodes are broken to around 1 μm and Fig. 1 shows the calibration of such an electrode after Ca^{2+} measurements in two cells (Alvarez-Leefmans et al., 1980). Against a background of 0.125 M K^+ the response to Ca^{2+} is Nernstian down to 1 μM (pCa 6) with 22 mV between pCa 6 and 7 and a useful response to pCa 8. There is minimal hysteresis. Interference from Mg^{2+} is seen to be negligible, as is that from H^+ in the range pH 8.4 to 6.4 (not shown). At pCa 7, 10 mmol/1 Na is seen to produce a slight interference which requires a small correction of the appar-

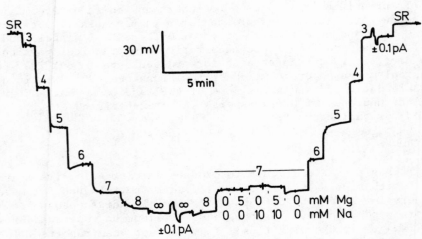

Fig. 1. Calibration of a 1 μm tip electrode containing PVC-gelled, neutral carrier sensor (Berridge, 1980). The numbers indicate the pCa, $-\log_{10}$ (free $[Ca^{2+}]/M$, of the test solutions which contained 0.125 M K^+.(See Tsien and Rink, 1980) S.R. denotes the basic bathing solution with 2 mmol/1 Ca^{2+}; pCa "∞" solution has 10 mmol/1 EGTA and no added Ca. In pCa 7, effects of adding 10 mmol/1 Na^+ and/or 5mmol/1 free Mg^{2+} are tested. Electrode resistance is tested twice by passing a current of $\pm$ 0.1 pA.

ent reading when measuring $[Ca^{2+}]_i$ in the 0.1 μM range. Above 1 μM Ca^{2+} effects of intracellular Na^+ cn be neglected. At least this much Na^+ interference is seen with the other Ca-sensors too, but has not always been considered or tested for. It is important to assess interference from any agents used in the experiments which could possibly get into the cells and influence the electrode. This is particularly important with lipophilic ions such as uncoupling agents which can give large signals with liquid, or PVC-gelled, sensors.

Our electrodes thus have satisfactory, though not yet ideal, performance for measuring cytoplasmic Ca^{2+} levels in the presence of the expected intracellular concentrations of K^+, Na^+, Mg^{2+} and H^+. Electrodes also need to be stable. Baseline drift does sometimes persist and a few millivolts per hour may have to be accepted. The performance, at low $[Ca^{2+}]$, is usually maintained much longer with the PVC-gelled sensor than with the liquid mixture but still it is usual to need new electrodes each day, and the lifetime still needs extending.

The performance of calcium-sensitive microelectrodes can vary from one to another, and with time. It is thus essential to calibrate each electrode in solutions of known, buffered Ca^{2+} levels encompassing the range of values to be measured and with a cationic background approximating to that inside cells. Extrapolation beyond the actually calibrated range is not permissible. It is also highly desirable to calibrate electrodes both before and after use in a cell.

GENERAL EXPERIMENTAL PROCEDURES AND PRECAUTIONS

It seems preferable to impale the cell first with the reference microelectrode, so that one is forced to observe whether subsequent impalement with the larger Ca-selective electrode causes any damage. This order of impalement has not often been adopted by workers with ion-selective electrodes but may be especially important with calcium where there is a huge inward electrochemical gradient, and we have seen that the basal $[Ca^{2+}]_i$ is readily elevated by repeated penetration, or by penetrations that produce sustained changes in membrane potential.

One should check that both electrodes are in the same cell, e.g. by passing outward current through the reference microelectrode and recording the resulting hyperpolarization with the calcium electrode. This manipulation also allows assessment of the input resistance of the cell.

Since the measurement of $[Ca^{2+}]_i$ requires the subtraction of the membrane potential from the potential recorded by the calcium electrode to give the differential signal, it is necessary for the reference microelectrode to record the same membrane potential as the calcium electrode. Within nerve cell bodies it can be assumed that the

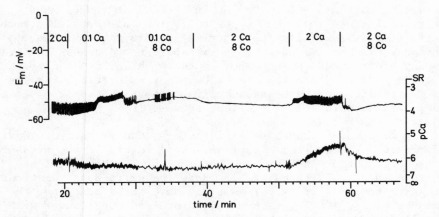

Fig. 2.   pCa, lower trace, and membrane potential (E_m), upper trace, in cell A of <u>Helix aspersa</u>. The basic bathing solution contained (mM): NaCl, 100; KCl, 4; $CaCl_2$, 2; $MgCl_2$, 3; Hepes 5; pH was 7.5; temp. 22 °C. External Ca^{2+} was changed between 2.0 and 0.1 mmol/l and 8 mmol/l cobalt chloride was added as indicated. The spikes appear truncated due to filtering of the voltage record.

cell interior is isopotential, but some test is necessary in cylindrical cells or syncytia where the space constant may be small relative to interelectrode distance. The ideal solution to this problem will be to produce double-barrelled microelectrodes.

Drift in the voltage record or generation of tip potentials, which in many types of experiment might be quite unimportant, could give rise to serious error in measurement of $[Ca^{2+}]_i$. Stable voltage recordings are therefore as important as stable calcium electrodes and in practice not always any easier to obtain (see Thomas, 1978).

It is desirable to show that the electrode responds appropriately inside the cells by imposing alterations of $[Ca^{2+}]_i$. We have seen the expected elevation of $[Ca^{2+}]_i$ with intracellular Ca injections. More important, EGTA injection produced the expected reduction of the indicated basal $[Ca^{2+}]_i$ down to approximately 10 nM (Alvarez-Leefmans et al., submitted for publication). This shows that unknown or untested components of the cytoplasm were not interfering with the electrodes. In many preparations this test will be difficult and to our knowledge it has not previously been performed.

Having finally obtained a reading one can believe one should consider that it represents only the free Ca level at the tip of the Ca electrode in that cell under the particular experimental conditions chosen.

INTRACELLULAR FREE CALCIUM IN HELIX NEURONES

Thireen impalements in different neurones from recently collected snails fulfilled the following stringent criteria: (a) membrane potential more negative than -45 mV; (b) no, or only transient, depolarization with the second impalement; (c) drift of differential signal $\leq$ 5 mV/hr; (d) adequate electrode response between pCa 7 and 8, before and after impalements. The mean basal pCa in these cells was 6.77 ± 0.07 (S.E.), corresponding to a free Ca^{2+} concentration of 0.17 μM.

We also examined factors which might affect $[Ca^{2+}]_i$. Changing external $[Ca^{2+}]$ had little effect on $[Ca^{2+}]_i$ of satisfactorily impaled silent cells which, incidentally, shows excellent sealing of the impaled membrane. In some spontaneously firing cells, such as cell A, that have a substantial inward Ca current during the spike (Standen, 1975) we sometimes saw marked changes in $[Ca^{2+}]_i$ with alterations of Ca gradient across the membrane and blockade of voltage dependent calcium entry. Fig. 2 shows records from such an experiment where reduction of external $[Ca^{2+}]$ to 0.1 mmol/l lowered $[Ca^{2+}]_i$. Subsequent application of 8 mmol/l cobalt, to block the Ca channels (Standen, 1975) stopped the cell firing and further lowered $[Ca^{2+}]_i$. In the now silent cell elevation of external $[Ca^{2+}]$ to 2 mmol/l had no effect, demonstrating the absence of non-specific Ca leaks. Removing the cobalt led to resumption of spiking with marked elevation of $[Ca^{2+}]_i$; readmitting cobalt abolished the spikes and again led to a lowering of $[Ca^{2+}]_i$.

Removal of external Na^+ is known to increase Ca uptake in axons, but had little effect on $[Ca^{2+}]_i$ in Helix nerve cell bodies.

The current interest in interactions between intracellular Ca^{2+} and H^+ prompted us to examine the effects of intracellular acidification with CO_2. Application of 5% CO_2, at constant external pH, never increased $[Ca^{2+}]_i$. In fact there was nearly always a decrease, which averaged 0.16 pCa units. Rather larger falls in $[Ca^{2+}]_i$, averaging 0.26 pCa units, were seen with 79% CO_2.

ACKNOWLEDGEMENTS

This work was supported by the Science Research Council.

REFERENCES

Alvarez-Leefmans, F.J., Rink, T.J., and Tsien, R.Y., 1980, Intracellular free calcium in Helix aspersa neurones, J. Physiol. (Lond.), 306:19P

Alvarez-Leefmans, F.J., Rink, T.J., and Tsien, R.Y., Measurement of free calcium concentration in neurones of Helix aspersa, using ion-sensitive microelectrodes, J. Physiol. (Lond.),(submitted for publication).

Berridge, M.J., 1980, Preliminary measurements of intracellular cal-
    cium in an insect salivary gland using a calcium microelectrode,
    Cell Calcium, (in press).
Coray, A., Fry, C.H., Hess, P., McGuigan, J.A.S., and Weingart, R.,
    1980, Resting calcium in sheep cardiac tissue and in frog skelet-
    al muscle measured with ion-selective micro-electrodes, J.
    Physiol. (Lond.), 305:60P.
Marban, E., Rink, T.J., Tsien, R.W., and Tsien, R.Y., 1980, Free
    calcium in heart muscle at rest and during contraction measured
    with a Ca^{2+}-sensitive microelectrode, Nature, Lond., in press .
Oehme, M., Kessler, M., and Simon, W., 1976, Neutral carrier Ca^{2+}-
    microelectrode, Chimia Aarau , 30:204.
Owen, J.D., and Brown, H.M., 1979, Comparison between free calcium
    selective microelectrodes and arsenazo III, in "Detection and
    Measurement of Free Ca^{2+} in Cells", C.C. Ashley and A.K.
    Campbell, eds., Elsevier/North Holland, Amsterdam, pp.395-408.
Rink, T.J., and Tsien, R., 1980, Calcium-selective microelectrodes
    with bevelled, sub-micron tips containing poly vinylchloride
    gelled neutral-ligand sensor, J. Physiol. (Lond.), 308 (in press)
Standen, N.B., 1975, Calcium and sodium ions as charge carriers in the
    action potential of an identified snail neurone, J. Physiol.
    (Lond.), 249:241.
Thomas, R.C., 1978, "Ion-sensitive intracellular microelectrodes",
    Academic Press, London.
Tsien, R., Rink, T.J., 1980, Neutral carrier ion-selective micro-
    electrodes for measurement of intracellular free calcium,
    Biochim. Biophys. Acta, 599:623.

INTRACELLULAR RECORDING OF POTASSIUM IN NEURONS OF THE MOTOR CORTEX OF AWAKE CATS FOLLOWING EXTRACELLULAR APPLICATIONS OF ACETYLCHOLINE

C.D. Woody and B. Wong

Depts. of Anatomy and Psychiatry
UCLA Medical Center
Los Angeles, CA 90024

Acetylcholine (ACh) is known to affect about half of the neurons of the cat motor cortex by causing an increase in the spontaneous rate of firing and input resistance (Krnjević et al, 1971; Woody et al, 1976; Woody et al, 1978). These effects can be prevented by local application of atropine, a muscarinic blocking agent (Swartz and Woody, 1979). The cells that respond in this way include pyramidal cells of Layer V, the neurons whose axons form the pyramidal tract (Crawford and Curtis, 1966; Krnjević and Phillis, 1963 a, b; Naito et al, 1969; Sakai and Woody, 1980; Spehlmann and Smathers, 1974).

Krnjevic and co-workers (1971) have suggested that these effects of acetylcholine may be mediated by a decrease in potassium conductance. An analogous action of acetylcholine has been postulated in the superior cervical ganglion (Weight and Votava, 1970); however, no direct measurements of [K+] have been made to see if the intracellular concentration of this ion changes after application of ACh. We have attempted to do this in neurons of the motor cortex of awake cats. Our preliminary findings, described herein, indicate that small increases in intracellular potassium ion concentration accompany the increased rates of firing found in cells responsive to ACh, without such changes being found in cells that fail to respond to ACh with increased rates of discharge.

METHODS

Ion-sensitive microelectrodes suitable for recording intracellularly from mammalian cortical neurons were prepared as described earlier by Wong and Woody (1978) after methods of Vyskočil and Kříž (1972) and Heyer and Lux (1973). Theta-type

glass capillaries were cleaned by boiling twice in methanol and were
then pulled to tips less than 0.5 μ. After bending 10-30 ° (Fig. 1),
the tips were dipped into a 0.3% solution of Siliclad (Clay Adams)
in 1-chloronaphthalene (1: 350, v/v) for 3 minutes.

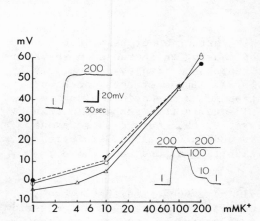
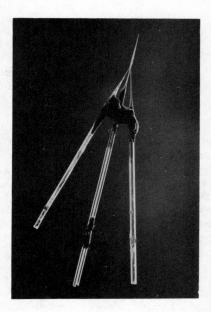

Fig. 1.   Left: In vitro calibration of a K+ ion-sensitive electrode.
          Filled circles are measurements made before in vivo recording;
          the question mark indicates the absence of values between
          1 and 100 mmol/l K+. The open circles are repetitions of
          these measurements made after in vivo recording; examples
          of these measurements (lower right) and of those made prior
          to recording (upper left) are illustrated. The time constant
          of most K+ electrodes was less than 1/2 sec and appears pro-
          longed due to a lag in changing calibrating solutions. A
          background of 200 mmol/l [Na+] was used as the competing ion
          (from Wong and Woody, 1978). Right: Multiple barrel micro-
          electrode used for recording intracellularly and extra-
          cellularly from neurons of the motor cortex. The outer (bent)
          electrodes also record [K+]. The inner (straight) electrodes
          are used for iontophoresis of acetylcholine. The outer
          electrodes are made from theta capillaries, 2 mm o.d.

After dipping, the electrodes were baked (tip up) for at least 1 h in an oven at 200 ^oC. One barrel was then back-filled with 1 mol/1 NaCl. Following this, sets of electrodes were dipped into potassium ion exchanger (Corning 477317) for 30 min or longer. Finally, the ion-sensitive barrel was back-filled with 0.5 mol/1 KCl.

The electrodes were then bonded to straight shanked double micro-pipettes (tips 1-2μ) that had been fused together by rotating under heat when pulled. The bonding was done with cyanoacrylate glue under a dissecting microscope using a Narishige microelectrode assembler (cf. Woody et al., 1976 for further details). The barrels of the straight micropipette were filled with 2 mol/1 ACh and 1 mol/1 NaCl, respectively. Sometimes another ion-sensitive electrode was added, with tip recessed 10-20μ to permit simultaneous extracellular re-cording and extracellular potassium measurement.

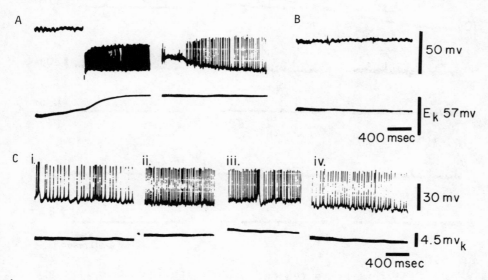

Fig. 2. Cell responding to acetylcholine (ACh) with increased firing and increased intracellular [K+]. A. Penetration of the cell. B. Exit from cell at end of experiment. C. Time period bet-ween A and B when ACh was iontophoresed for 30 sec. i) onset of iontophoresis, ii) 25 sec during iontophoresis, iii))10 set after end of iontophoresis iv 1/2 min after end of iontophoresis. In each case the DC recording of spike activi-ty is upper trace and the recording of [K+] is the lower trace. Calibrations are shown to the right for A-B and for C.

The electrodes were calibrated in known concentrations of K+ in a background of either 20 or 200 mmol/1 [Na+] before making the cortical recordings. An example is shown in Fig. 1. Further details and means for correcting the calibrations to 20 mmol/1 [Na+] have been described elsewhere (Wong and Woody, 1978).

Acetylcholine was applied extracellularly by iontophoresis (100-100 nA for 30 sec) after penetrating the cortical cells. The remaining procedures, including animal preparations and electrical recordings were as described earlier (Woody et al., 1978; Wong and Woody, 1978).

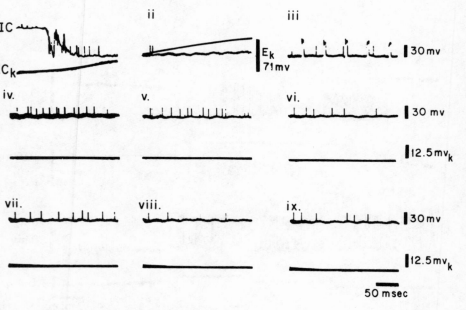

Fig. 3. Cell failing to respond to ACh with increased firing or increased intracellular [K+]. i) penetration of cell, ii)crest of intracellularly measured [K+] after penetration, iii) application of depolarizing current pulse to measure input resistance - spike height is reduced on current pulse applications, iv) during iontophoresis of ACh, v) immediately after cessation of ACh iontophoresis, vi) 1/2 min later, vii) 1 min later, viii) 2 min later, ix) 3 min later. Calibrations of recordings of spike activity and [K+] are shown to the right.

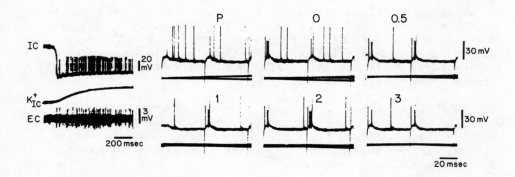

Fig. 4.   Another cell that failed to respond to ACh with either in-
          creased firing or increased intracellular [K+]. Penetration
          is shown to the left: IC - intracellular activity, K+ IC -
          intracellular [K+], EC - extracellular activity recorded
          simultaneously through an extracellular electrode (see
          Methods). The remaining traces show intracellular activity
          (upper trace) and intracellular [K+] (lower trace): P -
          prior to iontophoresis of ACh, 0 - at cessation of ACh, and
          then at 0.5, 1,2 and 3 min later. The E_k at penetration ex-
          ceeded 80 mV; the gain of the [K+]records (P, 0, 0.5, 1, 2,
          3) is ten times that at penetration.

RESULTS

     Recordings were obtained from 15 cortical neurons with resting
potentials averaging 50 $\pm$ 13 mV (S.D.) and E_k values averaging
-72 $\pm$ 23 mV. In seven of the cells it was possible to measure intracellular [K+] after iontophoresis of acetylcholine. Two of those cells
responded to ACh with an increase in firing rate. In both, an increase
in [K+] accompanied the increased rate of discharge. The remaining
five cells failed to show increased firing. Four showed no change or
a decrease in [K+].   One showed an increase in resistance and a variable increase in [K+]. Examples of these cell recordings are shown
in Figs. 2-4.

DISCUSSION

     The results, although preliminary, suggest that a small increase
in intracellular [K+] accompanies the increased rate of discharge
produced in some cortical neurons by acetylcholine. As shown in Fig.2,
the time course of the change in [K+] closely corresponds to that
of the change in firing rate. The increase in firing typically reaches a peak 30 sec to 1 min after iontophoresis of acetylcholine
(Woody et al., 1976). The hyperpolarizing effect of the small increase

in intracellular [K+] would not be sufficient to overcome the depo-larizing effect of an associated decrease in potassium conductance of the magnitude predicted empirically (Goldman, 1943; Hodgkin and Katz, 1949; Woody et al, 1978). Concentrations of ACh 10-100 times higher than those applied iontophoretically were required to produce cross-reactive alterations in the potential recorded through the K+ ion-sensitive electrodes.

ACKNOWLEDGEMENT

We thank E. Gruen for technical assistance and gratefully acknowledge the support of USPHS grant HD 5958 and NSF grant BNS 78-24146 in this research.

REFERENCES

Crawford, J.M.,and Curtis, D.R., 1966, Pharmacological studies on feline Betz cells, J. Physiol. (Lond.), 186:121.

Goldman, D.E., 1943, Potential, impedance, and rectification in membranes, J. Gen. Physiol., 27:37.

Heyer, E.,and Lux, H.D., 1973, Rapid changes of potassium concentra-tion at the outer surface of exposed single neurons during membrane current flow, J. Gen. Physiol., 61:385.

Hodgkin, A.L.,and Katz, B., 1949, The effect of sodium ions on the electrical activity of the giant axon of the squid, J. Physiol. (Lond.)108:37.

Krnjevic, K.,and Phillis, J.W., 1963(a), Acetylcholine-sensitive cells in the cerebral cortex, J. Physiol. (Lond.), 166:296.

Krnjevic, K.,and Phillis, J.W., 1963(b), Pharmacological properties of acetylcholine-sensitive cells in the cerebral cortex, J. Physiol. (Lond.), 166:328.

Krnjevic, K., Pumain, R.,and Renaud, L., 1971, The mechanism of excitation by acetylcholine in the cerebral cortex, J. Physiol., 215:247.

Naito, H., Nakamura, K., Kurosaki, T.,and Tamura, Y., 1969, Precise location of fast and slow pyramidal tract cells in cat sensori-motor cortex, Br. Res., 14:237.

Sakai, H.,and Woody, C., 1980 (in press), Identification of auditory responsive cells in coronal-pericruciate cortex of awake cats, J. Neurophysiol.

Spehlmann, R.,and Smathers, C.C., Jr., 1974, The effects of acetyl-choline and of synaptic stimulation on the sensorimotor cortex of cats. II. Comparison of the neuronal responses to reticular and other stimuli, Br. Res., 74:243.

Swartz, B.,and Woody, C., 1979, Correlated effects of acetylcholine and cyclic guanosine monophosphate on membrane properties of mammalian neocortical neurons, J. Neurobiol., 10:465.

Vyskočil, F.,and Kříž, N., 1972, Modifications of single and double-barrel potassium specific micro-electrodes for physiological experiments, Pflügers Arch., 377:265.

Weight, F.F.,and Votava, J., 1970, Slow synaptic excitation in sympathetic ganglion cells: evidence for synaptic inactivation of potassium conductance, Science, 170:755.

Wong, B.,and Woody, C., 1978, Recording intracellularly with potassium ion-sensitive electrodes from single cortical neurons in awake cats, Exp. Neurol., 61:219.

Woody, C.D., Carpenter, D.O., Gruen, E., Knispel, J.D., Crow, T.W., Black-Cleworth, P., February 1976, Persistent increases in membrane resistance of neurons in cat motor cortex, AFRRI Scientific Report, 1.

Woody, C.D., Swartz, B.E.,and Gruen, E., 1978, Effects of acetylcholine and cyclic GMP on input resistance of cortical neurons in awake cats, Br. Res., 158:373.

Woody, C.D., Sakai, H., Swartz, B., Sakai, M.,and Gruen, E., 1979, Responses of morphologically identified mammalian, neocortical neurons to acetylcholine (ACh), aceclidine (ACec), and cyclic GMP (cGMP), Soc. Neurosci. Abstr., 5:601.

POTASSIUM FLUXES OF ISOLATED NERVE ENDINGS MONITORED
BY A VALINOMYCIN-ACTIVATED ION-SELECTIVE MEMBRANE
ELECTRODE IN VITRO

András Csillag

First Department of Anatomy
Semmelweis University Medical School
1450 Budapest, Hungary

INTRODUCTION

Isolated nerve endings (synaptosomes) have proved useful model
systems for studying numerous aspects of synaptic function and of
other neuronal mechanisms. Their ability to build up and maintain
ionic gradients by active transport has been described by several
groups. Synaptosomes have been shown to have membrane potentials
(Blaustein and Holdring, 1975; Hanson et al., 1980) which could
primarily be regarded as potassium diffusion potential (Blaustein
and Goldring, 1975). In the present work, K^+-fluxes were monitored
in the course of the restoration of ionic equilibrium either in the
resting state of synaptosomes or under the effects of agents known
to alter the membrane potential and/or excitability of nervous elements. The use of an ion-selective electrode for measuring synaptosomal K^+-fluxes offers several advantages over other techniques. It
makes it possible to monitor time-dependent changes of the cation
continuously and without separating the particles from the suspending
medium. The K^+-sensitive valinomycin-electrode employed in this study
has also been used by our group in previous work (Csillag and Hajós,
1980).

MATERIALS AND METHODS

Synaptosomes were prepared from rat cerebral cortex by the
method of Hajós (1975).

Potassium movements were recorded in the suspending medium by
an OP-K-7113-D type of K^+-sensitive ion-selective membrane electrode
activated by valinomycin (Radelkis Electrochemical Instruments, Bu-

dapest). The ionophore is fixed to the membrane industrially and no reactivation is required within the lifetime of the membrane (3-4 months). Nor can valinomycin be released from the membrane during measurement. The electrode has a precision of 10^{-6} gion dm^3 and a selectivity coefficient for Na^+ of 2.6 x 10^{-4} (Havas et al., 1977). Changes in the order of 0.005 pK could be detected with a maximum response time of 10-30 s at 1 mmol/l K^+ as baseline, using 5-10 mg protein per measurement in a final volume of 5.5 ml. For the reference electrode a double-junctioned Ag/AgCl electrode with an outer filling solution of 0.1 mol/l $NaNO_3$ was used. The electrodes were immersed in a conical cell containing the medium, under continuous stirring. The system was calibrated by recording the response to 1 μmol/l K^+ after each measurement. As a routine, the medium contained 1 mmol/l K^+ and the ionic strength was below physiological in order to obtain maximal response amplitudes (although the system was also able to work in physiological media).

For flame photometry, samples of synaptosomes were rapidly spun in Eppendorf tubes on a bench centrifuge (12 000 x g, 30-60 s), the supernatants were removed by a Pasteur pipette and the tube walls were carefully wiped with a tissue tampon. The pellets were then extracted by 10 % trichloroacetic acid, resuspended by a Whirlimixer and recentrifuged for 3 min. The supernatants were used for K^+-determinations.

RESULTS AND DISCUSSION

On addition of synaptosomes to the medium, the K^+ level sharply rises after which it gradually decreases until a steady state is attained (Fig. 1). This corresponds to the restoration of intra-synaptosomal K^+-content. The initial phase shows a loss of K^+ from particles (in addition to what they have lost during preparation), whereas the second phase represents an accumulation of K^+. This latter phase has been found to depend on metabolic energy and on the integrity of the Na^+-K^+-transport system and also on the development of the morphological configuration typical of intact nerve endings in situ (Csillag and Hajos, 1980). On addition of various inhibitors (shown in Fig. 1) or by cooling, the curves had no influx phase and K^+-efflux was observed. The total amount of releaseable K^+ was in good agreement with the flame photometric data on K^+ contents (82.9 $\pm$ 6.8 nmol/mg).

Whereas blockers of energy-conservation and membrane transport caused an outflow of K^+ usually exceeding the value of initial ejection, another group of agents was found to decrease the uptake of K^+ without eliciting a loss of K^+ in excess to initial ejection. The K^+-uptake was strongly inhibited by the depolarising agent protoveratrine, a similar but less pronounced effect was found with GABA or L-glutamate and little or no effect with glycine or L-aspartate (Fig.2).

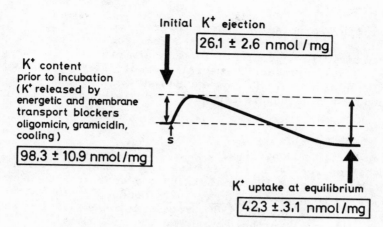

Fig. 1. A typical response curve of the K+-sensitive ion-selective membrane electrode recorded in the suspending medium of synaptosomes. The addition of synaptosomal fraction is indicated by 'S'. Medium: 160 mmol/l sucrose, 64 mmol/l NaCl, 0.8 mmol/l tris-HCl (pH 7.4), 1 mmol/l KCl, 1.25 mmol/l Na-pyruvate, 0.75 mmol/l malate and 0.5 mmol/l phosphate (both tris salts) in 5.5 ml final volume. Room temperature (21-23 °C). The mean ± S.E.M. values were calculated from 6-12 experiments on freshly prepared synaptosomes.

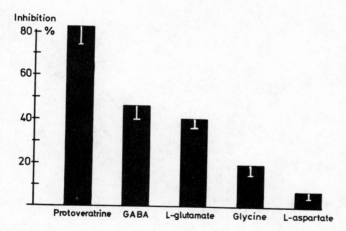

Fig. 2. The inhibition of synaptosomal K+-uptake by transmitter amino acids and protoveratine. The uptake values calculated from the influx phases of K+-electrode curves were divided by the average control values of the respective preparations. The mean ± S.E.M. of percentage data represent 3-9 experiments. The agents were present from the beginning of the measurements at 1 mmol/l concentrations except for glutamate (10 mmol/l) and protoveratrine A + B (50 µmol/l).

The transmitter amino acids and protoveratrine only acted in the range of the active K^+-uptake and did not affect the remainder (approx. 57 %) of diffusible K^+ content. The K^+ participating in the uptake phase might thus represent a special pool of diffusible synaptosomal K^+ (approx. 43 % at this K^+ concentration) most directly associated with changes of presynaptic membrane potential and/or excitability.

REFERENCES

Blaustein, M.P., and Goldring, J.M., 1975, Membrane potentials in pinched-off presynaptic nerve terminals monitored with a fluorescent probe: Evidence that synaptosomes have potassium diffusion potentials, J. Physiol. (Lond.), 247:589.

Csillag, A., and Hajós, F., 1980, Potassium movements in relation to synaptosomal morphology, J. Neurochem., 34:495.

Hajós, F., 1975, An improved method for the preparation of synaptosomal fractions in high purity, Brain Res., 93:485.

Hansson, E., Jacobson, J., Venema, R., and Sellström, A., 1980, Measurement of the membrane potential of isolated nerve terminals by the lipophilic cation [^{3}H] triphenylmethylphosphonium bromide, J. Neurochem., 34:569.

Havas, J., Kecskés, L., and Somodi, R., 1977, Potassium ion sensitive selective electrode and digital apparatus for potassium ion measurements, Orvos és Technika, 15(3):41.

SESSION III
ION ACTIVITIES IN THE SPINAL CORD
AND THEIR PHYSIOLOGICAL SIGNIFICANCE

EXTRACELLULAR K^+ ACCUMULATION IN THE SPINAL CORD

Eva Syková

Institute of Physiology
Czechoslovak Academy of Sciences
Vídeňská 1083, 142 20 Prague 4, Czechoslovakia

INTRODUCTION

Ionic changes in limited intra- and extracellular spaces are the consequence of the generation of every biopotential. A wide range of techniques has been used in recent years to show that normal neuronal activity causes K^+ to accumulate in the narrow clefts separating the cellular elements. However, it was not until the K^+ - selective microelectrodes with liquid ion exchanger - Corning code 477317 had been developed by J.L. Walker in 1971 that it has been possible to measure the dynamic changes of K^+ in the vicinity of active neurones and fibres. This development brought a new surge of interest in the functional significance of the transient K^+ accumulation in the nervous system. The two main questions at that time were:
1) What changes in $[K^+]_e$ occur during neuronal activity?
2) How might these changes of $[K^+]_e$ affect the functioning of the nervous system?

Needless to say, many new findings have become available, but the final answers to these questions remain open. In this paper I wish to present a short survey of the data about extracellular K^+ accumulation in the spinal cord and about its possible physiological significance, with special accent on the data obtained in our laboratory.

RESULTS

Extracellular K^+ accumulation and K^+ clearance in the spinal cord

In the first experiments performed in 1972, it was found that K^+ accumulates in the extracellular space of the rat spinal cord

139

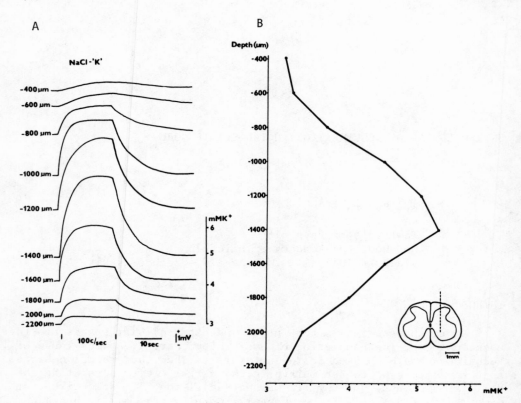

Fig. 1. Changes of $[K^+]_e$ produced by 100 Hz stimulation of the
posterior tibial nerve at various depths in the L7 spinal
segment of the cat. A. The depth of electrode insertion is
indicated for each record. The vertical bars below records
indicate the period of stimulation. In diagram B the depth
is indicated on the ordinate and increase of $[K^+]_e$ on the
abscissa (From Kříž et al., 1974).

during tetanic stimulation of the peripheral nerve and that the change of $[K^+]_e$ corresponds to several $mmol.1^{-1}$ (Vyklický et al., 1972;
Krnjević and Morris, 1972). Since then a large number of reports
have been performed in the mammalian as well as in the amphibian
spinal cord (Ten Bruggencate et al., 1974; Kříž et al., 1974; Somjen
and Lothman, 1974; Kříž et al., 1975; Krnjević and Morris, 1975a;
1975b; Lothman and Somjen, 1975; Vyklický et al., 1975; Somjen et

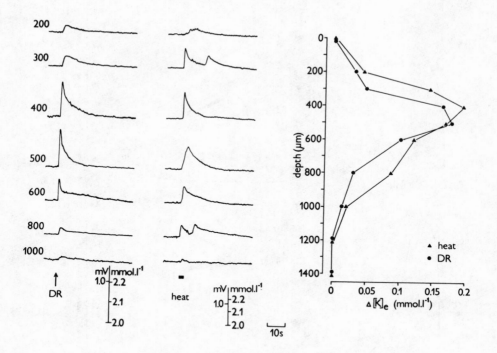

Fig. 2. Distribution of the changes in $[K^+]_e$ in the IXth spinal cord segment of the frog produced by single pulse electrical stimulation of the skin (DR) and by hot water application for 1-2 s (60 °C). DR - data from isolated spinal cord - hindlimb preparation, heat - from an experiment on spinal cord 'in situ'. Stimuli applied on the skin of the ipsilateral hindlimb.

al., 1976; Syková et al., 1976; Syková and Vyklický,1977; Syková and Vyklický, 1978; Nicoll, 1979; Syková et al., 1980). It was shown that K^+ accumulates preferably in deeper layers of the dorsal horn and in the intermediate region of the mammalian as well as the amphibian spinal cord following either single or tetanic electrical stimulation of peripheral nerves (Fig. 1), or adequate stimulation (Fig. 2). In this region, many primary afferents terminate and neuronal density is very high - about 6 neurones in 100 μm^3 (Aitken and Bridger, 1961; Kříž et al., 1974; Székely, 1976). The changes in $[K^+]_e$ in the upper dorsal horn or in the ventral horn following peripheral stimulation are negligible.

The accumulation of K^+ depends on the frequency and duration of stimulation. Its maximum at 100 Hz stimulation is usually reached after 10-15 s and does not exceed 10 $mmol.l^{-1}$. The stimulation at

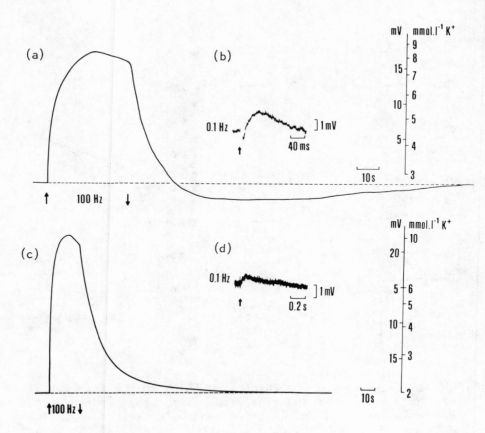

Fig. 3.   Changes in $[K^+]_e$ in the cat spinal cord (A,B) compared with those in the frog isolated spinal cord (C,D). A - tetanic stimulation (100 Hz) of the posterior tibial nerve; B - single volley applied to the posterior tibial nerve; C - tetanic stimulation (100 Hz) of the dorsal root IX; D - single volley applied to dorsal root IX. Records A and C from the ink recorder, B and D from the oscilloscope.

higher frequencies or of longer duration caused no further increase in $[K^+]_e$. However, even stimulation at 3 Hz increased $[K^+]_e$ by about 1 mmol.1^{-1} (Kříž et al., 1975). K^+ accumulation of up to 1 mmol.1^{-1} was also found under more physiological conditions, i.e. during adequate stimulation of skin nociceptors (Syková et al., 1980).

The level of increased $[K^+]_e$ is not sustained during the whole period of higher-frequency tetanic stimulation, but declines after its maximum is reached (Fig. 3). Furthermore, the process of redistribution of accumulated K^+ in the mammalian spinal cord does not

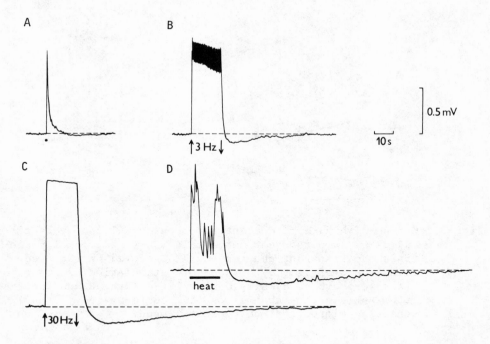

Fig. 4. Dorsal root hyperpolarization following a single electrical shock (A), tetanus at 3 Hz (B) at 30 Hz (C) and hot water (60 °C) application (D) on the skin of the hindlimb. Experiment on isolated frog spinal cord - hindlimb preparation.

stop after the original resting level is reached, but $[K^+]_e$ continues to decrease below the initial resting level (Fig.3A). This decrease of $[K^+]_e$ during the stimulation as well as the undershoot apparently reflect the active processes which participate in the redistribution of accumulated K^+. In the frog spinal cord the depolarization of the dorsal root fibres in response to electrical as well as adequate stimulation was followed by hyperpolarization (Fig. 4). The amplitude and duration of hyperpolarization correlated with the magnitude and time course of elevated $[K^+]_e$ (see Fig. 16). The undershoot as well as dorsal root hyperpolarization (DRH) were highly sensitive to anoxia; the DRH in the isolated frog spinal cord was eliminated by the application of ouabain and by the replacement of Na^+ in the Ringer solution for Li^+ (Kříž et al., 1975; Syková, unpublished observations). There are good reasons to believe that the undershoot and DRH are the result of active K^+ uptake by stimulation of the Na-K pump in neurones as well as in the primary afferent fibres themselves (Davidoff and Hackman, 1980; Syková et al., in preparation). In fact, the ATPase activity of these neurones and fibres will be stimulated

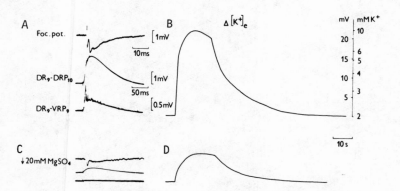

Fig. 5. Effect of high Mg^{2+} concentration on dorsal root potentials
         (DR-DRPs), ventral root potentials (DR-VRPs), focal poten-
         tials and transient changes in $[K^+]_e$ evoked in isolated
         spinal cord of frog by orthodromic stimulation. Focal poten-
         tials were evoked by single stimuli in IXth DR and recorded
         with the reference channel of the double-barrel, potassium-
         sensitive microelectrode against ground.

by both the increased $[K^+]_e$ and the Na^+ load of the cells. Because
the 'undershoot' was only found to be pronounced in the close vicinity
of discharging neurones, it is likely that the neurones and not the
glial cells are responsible for the active reabsorption of accumulated
K^+ (Kříž et al., 1975). On the other hand, for the restoration of
normal $[K^+]_e$ levels presumably other mechanisms contribute besides
active K^+ uptake by the Na-K pump in active elements, such as passive
diffusion in the extracellular space, dispersal across the blood-brain
barrier and passive or active dissipation via glial cells (see
Gardner-Medwin; Nicholson; Somjen et al.; in this volume). The answer
to the question whether they play any significant role in the clearance of accumulated K^+ from the extracellular space is not yet entirely clear.

The role of K^+ accumulation in the mechanism of PAD

The finding that K^+ accumulates preferentially in the deeper
layers of the dorsal horn has led to the reinvestigation of the original hypothesis of Barron and Matthews (1938) suggesting that alteration in ionic concentrations following neuronal impulses causes
depolarization of primary afferent fibres. Generally speaking, it is

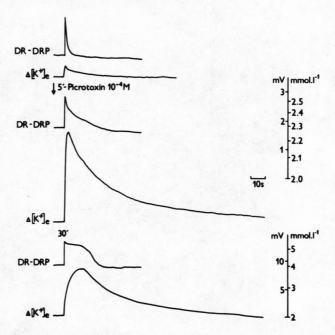

Fig. 6. The effects of picrotoxin (10^{-4} mol.1^{-1}) on the dorsal root potentials (DR-DRPs) and changes in $[K^+]_e$ in the isolated frog spinal cord. Note the prolongation of DR-DRPs 5 s and 30 s after picrotoxin and the corresponding increase of $[K^+]_e$. N.B. that the calibration is different for $[K^+]_e$ after 30 s.

widely accepted at the present time that primary afferent depolarization PAD is the mechanism underlying presynaptic inhibition (Eccles, 1964) and consists of at least two components which operate by different mechanisms. One component of PAD results from a change in the ionic permeability of primary afferent terminals produced by the action of a specific depolarizing transmitter - GABA - released at axo-axonic synapses (for review see Schmidt, 1971; Levy, 1977). Recently, evidence has been accumulating which supports the idea that the second component of PAD is caused by K^+ accumulation in the spinal cord especially after repetitive or prolonged stimulation.

The so-called 'dual' mechanism of the origin of the dorsal root potentials DRPs was supported by the experiments in the isolated spinal cord of the frog. When 20 mmol.1^{-1} $MgSO_4$ was added to the Ringer solution to block synaptic transmission, the ventral root discharge and focal potentials evoked by a single volley in the dorsal root disappeared, but the DRPs were not eliminated (Vyklický et al., 1976; Syková and Vyklický, 1977). DR-DRPs diminished in amplitude to about 10 % of the control and also the K^+ transient, evoked

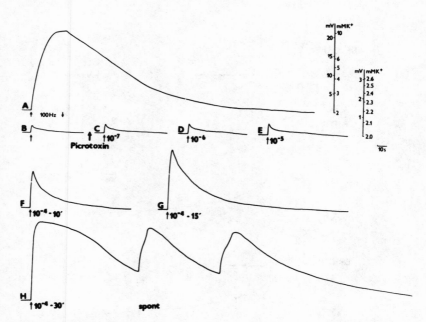

Fig. 7. The effect of various concentrations of picrotoxin on $[K^+]_e$. (A), Changes in $[K^+]_e$ recorded in the intermediate region of the IXth spinal cord segment when DR_9 was stimulated at 100 Hz for 35 s (arrows); (B), changes in $[K^+]_e$ evoked by a single stimulus; (C-E), $[K^+]_e$ evoked by a single stimulus when picrotoxin was applied continuously at concentrations of 10^{-7}, 10^{-6} and 10^{-5} mol.l^{-1} for 30 min; (F-H), $[K^+]_e$ evoked by a single stimulus when picrotoxin (10^{-4} mol.l-1) was applied for 10 min in F, 15 min in G and 30 min in H. Note spontaneous elevations of $[K^+]_e$ in H. Calibration on the right applies to B-G, on the left to A and H. (From Syková and Vyklický, 1978).

by 100 Hz stimulation, decreased to about 10-15 % of its original values (Fig. 5). The Mg^{2+} resistant DR-DRPs have been called 'asynaptic' and the most likely explanation for their origin is the depolarization by K^+ released from the stimulated primary afferent fibres. They were found to exhibit non-linear summation (Syková and Vyklický, 1977; Nicoll, 1979), similar to that occurring in glial cells during repetitive stimulation (Kuffler et al., 1966). It is reasonable to assume that the K^+ released from the postsynaptic neurones during their activation also significantly contributes to PAD when synaptic transmission is intact and that the K^+ component in normal DR-DRPs evoked by a single afferent volley should therefore be more than 10 %.

Further evidence for the fact that DRPs have a K^+ component was the finding that only the 'early' component of the DRPs with the

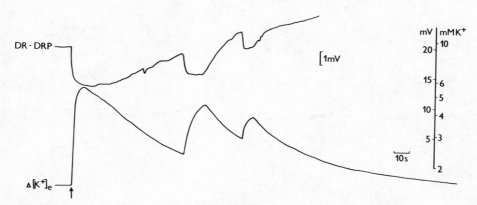

Fig. 8.   Records of evoked and spontaneous dorsal root potentials
and changes in $[K^+]_e$ when picrotoxin 5×10^{-4} $mol.l^{-1}$ was
applied. DR-DRPs, dorsal root potentials evoked by a single
pulse applied to DR_9 and recorded from DR_{10}. Negativity
downwards . $[K^+]_e$, elevations of $[K^+]_e$ recorded simultaneously with DR-DRPs from the intermediate region of the
IXth spinal cord segment. Note spontaneous changes in $[K^+]_e$
and the corresponding DRPs (From Syková and Vyklický, 1978).

shorter latency is depressed by the GABA-antagonists picrotoxin and
bicuculline (Barker et al., 1975; Lothman and Somjen, 1976; Syková
and Vyklický, 1978; Davidoff et al., 1980), while the longlasting,
'late' component of the DRPs is augmented and accompanied by a substantial increase in $[K^+]_e$. As is demonstrated in Fig. 6, picrotoxin
in concentrations 10^{-4} $mol.l^{-1}$ depressed the 'early' component of
DR-DRPs to about 60 % of the control, but it prolonged and enhanced
the 'late' phase of DR-DRPs and increased $[K^+]_e$ from 0.05 $mmol.l^{-1}$
to 4 $mmol.l^{-1}$. It is evident that the duration and amplitude of the
'late' DRP corresponds to the increase in $[K^+]_e$.

The shift in the time course of $[K^+]_e$ changes, when compared
with that of evoked DRPs, is apparently due to the fact that the
diffusion time for K^+ released from the secondary neurones to reach
primary afferent terminals will be much shorter than to reach the tip
of the microelectrode. The primary afferent terminals are separated
from secondary neurones only by a narrow cleft of about 15 nm width,
while the K^+ selective microelectrode with a 2-4 μm tip diameter
cannot be placed anywhere as close to the surface of a neurone. The
K^+ selective microelectrode therefore reflects changes of $[K^+]_e$ in
a relatively large volume of intracellular space to which many neurones and fibres contribute by releasing K^+ during their spike activity
(Neher and Lux, 1973; Kříž et al., 1975).

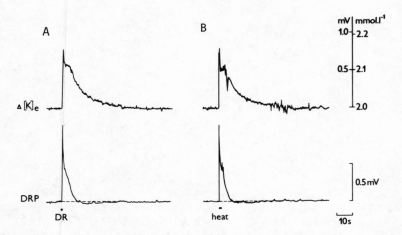

Fig. 9. Transient increases of $[K^+]_e$ in IXth spinal cord segment of the frog and dorsal root potentials recorded from the Xth dorsal root in the isolated spinal cord - hind limb preparation. A - response to a single shock applied to the skin, B - response to stimulation with hot water (1-2 s, 60 °C). A and B are from one experiment, microelectrode at a depth 400 μm.

The effect of picrotoxin on changes of $[K^+]_e$ recorded in the intermediate region of the lumbal spinal cord when DR was stimulated was found to be dose dependent. A slight effect was found when picrotoxin was applied in concentrations from 10^{-7} to 10^{-5} mol.1^{-1}. At 10^{-4} mol.1^{-1}, changes of $[K^+]_e$ in response to a single volley were about 10 mmol.1^{-1}, i.e. about 100 times greater than in the Ringer solution (Fig. 7). At this and higher concentrations of picrotoxin, paroxysmal changes in $[K^+]_e$ tended to develop spontaneously, usually after preceding stimulation. The records in Fig. 8 demonstrate that the evoked and spontaneous changes in $[K^+]_e$ correlated well with the DRPs. The intracellular recordings from motoneurones before and after addition of picrotoxin proved that these large K^+ transients as well as enhanced field potentials after addition of picrotoxin were produced by enhanced neuronal firing (Syková and Vyklický, 1978).

The 'late',presumably K^+ component was found even in normal DRPs evoked by single supramaximal shocks applied to the skin of the hindlimb and especially in those evoked by nociceptive stimulation (Fig. 9). The 'late' component with the slower time course may be recognized as a hump on the decay phase of these DRPs. When the activity of dorsal horn neurones in the frog was studied in response to nociceptive stimulation of the skin with hot water (50-60 °C applied for 1-2 s) it was found to produce longlasting, high-frequency repetitive

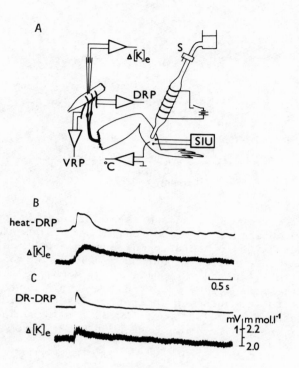

Fig. 10.   Responses of the frog spinal cord to nociceptive stimulation.
A: schema of the experimental arrangement. In various combinations, two of the following inputs were led to a dual-
beam oscilloscope or a two-channel ink writer: dorsal
root potentials recorded from dorsal root VIII or IX (DRP),
ventral root potentials recorded from ventral root IX or X
(VRP), temperature monitored by a thermocouple placed on
the surface of the stimulated skin ($^{\circ}$C) and potassium selective microelectrode ($\Delta[K^+]_e$).'Heat responses' were evoked
by a flow of previously heated water by opening a stopcock
(S). SIU, stimulation isolation unit. B: responses to single
volley electrical stimulation of the skin (DR-DRP and
$\Delta[K^+]_e$) recorded in another frog. C: heat-DRP and $\Delta[K^+]_e$
from the same places (hot water applied for 2 s, temperature 60 $^{\circ}$C).

firing (0.5-2 s; 50-200 Hz) in neurones in the dorsal horn and intermediate region of the cord. A single volley applied to the skin u-
sually evoked only 2-5 spikes (Czéh et al., 1980). The usually longer-
lasting 'late' component of DRPs evoked by nociceptive stimulation
could therefore be produced by greater K^+ accumulation arising from
longlasting neuronal firing leading to a greater and longer increase

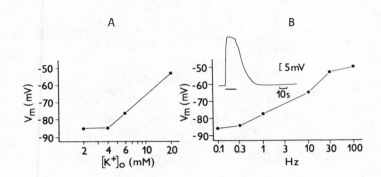

Fig. 11.   Effect of $[K^+]_e$ and dorsal root stimulation on membrane
           potential of a motoneuron. All measurements are from a
           maintained penetration of a single neurone. A. Steady state
           membrane potential during perfusion of the spinal cord
           with 2,4,6 and 20 $mmol.1^{-1}$. B. Membrane potential of the
           same motoneurone 0.5 s following a 15 s dorsal root tetanus
           at the frequencies indicated. Inset record obtained with
           tetanic stimulation of 100 Hz for 15 s. The time constant
           of the pen recorder was about 0.2 s (From Syková and Orkand,
           1980).

in $[K^+]_e$ (Fig. 10), similarly, as had previously been described to
cause sustained DRPs during tetanic electrical stimulation (Lothman
and Somjen, 1975; Syková and Vyklický, 1977; Nicoll, 1979; Davidoff
et al., 1980; Syková et al., 1980). It is assumed that a part of the
K^+ component in these DRPs gradually increases with the frequency
and duration of stimulation up to about 90 % (Nicoll, 1979). $[K^+]_e$
changes produced by the nociceptive stimulation can be compared with
those evoked by tetanic stimulation rather than by a single volley
and the K^+ component could therefore be of greater physiological
significance than has hitherto been believed.

The effects of increased $[K^+]_e$ on synaptic transmission

        An increase in $[K^+]_e$ should affect synaptic transmission, be-
cause of changes in the amount of transmitter released and alteration
in the membrane potential of both pre- and postsynaptic elements.
To examine the effects of extracellular K^+ accumulation resulting
from prior activity, the electrophysiological changes in spinal cord
transmission were recorded in the isolated frog spinal cord following
stimulation of dorsal roots and compared to those induced by increasing $[K^+]_e$ when K^+ enriched Ringer was applied to the cord (Sy-

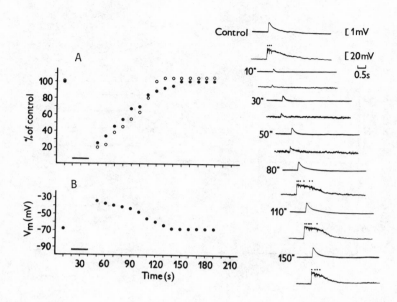

Fig.12.   Effect of elevated $[K^+]_e$ on dorsal root potentials and
motoneurone membrane potential, EPSP and spontaneous synaptic activity. Top: Motoneurone resting potential with
change in $[K^+]_e$ from 2 to 20 and back to 2 mmol.l^{-1} (flow
rate about 2 ml/min). The membrane was more depolarized
about 5 min after changing to 20 mmol.l^{-1} K$^+$ than at 6 min
due to increased neuronal activity resulting from elevated
K$^+$. Bottom: a - e, upper record is the potential recorder
extracellularly from the dorsal root following a single
volley in an adjacent dorsal root, lower record is the intracellularly recorded EPSP produced by the same stimulus.
a, control; b, 2 min after 20 mmol.l^{-1} K$^+$; c, 6 min after
20 mmol.l^{-1} K$^+$; d, 4 min after 2 mmol.l^{-1} K$^+$; e, 7 min
after 2 mmol.l^{-1} K$^+$. Bottom right: records of spontaneous
synaptic activity recorded intracellularly from motoneurone
at indicated membrane potentials (From Syková and Orkand,
1980).

ková and Orkand, 1980). It was found that many of the after-effects
of tetanic dorsal root stimulation could be mimicked by increasing
$[K^+]_e$. These include the depolarization of neurones and neuroglia,
prolongation and depression of excitatory postsynaptic potentials
(EPSPs), depression of DRPs, facilitation and depression of VRPs,
depression of antidromic spikes recorded from motoneurones as well
as increased spontaneous synaptic activity (Fig.11,12,13). The
correlation between the depression of DR-DRPs and the K$^+$ elevation

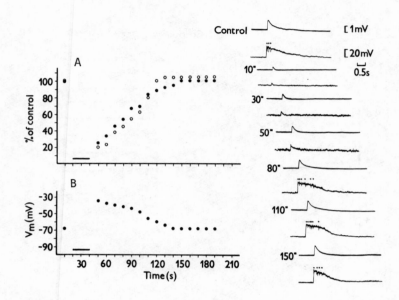

Fig.13.   Inhibition of dorsal root potentials and EPSP following
          a dorsal root tetanus. A: Amplitudes of DR-DRP ($\bullet$) and
          EPSP (o) after tetanic stimulation of the adjacent dorsal
          root at 100 Hz for 20 s. B: Graph of motoneurone resting
          potential under same conditions as above. Records are pairs
          of tracings of DRP (upper) and EPSP (lower) at times after
          tetanus indicated. Dots above EPSP indicate occurrence of
          motoneurone spikes which are too brief to be visible at the
          slow sweep speed. Note prolongation of EPSP and increased
          numbers of spikes during recovery. (From Syková and Orkand,
          1980).

after tetanic stimulation has already been shown in our earlier experiments on the frog isolated spinal cord (Fig. 14). Even though
increased $[K^+]_e$ in the bathing fluid can simulate, to a remarkable
extent, electrophysiological changes in both neurones and glia which
occur in the isolated spinal cord of the frog after repetitive stimulation of dorsal root, it is difficult to assess whether all these
changes resulting from peripheral stimulation could be attributed to
K^+ accumulation. Nevertheless, $[K^+]_e$ does increase during neuronal
activity under natural conditions (Orkand et al., 1966; Baylor and
Nicholls, 1969; Singer and Lux, 1975; Syková et al., 1974; 1980) and
undoubtedly under pathological states such as epilepsy (Prince, 1978).
If one uses the data from Fig. 11, dorsal root stimulation at 1 Hz
would lead to the accumulation of an additional 4 mmol.1^{-1} K^+ and
30-100 Hz about 20 mmol.1^{-1} K^+. These estimates are based on using

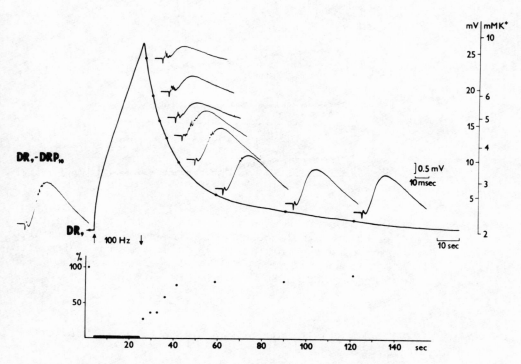

Fig.14. Depression of DRPs associated with increased $[K^+]_e$ induced in the IXth segment by stimulation of DR_9 at 100 Hz. Full circles in the record of changes in $[K^+]_e$ indicate when the $DRPs_{10}$ were recorded in response to a single volley in DR_9. The stimulation of DR_9 at 100 Hz lasted 20 s and is indicated by arrows and a thick line in the diagram. The amplitudes of $DRPs_{10}$ were plotted as percentage of the control at various intervals after the end of DR_9 stimulation. The microelectrode was inserted into the IXth spinal segment. (From Syková et al., 1976).

neurones as K^+ detectors. The situation is therefore more complicated because of the number of other factors which may alter neuronal membrane potential. On the other hand, the finding that glial cell depolarization after dorsal root stimulation in the isolated spinal cord of the frog corresponds to the K^+ accumulation measured by K^+ selective microelectrodes (Nicoll, 1979; Syková and Orkand, 1980) does not exclude the possible underestimation of increased $[K^+]_e$ in the close vicinity of active neurones. It was shown that glial cells are accurate K^+ electrodes only when entirely surrounded by uniform K^+ (Kuffler et al., 1966) and their membrane potential only indicates an average K^+ when the K^+ differs around various parts of the glial syncytium

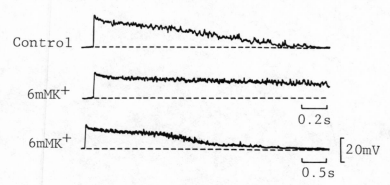

Control

6mMK$^+$

0.2s

6mMK$^+$

20mV

0.5s

Fig.15. Prolongation of EPSP with raised $[K^+]_e$. Intracellular recording from a single motoneurone in 2 mmol.1^{-1} K$^+$ (control) and after elevation of the $[K^+]_e$ in the perfusion fluid to 6 mmol.1^{-1}. Lowest trace at 2.5x slower sweep speed. (From Syková and Orkand, 1980).

(Futamachi and Pedley, 1976; Syková and Orkand, 1980; Orkand et al., in this volume).

There are sufficient indications that the large increase of $[K^+]_e$ exceeding 6 mmol.1^{-1} tends to inhibit transmission in the spinal cord (Krnjevič and Morris, 1976; Somjen, 1979; Syková and Orkand, 1980; Vyklický and Syková, this volume), by causing significant depolarization of the membrane (Fig. 11), alterations in synaptic function and changes in a variety of biochemical processes. But even small changes in $[K^+]_e$ should affect the functional properties of neurones, i.e. the threshold, the rate and amount of spontaneous activity and the amount of transmitter release at synapses. In the frog spinal cord, changes in $[K^+]_e$ in the range 0.5 - 6.0 mmol.1^{-1} gave an increase in spontaneous as well as evoked activity (Fig. 12, 13), a prolongation of motoneuronal EPSP (Fig. 15), and facilitation of reflex activity (Syková and Orkand, 1980; Nicoll, 1979; Vyklický and Syková, this volume).

In experiments where adequate stimulation was used, spontaneous DRPs, ventral root potentials (VRPs) and changes in $[K^+]_e$ were frequently observed at various intervals after preceding electrical and adequate stimulation, but mainly during the period in which the elevated $[K^+]_e$ was returning to the control level, as measured by K$^+$-selective microelectrodes (Fig. 16). This suggests that there occurs a period of increased excitability due to partial depolarization of neurones which can make them more excitable. It also supports the

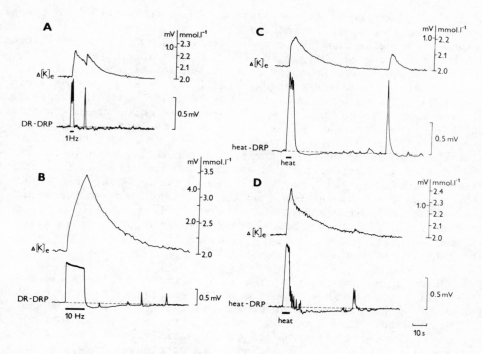

Fig.16. Evoked and spontaneous changes in $[K^+]_e$ and dorsal root potential in IXth spinal segment of the frog. A and B - electrical stimulation of the skin, C and D - nociceptive stimulation with hot water (60 °C) applied to the skin of the hindlimb. A,B and D - from the experiment on spinal cord 'in situ', C - from isolated spinal cord - hindlimb preparation.

idea that a relatively small increase in $[K^+]_e$, up to about 6 mmol.1^{-1} exerts an overall facilitatory effect on spinal cord transmission (Nicoll, 1979; Syková and Orkand, 1980; Vyklický and Syková, this volume).

CONCLUSIONS

There is no doubt that K^+ accumulation resulting from prior activity in the spinal cord does occur even under physiological conditions. The principal question which remains is whether the changes in $[K^+]_e$ are sufficiently large to affect appreciably spinal cord transmission. It is believed that the changes in $[K^+]_e$ during prolonged high-frequency stimulation are not seriously underestimated when measured with ISMs because of the 'steady state' achieved. Thus the situation is less clear during adequate stimulation of the skin (nociceptive, tactile), short electrical low-frequency tetanic sti-

mulation of peripheral nerves or stimulation with single electrical
pulses. The dead space created by the microelectrode, destruction or
neighbouring cells and fibres necessarily causes an underestimation
of the real value of changes in $[K^+]_e$. The local changes of $[K^+]_e$
in response to single shock or adequate stimulation may therefore
substantially exceed the changes established by K^+ selective microelectrodes, i.e. $0.5 - 1$ mmol.1^{-1}. On the other hand, the decrease
of presynaptic spike amplitude which requires more extreme changes
in $[K^+]_e$ is not the only effect which can rise from the increased
$[K^+]_e$. The K^+ accumulation may significantly influence the excitability of neurones as well as intraspinal terminals, even in the range
of small $[K^+]_e$ changes. Instead of any 'direct' effects of K^+ accumulation, shifts in $[K^+]_e$ may alter both $[Ca]_e$ and $[Ca]_i$ and these
should have a strong influence on the release of transmitters and
lead to excitability changes. Besides that, K^+ accumulation may exert
an 'indirect' effect on spinal cord transmission by stimulation of
oxygen consumption and a variety of other biochemical processes and
the rate of protein synthesis.

However, on the basis of the data available at the present time,
it is still not possible to estimate the precise site at which changes of $[K^+]_e$ influence synaptic transmission. The conclusion that K^+
acumulation resulting from neuronal activity under physiological conditions has a small (if any) effect is probably an underestimate.
Besides the role of the $[K^+]_e$ changes in pathophysiology, the main
question concerns its role in normal nervous functions. The idea that
K^+ may modulate nervous system activity, in a manner analogous to
that proposed for local hormones, deserves further attention.

REFERENCES

Aitken, J.T., and Bridger, J.E., 1961, Neuron size and neuron popu-
    lation density in the lumbosacral region of the cat's spinal
    cord, J. Anat., 95:38.
Barker, J.L., Nicoll, R.A., and Padjen, A., 1975, Studies on con-
    vulsants in the isolated frog spinal cord. II. Effects on root
    potentials. J. Physiol. (Lond.), 245:537.
Barron, D.H., Matthews, B.H.C., 1938, The interpretation of potential
    changes in the spinal cord, J. Physiol. (Lond.), 92:276.
Baylor, D.A., and Nicholls, J.G., 1969, Changes in extracellular po-
    tassium concentration produced by neuronal activity in the
    central nervous system of the leech, J. Physiol. (Lond.), 203:555
Bruggencate Ten, G., Lux, H.D., and Liebl, L., 1974, Possible re-
    lationship between extracellular potassium activity and pre-
    synaptic inhibition in the spinal cord of the cat, Pflügers
    Arch.ges.Physiol., 349:301.
Czéh, G., Syková, E., and Vyklický, L., 1980, Neurones activated from
    nociceptors in the spinal cord of the frog, Neuroscience Lett.,
    16:257.

Davidoff, R.A., and Hackman, J.C., 1980, Hyperpolarization of frog primary afferent fibres caused by activation of a sodium pump, J. Physiol. (Lond.), 302:297.

Davidoff, R.A., Hackman, J.C., and Osorio, I., 1980, Amino acid antagonists do not block the depolarizing effects of potassium ions on frog primary afferents, Neuroscience, 5:117.

Eccles, J.C., 1964, Presynaptic inhibition. In: "The Physiology of Synapse", chap. XV, pp. 220-238, Berlin: Springer Verlag.

Futamachi, K., and Pedley, T.A., 1976, Glial cells and potassium: their relationship in mammalian cortex, Brain Res., 109:311.

Kříž, N., Syková, E., Ujec, E., and Vyklický, L., 1974, Changes of extracellular potassium concentration induced by neuronal activity in the spinal cord of the cat, J. Physiol. (Lond.), 238:1.

Kříž, N., Syková, E., and Vyklický, L., 1975, Extracellular potassium changes in the spinal cord of the cat and their relation to slow potentials, active transport and impulse transmission, J. Physiol. (Lond.), 249:167.

Krnjević, K., and Morris, M.E., 1972, Extracellular K^+ activity and slow potential changes in spinal cord and medulla, Can. J. Physiol. Pharmacol., 50:1214.

Krnjević, K., and Morris, M.E., 1975a, Correlation between extracellular focal potentials and K^+ potentials evoked by primary afferent activity, Can. J. Physiol. Pharmacol., 53:912.

Krnjević, K., and Morris, M.E., 1975b, Factors determining the decay K^+ potentials in the central nervous system, Can. J. Physiol. Pharmacol., 53:923.

Krnjević, K., and Morris, M.E., 1976, Input-output relation of transmission through cuneate nucleus, J. Physiol. (Lond.), 257:791.

Kuffler, S.W., Nicholls, J.G., and Orkand, R.K., 1966, Physiological properties of glial cells in the central nervous system of amphibia, J. Physiol. (Lond.), 29:768.

Levy, R.A., 1977, The role of GABA in primary afferent depolarization, Prog. Neurobiol., 9:211.

Lothman, E.W., and Somjen, G.G., 1975, Extracellular potassium activity, intracellular and extracellular potential responses in the spinal cord, J. Physiol. (Lond.), 252:115.

Neher, E., and Lux, H.D., 1973, Rapid changes in potassium concentration at the outer surface of exposed single neurons during membrane current flow, J.gen.Physiol., 61:385.

Nicoll, R.A., 1979, Dorsal root potentials and changes in extracellular potassium in the spinal cord of the frog, J. Physiol. (Lond.), 290:113.

Orkand, R.K., Nichools, J.G., and Kuffler,S.W., 1966, Effect of nerve impulses on the membrane potential of glial cells in the central nervous system of amphibia, J. Neurophysiol., 29:788.

Prince, D.A., 1978, Neurophysiology of epilepsy, Ann.Rev.Neurosci., 1:395.

Schmidt, R.F., 1971, Presynaptic inhibition in the vertebrate central nervous system, Ergebn. Physiol., 63:21.

Singer, W., and Lux, H.D., 1975, Extracellular potassium gradients and visual receptive fields in the cat striate cortex, Brain Res., 96:378.

Somjen, G.G., 1979, Extracellular potassium in the mammalian central nervous system, Ann.Rev.Physiol., 41:159.

Somjen, G.G., and Lothman, E.W., 1974, Potassium sustained focal potential shifts and dorsal root potentials of the mammalian spinal cord, Brain Res., 69:153.

Syková, E., Czéh, G., and Kříž, N., 1980, Potassium accumulation in the frog spinal cord induced by nociceptive stimulation of the skin, Neurosci. Lett.,17:253.

Syková, E., and Orkand, R.K., 1980, Extracellular potassium accumulation and transmission in frog spinal cord, Neuroscience, 5:1421.

Syková, E., Rothenberg, S., and Krekule, I., 1974, Changes of extracellular potassium concentration during spontaneous activity in the mesencephalic reticular formation of the rat, Brain Res., 79:333.

Syková, E., Shirayev, B., Kříž, N., and Vyklický, L., 1976, Accumulation of extracellular potassium in the spinal cord of frog, Brain Res., 106:413.

Syková, E., and Vyklický, L., 1977, Changes of extracellular potassium activity in isolated spinal cord of frog under high Mg^{2+} concentration, Neurosci. Lett., 4:161.

Syková, E., and Vyklický, L., 1978, Effects of picrotoxin on potassium accumulation and dorsal root potentials in the frog spinal cord, Neuroscience, 3:1061.

Székely, G., 1976, The morphology of motoneurons and dorsal root fibers in the frog's spinal cord, Brain Res., 103:275.

Vyklický, L., Syková, E., Kříž, N., and Ujec, E., 1972, Post-stimulation changes of extracellular potassium concentration in the spinal cord of the rat, Brain Res., 45:612.

Vyklický, L., Syková, E., and Kříž, N., 1975, Slow potentials induced by changes of extracellular potassium in the spinal cord of the cat, Brain Res., 87:77.

Vyklický, L., Syková, E., and Mellerová, B., 1976, Depolarization of primary afferents in the frog spinal cord under high Mg^{2+} concentrations, Brain Res., 117:153.

Walker, J.L., 1971, Ion specific liquid ion exchanger microelectrodes, Analyt. Chem., 43:89A.

EXTRACELLULAR POTASSIUM AND CALCIUM ACTIVITIES IN THE MAMMALIAN SPINAL CORD, AND THE EFFECT OF CHANGING ION LEVELS ON MAMMALIAN NEURAL TISSUES

G. Somjen[1], R. Dingledine[2], B. Connors[3], and B. Allen[1]

[1]Department of Physiology, Duke University
Durham, North Carolina, USA
[2]Department of Pharmacology, University of North Carolina
Chapel Hill, North Carolina, USA
[3]Department of Neurology, Stanford University
Stanford, California, USA

INTRODUCTION

The spinal cord was one of the first mammalian tissues to be examined with potassium-selective microelectrodes (Vyklicky et al., 1972; Krnjević and Morris, 1972). Since then data have steadily been accumulating concerning the behavior of extracellular potassium ($[K^+]_o$) in the spinal cord and in other regions of gray matter and, more recently, concerning extracellular calcium activity ($[Ca^{2+}]_o$). In this short review we will summarize the work done in our laboratory at Duke University, and related works of other authors, with some emphasis on the more recent findings, and will try to assess the significance of transient variations of $[K^+]_o$ and $[Ca^{2+}]_o$ for the functioning of neuronal tissue. To this end we will compare the changes of ion activity observed in mammalian central gray matter in situ, with the effects of deliberately imposed changes of ion levels in bathing media upon mammalian neural tissues maintained in vitro.

Sustained potential (SP) shifts and responses of $[K^+]_o$

Repetitive stimulation of a large peripheral nerve of mixed function evokes in the spinal cord shifts of the electric potential, which can be recorded with extracellularly placed microelectrodes and direct coupled amplification. These SP shifts occur if ventral roots have been cut, but not if input through dorsal roots has been interrupted. When a large mixed-function

nerve is stimulated, the electric potential usually shifts in the
negative direction throughout the entire gray matter. If a cuta-
neous nerve is used, the maximum occurs in a more dorsal position
than when a muscle nerve is stimulated. By distribution, time-
course, and input-output function, these SP shifts differ from
focally recorded synaptic potentials, and from the potentials
associated with primary afferent depolarization. SP shifts
roughly mirror glial depolarization in timecourse, maximal amplitude, and spatial distribution; they have no identifiable counter-
part in electric responses generated by neurons (Somjen, 1969,
1970).

These observations seemed to indicate that SP shifts of the
spinal cord are, in large part, the product of glial depolarization, with neurons adding but little (Somjen, 1969, 1970, 1973).
From the known influence of $[K^+]_o$ on the glial membrane potential,
discovered in neural tissue of cold-blooded animals (Kuffler and
Nicholls, 1966) it seemed that the depolarizing response of glial
cells in the mammalian spinal cord could also be caused by the
rising tide of $[K^+]_o$. With the application of potassium-selective
microelectrodes to spinal tissue, the extent of the responses of
$[K^+]_o$ during afferent stimulation became clear (Vyklicky et al.,
1972; Krnjevic and Morris, 1972). Moreover, the responses of
$[K^+]_o$ turned out to be closely related to the SP shifts, recorded
simultaneously and from the same locations in the tissue (Fig. 1
& 2) (Somjen and Lothman, 1974; Lothman and Somjen, 1975;
Cordingley and Somjen, 1978), and the membrane potential of
spinal glial cells was shown to be governed by the Nernst equation
for K^+ (Lothman and Somjen, 1975). Thus there exists a three-way
correlation between responses of $[K^+]_o$, of glial membrane potential, and extracellular SP shifts.

Sources of the rising $[K^+]_o$

The sequence of events, thus, appears to be: during excitation K^+ ions enter the interstitial space, and the rising $[K^+]_o$
causes depolarization of glial cells; this in turn sets up a
gradient of potential causing current to flow in extracellular
space, registered as an SP shift. The question then is, where
exactly do the extra K^+ ions come from?

It has been accepted since several decades that the conduction of impulses along nerve fibers is associated with the exit
of K^+ ions from axoplasm, and Frankenhaeuser and Hodgkin (1956)
inferred from detailed examination of the membrane phenomena which
follow impulse discharge that K^+ ions may accumulate in the periaxonal spaces of peripheral nerve. Some of the excess K^+ accumulating during excitation in the spinal interstitium may likewise
come from nerve fibers. Probably more K^+ comes from unmyelinated

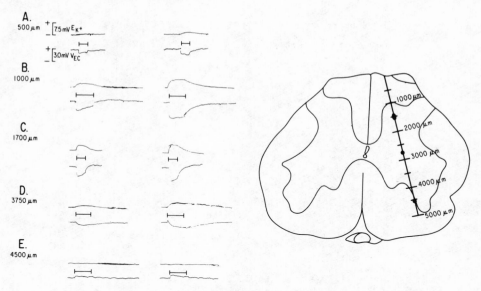

Fig. 1. Potassium responses and sustained potential shifts evoked by repetitive stimulation of an efferent nerve. E_K: potential of a potassium-selective microelectrode; V_{EC}: potential recorded from its "reference" barrel. Electrode track indicated on the outline drawing of a cross section of the spinal cord, with indications of the three points where pontamine blue die marks have been deposited. Stimulation intensity for the left hand column of tracings was just maximal for A-fibers; for the stimuli of the right-hand column C-fibers were also recruited. (From: Lothman and Somjen, 1975, by permission of the Publisher).

fibers than from myelinated fibers, because the latter exchange ions only at the Nodes of Ranvier. Accordingly in the white matter, near the entry zone of a dorsal root, $[K^+]_0$ is rising only when C-fibers are excited (Fig. 1A, Lothman and Somjen, 1975; Galvan; and Smith: this volume). Within the gray matter the presynaptic terminal arborization of all fibers is, of course, unmyelinated. That such presynaptic elements contribute a part of the $[K^+]_0$ responses in gray matter has indeed been demonstrated by blockade of synaptic transmission by raising $[Mg^{2+}]_0$ in frog spinal cord (Syková and Vyklický, 1977) and also by applying Mn^{2+} to the cerebellar cortex (Nicholson et al., 1978). In both these preparations, blockade of synaptic transmission did depress $[K^+]_0$ responses, but did not abolish them.

Less clear is the contribution of the soma-dendritic expanse of neuronal membranes to the rise of $[K^+]_0$. Krnjević and

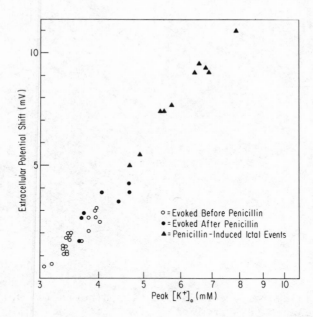

Fig. 2. Correlation of maxima of extracellular potassium activity,
         calculated from potassium electrode measurements, and
         amplitudes of extracellular sustained potential (SP)
         responses. From recordings similar to those illustrated
         in Fig. 1, before and after the i.v. administration of
         a convulsant dose of penicillin; triangles indicate
         measurements during spontaneous paroxysmal discharges.
         (From: Lothman and Somjen, 1976, by permission).

Morris (in press) have argued that it is small compared to that
of the presynaptic arbor, for two reasons. First, because unmyelinated presynaptic terminals present a larger surface than
dendritic processes; and second, because the invasion of motoneurons by antidromic impulses is not accompanied by detectable
rise of $[K^+]_o$ in the ventral horns (Somjen and Lothman, 1974;
Nicoll, 1979). One must consider, however, that antidromically
travelling impulses may not invade finer dendritic branches,
where much of the orthodromic synaptic activity is taking place;
and whatever dendritic surfaces may be lacking in surface area,
could be compensated for by the extended duration of synaptic
currents. Prolonged depolarization, no matter how caused, could
drive K^+ outward in two ways: first, because depolarization moves
the membrane potential away from the equilibrium level for K^+
ions; and second, by the activation of voltage-dependent K^+ conductance. Deschenes and Feltz (1976) have in fact shown that the
depolarization of dorsal root ganglion cells caused by GABA is

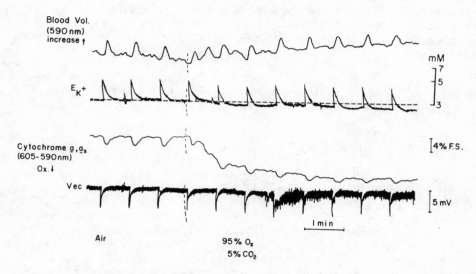

Fig. 3. Recordings of the relative amount of hemoglobin ("blood volume") and the relative oxidation of cytochrome a, a_3 (for optical recording techniques see: Jöbsis et al., 1977; Rosenthal et al., 1979), potassium potential and focal extracellular potential recorded as in Fig. 1. At the vertical marks the respired gas was changed from room air to 95% O_2 with 5% CO_2: note vasodilatation, relative oxidation of cytochrome a, a_3, and decrease of potassium level. Note also responses of all four variables to repeated trains of stimuli, evoked as in Fig. 1, but shown here on a more compressed timescale. (Experiment by LaManna, Rosenthal, Younts, and Somjen; illustration from: Somjen, 1978 a).

associated with a rise of $[K^+]_o$, even though the depolarization itself is believed to be due to an increase of Cl^- conductance (Deschenes et al., 1976). Glutamate and any other excitatory transmitters can similarly cause the release of K^+ into interstitial fluid without necessarily affecting K^+-permeability (e.g. Bührle and Sonnhof, this volume). In addition there are indications that specific increases of K^+-conductance by some transmitters also do occur (e.g. Segal and Gutnick, in press). And, finally, Karwoski and Proenza (unpublished) treated isolated retinae of necturus with tetrodotoxin to block impulse conduction. When a retina so treated was stimulated by flashing light, sub-

stantial amounts of K^+ ions were still released into the extracellular space in the distal layers. Even in the absence of TTX
the distal short-axon neurons of Necturus retina normally do not
generate impulses, only graded and electrotonically conducted potentials.

In sum, there are good reasons to believe that significant
amounts of K^+ are released not only with action currents, but also
with synaptic currents.

The reuptake of released K^+

Activation of the spinal gray matter by afferent nerve stimulation is accompanied by a metabolic reaction which can be recorded
as an oxidation of cytochrome a, a_3 in the intact tissue (Fig.3)
(Rosenthal et al., 1979). Also associated with such responses is
a detectable increase of hemoglobin, indicating dilatation of
small blood vessels and hence presumably increased blood flow.
Measurements in hippocampus, cerebral cortex and spinal cord revealed a consistent correlation between the increase of $[K^+]_o$ and
the oxidative metabolic responses of the tissue (Lewis and Schuette,
1975; Lothman et al., 1975, Rosenthal et al., 1979). The oxidative
responses of cytochrome a, a_3 are also proportional to the vasodilatation (Rosenthal et al., 1979). It seems, then, that excess
$[K^+]_o$ represents a load which calls for proportionate expenditure
of oxidative energy, and the call for increased energy is matched
by increased delivery of oxygen by the circulation.

Excitable cells maintain a high intracellular content of K^+,
and exclude Na^+, with the aid of a reciprocal Na^+, K^+ transport
system, fuelled by the breakdown of ATP, recovery of which requires
energy supplied by oxidative metabolism (Skou, 1975). Since neurons which have lost K^+ also gain Na^+ as a rule, their Na^+, K^+-
ATPase will be stimulated both by $[K^+]_o$ and $[Na^+]_i$. Activation
of membrane transport enables rapid retrieval of the lost K^+, and
the extrusion of the Na^+ gained, and thus makes prolonged repetitive neuronal excitation possible.

Since, however, the excess of $[K^+]_o$ built up locally near excited neurons creates a gradient in the interstitial spaces, some
of the excess K^+ may be dispersed through the tissue and, initially,
escape recapture by neurons. Some of it may also be taken up by
glial cells, because certain observations indicate that a K^+ _up-
take mechanism of glial cells is stimulated at the levels of $[K^+]_o$
encountered in stimulated central nervous tissue (e.g. Hertz, 1978).
The relative importance of the several modes of K^+ dispersal in
tissue is not accurately determined. Views and observations per-
taining to this circle of problems have recently been reviewed
(Somjen, 1979 a;in press: b, c; Gardner-Medwin, in press).

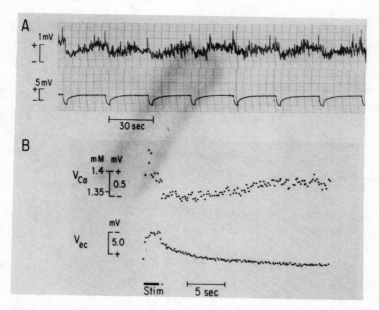

Fig. 4.   Responses recorded with a Ca^{2+} selective microelectrode,
upper traces, (V_{Ca}); and from its "reference" barrel,
(V_{ec}); from the dorsal horn of a spinal cord. A: polygraph tracings; B: electronically computed average of 8
responses. Stimulation of a large mixed afferent nerve
by trains of stimuli, as in Fig. 1. The sharp upward
deflections at the onset of each stimulus train in the
recording of Ca^{2+} -potential are electric artefacts
(from: Somjen, in press b, by permission).

Responses of calcium in spinal gray matter

        The activity of other ions besides potassium may be perturbed
by neuronal excitation. Na^+ ions disappear from interstitial
space as nerve impulses are conducted but changes of $[Na^+]_0$ may be
small compared to its resting level, since Na^+ is the principal
extracellular cation. $[Ca^{2+}]_0$ has, however, been shown to change
during excitation of several parts of the CNS (Heinemann et al.,
1977; Nicholson et al., 1978) and the spinal cord turned out to
be no exception (Somjen, 1979 b; in press: a).

        In the dorsal horn of the spinal cord, where the responses of
$[K^+]_0$ to stimulation of a peripheral nerve are maximal, one also
usually records a decline of $[Ca^{2+}]_0$. The decrease of $[Ca^{2+}]_0$ is
of a slower timecourse than the rise of $[K^+]_0$ and, if relatively
short trains of stimuli are used, $[Ca^{2+}]_0$ may sink to a minimum
only after stimulation has ceased (Fig. 4). If the same pulse

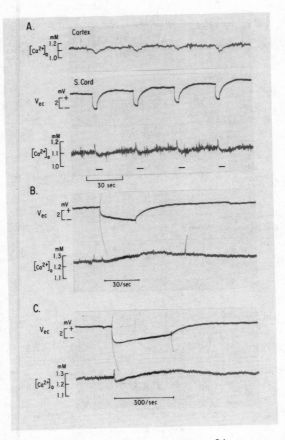

Fig. 5. A: Simultaneous recording of Ca^{2+} potential in the somatosensory receiving area of the cerebral cortex, and in
the spinal dorsal horn, evoked by trains of stimuli
applied to a mixed function afferent nerve in the leg.
Recording in spinal cord at a depth of 1.5mm from the
dorsal surface. B and C: Responses recorded at a depth
of 1.25 mm, with two different stimulus frequencies,
illustrating rise of $[Ca^{2+}]_o$ (in B) and biphasic response (in C) (from Somjen, in press a, by permission).

train is repeatedly applied to an afferent nerve, the amplitude
of the successive $[Ca^{2+}]_o$ responses usually diminishes greatly.
In a minority of spinal cords $[Ca^{2+}]_o$ shows a very slow rise instead of the decrease (Fig. 5) and it can happen that in the span
of several hours the one type of response converts to the other,
without deliberate change of experimental conditions.

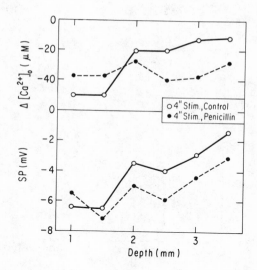

Fig. 6. Amplitude of responses of extracellular calcium activity $[Ca^{2+}]_0$, computed from recordings such as the ones illustrated in Fig. 3 and 4, and extracellular SP shifts, recorded at varying depths from dorsal surface of the spinal cord, along an electrode track similar to that shown in Fig. 1., before and after the i.v. administration of a convulsant dose of penicillin. Note that the depression of the Ca^{2+} responses at 1 and 1.5 mm depth was probably not caused by the penicillin, but was an expression of the usual tendency for Ca^{2+} responses to diminish with time; the enhancement of the Ca^{2+} response seen at 2.5 mm and deeper was, however, due to penicillin, for it has never been observed without such treatment (from: Somjen, in press a, by permission).

In the ventral horn $[Ca^{2+}]_0$ is changed only little or not at all by stimulus trains which evoke appreciable responses in the dorsal gray matter. This stability is, however, broken after the administration of a convulsant dose of penicillin. Following such an injection stimuli which previously had little effect evoke very large responses of $[Ca^{2+}]_0$. This enhancement of stimulus-evoked $[Ca^{2+}]_0$ responses occurs only in ventral, not in dorsal gray matter and is in excess of the simultaneously occurring enhancement of the SP shifts (Fig. 6). Spontaneous paroxysmal discharges are also

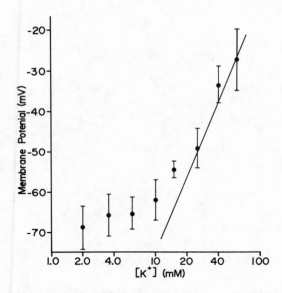

Fig. 7.   The membrane potential of dorsal root ganglion cells as
          a function of the potassium concentration in the bathing
          solution.   Each point the mean of data from 4 to 9 neurons
          vertical bars show standard deviation. Na^+ was deleted
          as K^+ was added to keep total ionic strength constant.
          Temperature :   33 to 36° C in different experiments.

associated with large decreases of $[Ca^{2+}]_o$ in the ventral, but not
in the dorsal horns.

That $[Ca^{2+}]_o$ should decline during neuronal activity, at least
in certain layers of the gray matter, was not entirely unexpected
because it had been the belief that Ca^{2+} ions enter presynaptic
nerve terminals in the course of synaptic transmission (Katz and
Miledi, 1967; 1969).   More recently Ca-dependent self-regenerative
potential responses of dendritic and somatic membranes have also
been described (Barrett and Barrett, 1976; Llinas et al., 1977;
Yoshida et al., 1978; Wong and Prince, 1978; Lux and Hofmeier, 1978;
McAfee and Yarowsky, 1979; Schwindt and Crill, 1980).   Less obvious
is the source of the excess $[Ca^{2+}]_o$ when it is seen to rise.   There
are three possible causes for such an increase: (1) Discharge
from cells, from sequestered intracellular storage sites; (2) Transfer from blood, perhaps by a neurally or glially regulated mechanism operating at the blood-brain barrier and coupled in some way
to neuronal activation; (3) Restriction of the solvent volume, due

to the entry of water and NaCl into cells, leaving Ca^{2+} ions behind (the latter mechanism suggested by C. Nicholson, personal communication).

The effect of changing $[K^+]_0$ levels on neurons

Variations of both $[K^+]_0$ and of $[Ca^{2+}]_0$ are known to influence neuronal function. Therefore, one set of nerve cells could, in principle, influence another set by the release of these ions. To find out whether the changes of $[K^+]_0$ which actually occur in the spinal cord could indeed have such an effect, one must know by how much $[K^+]_0$ changes normally, without experimental interference, and one must also have an accurate estimate of the sensitivity of neurons to variations of $[K^+]_0$. Responses evoked by massive electrical stimulation cannot be regarded as representative of a condition occurring in undisturbed nervous systems. Scarce and scattered data are available concerning $[K^+]_0$ changes under the influence of more physiological stimuli in several parts of the vertebrate CNS, including the spinal cord (references quoted in Somjen, 1979, a; see also Syková, this volume; Krnjević and Morris, in press). Withal it seems that, with the possible exception of the hippocampus, $[K^+]_0$ would rarely rise above 4.0 mM in a healthy intact CNS and probably never above 5.0 mM.

In this range, between 3.0 and 5.0 mM, neuronal membranes are relatively insensitive to changes of $[K^+]_0$. For the squid axon, the isolated Node of Ranvier of myelinated nerve fibers of frogs, and neurons of leech ganglia, the dependence of the membrane potential upon $[K^+]_0$ has long been determined (Curtis and Cole, 1942; Huxley and Stämpfli, 1951; Kuffler and Nicholls, 1966). For central neurons of the mammalian nervous system such data are however lacking. It is for this purpose not enough to have measured the membrane potential of a neuron and also $[K^+]_0$ near it, (Lothman and Somjen, 1975) because of the overriding influence exerted by synaptic input over the membrane potential of central neurons. Nor would the use of isolated tissue slices, with synaptic activity blocked by high Mg^{2+}, be entirely satisfactory, for the excess Mg^{2+} may well influence the very properties of the neuronal membrane we are interested in. Dorsal root ganglion cells are however devoid of synapses and even if they are not central neurons, they are close relatives.

The dependence of the membrane potential of dorsal root ganglion cells upon the prevailing $[K^+]_0$ is shown in Fig. 7. In spite of the considerable statistical variation inherent in, and due to, the technical difficulties of such experiments, the mean of the measured values agrees well with those reported for the other neural membranes which were investigated under better controlled conditions (references in previous paragraph). As long as

$[K^+]_o$ remains within physiological limits, its variations affect the membrane potential of dorsal root ganglion cells only little. A steep dependence of membrane potential on $[K^+]_o$ is beginning to be manifest only when $[K^+]_o$ approaches 10 mM. The electrical excitability, measured by intracellular current injection, also changed little as long as $[K^+]_o$ was kept between 3.0 and 5.0 mM.

It seems safe to conclude that the variations of $[K^+]_o$ which occur with the normal activity of the healthy spinal cord do not significantly perturb neuronal function. The situation must however be different in those pathologic conditions, such as paroxysmal discharges and hypoxia, under which $[K^+]_o$ can rise to truly high levels.

The effect of changing $[Ca^{2+}]_o$ on neuronal function in the mammalian central nervous system

Deposition of Ca^{2+} near neurons in the mammalian CNS by microiontophoresis depresses their excitability without affecting synaptic potentials, resting membrane potential, or resting membrane resistance (Kato and Somjen, 1969; Kelly et al., 1969); and the removal of Ca^{2+} by chelating agents enhances neuronal excitability (Curtis et al., 1960). When Ca^{2+} was administered by iontophoresis the actual levels of $[Ca^{2+}]_o$ could not be measured. We have now tried to determine the changes of membrane properties of dorsal root ganglion cells in vitro, while changing $[Ca^{2+}]$ in the bathing solution. The results are incomplete at the time of this writing, but it seems that varying Ca^{2+} between 0.5 to 2.0 mM resulted in changes of rheobase and also in the ability of the cells to fire repetitively in response to prolonged electric current, without consistent changes of resting membrane resistance or of resting membrane potential.

$[Ca^{2+}]_o$ is however known to enhance synaptic transmission across many neural junctions (Dodge and Rahamimoff, 1967; Katz and Miledi, 1967; Bracho and Orkand, 1970; Richards and Sercombe, 1970; Llinas et al., 1976) and the absence of a detectable similar effect when Ca^{2+} was deposited by iontophoresis (Kato and Somjen, 1969; Kelly et al., 1969) had seemed anomalous.

To determine the influence of $[Ca^{2+}]_o$ on synaptic transmission in mammalian central nervous tissue more reliably, we therefore recorded synaptic potentials in slices of hippocampal tissue maintained in vitro (Dingledine and Somjen, in press). With a capillary microelectrode placed in the stratum radiatum in CA1 region in an extracellular position we recorded simultaneously the compound presynaptic spike, and the compound synaptic potential (EPSP) of pyramidal cells. A tungsten microcathode was used for punctate focal stimulation of afferent fibers. By varying the stimulus

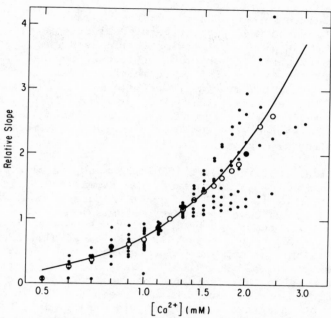

Fig. 8. The strength of synaptic transmission as a function of $[Ca^{2+}]_0$ in a slice of rat hippocampal tissue in vitro. Ordinate: slope of input-output function of extracellular EPSP, as explained in text; abscissa: Ca^{2+} activity measured in the tissue with ion-selective microelectrode, the "reference" barrel of which served for the focal electric recording. Input-output functions were normalized to that obtained in 1.2 mM $[Ca^{2+}]_0$, the control level. Filled circles: individual experiments (some points obtained by interpolation); open circles: mean of all data. $[Ca^{2+}]_0$ was changed by changing calcium concentration of bathing solution, and measurements obtained while tissue $[Ca^{2+}]_0$ was slowly "catching up" with bathing solution (see text). (From: Dingledine and Somjen, in press, by permission).

intensity, and measuring the amplitudes of the presynaptic volley and of the extracellular EPSP, (the time interval for the measurement of the EPSP being chosen so as not to be contaminated by the post-synaptic population spike), an input-output function could be plotted. If only stimulus intensities of moderate strength were used, the input-output function i.e. the growth of aggregate post-synaptic current plotted as a function of the recruitment of presynaptic afferent fibers) could be represented by a straight line. Its slope was taken to indicate synaptic efficiency.

$[Ca^{2+}]_0$ was caused to vary in these experiments by changing the solution perfusing the tissue chamber. We found, however, that

it is essential to measure $[Ca^{2+}]_o$ in the tissue. We used therefore double-barreled Ca^{2+} -selective microelectrodes, the reference
barrel of which supplied the focal electric recordings. After a
sudden change of perfusion solution it took an average of 30 to
60 minutes for the tissue $[Ca^{2+}]_o$ to reach the same level as the
bath $[Ca^{2+}]$ or about 9 minutes to achieve half the desired change.
A summary of the results of this study are shown in Fig. 8. Although our experimental design differed, our findings and conclusions agree in essence with those of Richards and Sercombe (1970)
concerning olfactory cortex.

It is clear that, at least in hippocampus and olfactory cortex, transmission across synapses of the mammalian CNS is a continuous function of $[Ca^{2+}]_o$. The question then arises, why a
corresponding influence on synaptic transmission was not noted when
Ca^{2+} (or Mg^{2+}) was deposited by iontophoresis in the vicinity of
central neurons (Kato and Somjen, 1969; Kelly et al., 1969). The
first explanation that comes to mind is, that the iontophoresis
pipettes were positioned near cell bodies, and the material released did not reach the presynaptic terminals scattered over a
wide expanse of dendritic surface. This explanation is however
not entirely satisfactory. The first discrepancy is, that intracellularly recorded IPSPs were also not considerably affected by
iontophoretic deposition of the divalent cations; inhibitory terminals are believed to be nearer to the recording site in the cell
body than excitatory terminals. Similarly puzzling are the older
observations that salts of both Ca^{2+} and Mg^{2+} act as depressants,
when administered into the cerebral ventricles, (Leusen, 1950;
Feldberg and Sherwood, 1957; Feldberg, 1958). Moreover, instead
of an antagonistic effect, these two cations reinforce one another's
action in causing coma when administered by this route (Somjen,
unpublished). When diffusing into the gray matter from the cerebral ventricles, neuropil and synaptic regions should be affected
as well as cell body layers. Under these conditions it is not clear
why Ca^{2+} did not antagonize the synaptic blocking action of Mg^{2+}

All of which forces us to admit that we still do not have the
complete picture concerning the effects of divalent cation. The
differential sensitivity of various synaptic systems, and of the
impulse generators of various types of neurons will have to be investigated further before the reactions of the system as a whole
can be predicted from the effects of these ions on its various
components.

Finally we should emphasize, that variation of $[Ca^{2+}]_o$ occurring in healthy tissue under normal conditions probably do not exceed 0.02 mM above and below the "resting" baseline level at least
in the cerebral neocortex and in the spinal cord (Somjen, in press
a). As with K^+ so also with Ca^{2+}, interactions of extracellular ion

activity and neuronal function are of greater relevance to patho-physiology than to the normal working of the CNS.

Some remarks relating to dorsal root potentials (DRP)

The controversy concerning the role of K^+ ions in the genera-tion of the negative DRP (Vyklicky, 1978; Somjen, 1978 b) seems to have been resolved. A consensus seems to have developed, that the DRP evoked by a single synchronous volley is transmitted mainly by an agent other than K^+, possibly GABA; but that in causing the sustained DRP in response to prolonged repetitive stimulation, K^+ may play a gradually increasing part (Lothman and Somjen, 1975; Syková and Vyklický, 1977; Syková et al., 1980; Davidoff et al., 1980). During prolonged stimulation the GABA output from presynap-tic terminals can be subject to "fatigue", and the post-junctional effect of GABA is known to be subject to desensitization (Deschenes et al., 1976). Neither of these two effects would be manifest with depolarization caused by K^+.

Some of our recent findings are in good agreement with this compromise interpretation (Kinnes et al., 1980). The depolariza-tion of dorsal root ganglion cells evoked by GABA can be suppressed by penicillin; and penicillin administered intravenously also de-presses the negative DRP, and slows its timecourse (see also David-off, 1972). This is as it should be if GABA is the main transmitter agent of the DRP evoked by single shock stimuli. When repetitive trains of stimuli were used, the depressant effect of penicillin on the sustained plateau phase of the DRP was, in some experiments at least, clearly less than on the single-pulse-evoked DRP. This is expected, if K^+ has a greater role in transmitting the sustained DRP, than in the single-shock-DRP, since the depolarizing effect of high $[K^+]_o$ would not be blocked by penicillin.

But while the agents responsible for transmitting the DRP are seemingly being clarified, the relationship between primary afferent depolarization and the synaptic inhibitory effect deemed "presynaptic" has become rather more confused. In the studies just quoted (Lothman and Somjen, 1976; Davenport et al., 1978; Kinnes et al.,1980) it turned out that intravenous administration of penicillin did not block the inhibitory effect customarily called presynaptic, even though it did depress the DRP recorded in the same preparation. This dissociation was noted whether inhibition was gauged from the amplitude of the monosynaptic reflex, or the amplitude of the EPSP conducted electrotonically into a ventral root. Administration of ammonium acetate seems to bring about a similar dissociation, depressing the negative DRP, but not the primary afferent depolarization detected by focal microstimulation, nor the "presynaptic" inhibition of EPSPs (Iles et al, 1979).

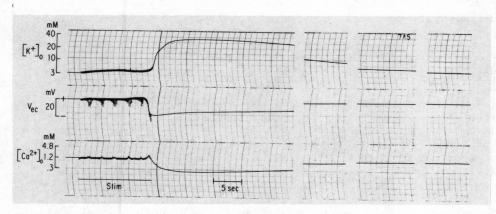

Fig. 9.   Spreading depression in a slice of rat hippocampal tissue in vitro, provoked by intense repetitive punctate focal stimulation. $[K^+]_o$ and $[Ca^{2+}]_o$ recorded with two ion-selective microelectrodes, both in stratum radiatum, near one another; extracellular potential from "reference" barrel of Ca^{2+}-selective electrode.

Ion changes and pathophysiology of the spinal cord

The bearing of ion changes upon the mechanism of seizures has been and will again be reviewed elsewhere (Somjen, 1980; in press a; Somjen et al., in press; also : Prince, 1978). Briefly, during epileptiform paroxysmal activity $[K^+]_o$ rises to a level around 8 or 10 mM in spinal cord. At the same time $[Ca^{2+}]_o$ in ventral horn drops from 1.2 to 1.1 or 1.0 mM. Both these changes in ionic activity will tend to interfere in the same sense with neuronal function. The decrease of $[Ca^{2+}]_o$ and the increase of $[K^+]_o$ will both reduce the output of synaptic transmitter, the former by depressed excitation-secretion coupling, the latter by presynaptic depolarization and consequent decrease of presynaptic spike size. Both will also enhance neuronal excitability: the decreased $[Ca^{2+}]_o$ by de-stabilizing neuronal membranes, and the high $[K^+]_o$ by depolarizing neurons. It should be added, however, that elevated $[K^+]_o$ tends to enhance "accommodation" and reduce the capability of neurons to fire repetitively, but low $[Ca^{2+}]_o$ tends to counteract "accommodation", and favor repetitive firing. In this one respect, therefore, the two changes, elevated $[K^+]_o$ and decreased $[Ca^{2+}]_o$, are antagonistic. Nevertheless, the net effect of the changed extracellular ion activities will be to insulate neural assemblies from synaptic input, and to favor spontaneous excitatory waves and non-synaptic interactions between adjacent neural groups.

It should be emphasized, however, that while the observed changes of extracellular ion activity are large enough to influence

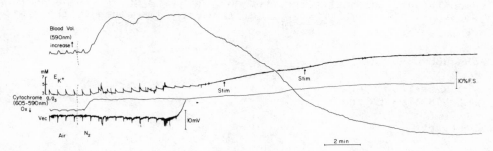

Fig. 10.   Agonal changes in a decapitate spinal cord. Recording
conditions similar to Fig. 3. At vertical marks respiratory gas changed from room air to nitrogen (experiment
by LaManna, Rosenthal, Younts and Somjen; from: Somjen,
1978, by permission).

the course of seizures, neither their magnitude nor their timecourse
is consistent with the suggestion that they actually cause, or
trigger, paroxysmal activity. On the other hand there are reasons
to believe that changes in the transmembrane flux of Ca^{2+} ions (but
not in their extracellular activity) may have a causal role in the
chain of events leading to seizure discharges (Heinemann et al.,
1978; Somjen et al., 1978; Somjen, in press a).

The spinal cord takes a special place amongst neural tissues
in that it seeems to be immune to spreading depression. This phenomenon can be provoked not only in practically all parts of the
brain in situ (Bureš et al., 1974) but also in isolated slices of
hippocampal tissue (Fig. 9). By contrast, the changes occurring
in various spinal functions during agonal anoxia can be seen in
Fig. 10. There is a gradual extinction of SP shifts and stimulus-
evoked $[K^+]_0$ responses, associated with reduction of cytochrome a,
a_3, an initial increase of the volume of blood due to reactive vasodilatation, followed by drainage of blood when the heart fails. At
no time is there the explosive increase of $[K^+]_0$ and the very large
and sudden negative shift of the electric potential so characteristic of cortical hypoxia. $[Ca^{2+}]_0$ also drifts to its final post-
mortem level in the spinal cord (Somjen, in press: a) without the
violent swings exhibited in cerebral cortex.

There is thus a peculiar contrast between the cerebellar cortex, which is capable of spreading depression but does not exhibit
true paroxysmal activity, and the spinal cord which is readily pro-

voked into seizure discharge, but does not undergo spreading depression. Hidden in this contrast there may lie clues to the basic mechanism of both processes.

ACKNOWLEDGEMENTS

Research reported here was supported by PHS grant NS 11933. We would like to thank Mrs. Marjorie Andrews for editing and typing.

REFERENCES

Barrett, E.F., and Barrett, J.N., 1976, Separation of two voltage-sensitive potassium currents and demonstration of a tetrodotoxin-resistant calcium current in frog motoneurons, J. Physiol. (Lond.), 255:737.

Bracho, H., and Orkand, R.K., 1970, Effect of calcium on excitatory neuromuscular transmission in the crayfish, J. Physiol., 206:61.

Bureš, J., Burešová, O., and Křivánek, J., 1974, "The Mechanism and Applications of Leao's Spreading Depression of Electroencephalographic Activity", Academia, Prague.

Cordingley, G.E., and Somjen, G.G., 1978, The clearing of excess potassium from extracellular space in spinal cord and cerebral cortex, Brain Res., 151:291.

Curtis, H.J., and Cole, K.S., 1942, Membrane and action potentials from the squid giant axon, J. Cell. Comp.Physiol., 19:135.

Curtis, D.R., Perrin, D.D., and Watkins, J.C., 1960, The excitation of spinal neurones by the iontophoretic application of agents which chelate calcium, J.Neurochem., 6:1.

Davenport, J., Schwindt, P.C., and Crill, W.E., 1978, Presynaptic and long-lasting postsynaptic inhibition during penicillin-induced spinal seizures, Neurology, 23:592.

Davidoff, R.A., 1972, Penicillin and inhibition in the cat spinal cord, Brain Res., 45:638.

Davidoff, R.A., Hackman, J.C., Osorio, I., 1980, Amino acid antagonists do not block the depolarizing effects of potassium ions on frog primary afferents, Neuroscience, 5:117.

Deschenes, M., and Feltz, P., 1976, GABA-induced rise of extracellular potassium in rat dorsal root ganglia: an electrophysiological study in vivo, Brain Res., 118:494.

Deaschenes, M., Feltz, P., and Lamour, Y., 1976, A model for an estimate in vivo of the ionic basis of presynaptic inhibition: an intracellular analysis of the GABA-induced depolarization in rat dorsal root ganglia, Brain Res., 118:486.

Dingledine, R., and Somjen, G., in press, Calcium dependence of synaptic transmission in the hippocampal slice, Brain Res.

Dodge, F.A., and Rahamimoff, R., 1967, Cooperative action of calcium ions in transmitter release at the neuromuscular junction, J. Physiol., 193:419.

Feldberg, W., 1958, Anaesthesia and sleep-like conditions produced by injection into the cerebral ventricles of cats, J. Physiol., 140:20.

Feldberg, W., and Sherwood, S.L., 1957, Effects of calcium and potassium injected into the cerebral ventricles of the cat, J. Physiol., 139:408.

Frankenhaeuser, B., and Hodgkin, A.L., 1956, The after-effects of impulses in the giant nerve fibers of Loligo, J. Physiol.,131:341.

Gardner-Medwin, A.R., in press, Membrane transport and solute migration affecting the brain cell microenvironment, in: Dynamics of the brain cell microenvironment (Nicholson, C.) Neuroscience Res. Prog. Bull.

Heinemann, U., Lux, H.D., and Gutnick, M.J., 1977, Extracellular free calcium and potassium during paroxysmal activity in the cerebral cortex of the cat, Exp.Brain Res., 27:237.

Heinemann, U., Lux, H.D.,and Gutnick, M.J. 1978, Changes in extracellular free calcium and potassium activity in the somatosensory cortex of cats, in: "Abnormal Neuronal Discharges", N. Chalazonitis and M. Boisson eds., Raven Press, New York.

Hertz, L., 1978, An intense potassium uptake into astrocytes, its further enhancement by high potassium, and its possible involvement in potassium homeostasis at the cellular level, Brain Res., 145:202.

Huxley, A.F., and Stämpfli, R., 1951, Effect of potassium and sodium on resting and action potentials of single myelinated nerve fibers, J. Physiol., 112:496.

Iles, J.F., Jack, J.J.B., and Lewis, G.H., 1979, Dorsal root potentials and presynaptic depolarization: actions of ammonia, J. Physiol., 296:98p.

Jöbsis, F.F., Keizer, J., LaManna, J.C., and Rosenthal, M., 1977, Reflectance spectrophotometry of the intact cerebral cortex. I. Dual wavelength technique, J. appl. Physiol., 43:858.

Kato, G., and Somjen, G.G., 1969, Effects of micro-iontophoretic administration of magnesium and calcium on neurones in the central nervous system of cats, J. Neurobiol., 1:181.

Katz, B., and Miledi, R., 1967, The timing of calcium action during neuromuscular transmission, J. Physiol. (Lond.), 189:535.

Katz, B., and Miledi, R., 1969, Tetrodotoxin resistant activity in presynaptic terminals, J. Physiol. (Lond.), 203:459.

Kelly, J.S., Krnjević, K., and Somjen, G., 1969, Divalent cations and electrical properties of cortical cells, J. Neurobiol., 197:208.

Kinnes, C.G., Connors, B., and Somjen, G., 1980, The effect of convulsant doses of penicillin on primary afferents, dorsal root ganglion cells, and on "presynaptic" inhibition in the spinal cord, Brain Res., 192:495.

Krnjević, K., and Morris, M.E., 1972, Extracellular K^+ activity and slow potential changes in spinal cord and medulla, Canadian J. Physiol. Pharmacol., 50:1214.

Krnjević, K., and Morris, M., in press, Electrical and functional correlates of changes in transmembrane ionic gradients produced by neural activity in the central nervous system. in: "The Application of Ion-selective Electrodes", T. Zeuthen, ed., Elsevier, Amsterdam.

Kuffler, S.W., and Nicholls, J.G., 1966, The physiology of neuroglial cells, Ergeb. Physiol., 57:1.

Leusen, I., 1950, The influence of calcium, potassium and magnesium ions in cerebrospinal fluid on vasomotor system, J. Physiol., 110:319.

Lewis, D.V., and Schuette, W.H., 1975, NADH fluorescence and $[K^+]_o$ changes during hippocampal electrical stimulation, J. Neurophysiol., 38:405.

Llinas, R., Steinberg, I.Z., and Walton, K., 1976, Presynaptic calcium currents and their relation to synaptic transmission: Voltage clamp study in squid giant synapse, and theoretical model for calcium gate, Proc. Nat. Acad. Sci. (USA), 73:2918.

Llinas, R., Sugimori, M., and Walton, K., 1977, Calcium dendritic spikes in the mammalian Purkinje cells, Neuroscience Abstracts, 3:58.

Lothman, E., LaManna, J., Cordingley, G., Rosenthal, M., and Somjen, G., 1975, Responses of electrical potential, potassium levels, and oxidative metabolic activity of the cerebral neocortex of cats, Brain Res., 88:15.

Lothman, E.W., and Somjen, G.G., 1975, Extracellular potassium activity, intracellular and extracellular potential responses in the spinal cord, J. Physiol., 252:115.

Lothman, E.W., and Somjen, G.G., 1976, Functions of primary afferents, and responses of extracellular K^+ during spinal epilep iform seizures, Electroencephalogr. Clin. Neurophysiol., 41:253.

Lux, H.D., and Hofmeier,G., 1978, Kinetics of the calcium dependent potassium current in helix neurons, Pflüg.Arch., 373:R47

McAfee,D.A., and Yarowsky, P.J., 1979, Calcium-dependent potentials in the mammalian sympathetic neurone, J. Physiol., 290:507.

Nicholson, C., Bruggencate,G. Ten, Stöckle, H., and Steinberg, R., 1978, Calcium and potassium changes in extracellular microenvironment of cat cerebellar cortex, J. Neurophysiol., 41:1026.

Nicoll, R.A., 1979, Dorsal root potentials and changes in extracellular potassium in the spinal cord of the frog, J. Physiol., 290:113.

Prince, D., 1978, Neurophysiology of epilepsy, Ann. Rev. Neurosci., 1:395.

Richards, C.D., and Sercombe, R., 1970, Calcium, magnesium and electrical activity of guinea pig olfactory cortex in vitro, J. Physiol., 211:571.

Rosenthal, M., LaManna, J., Yamada, Y., Younts, W., and Somjen, G., 1979, Oxidative metabolism, extracellular potassium, and sustained potential shifts in cat spinal cord in situ, Brain Res., 162:113.

Schwindt, P.C., and Crill, W.E., 1980, Properties of a persistent inward current in normal and TEA-injected motoneurons, J. Neurophysiol., 43:1700.

Segal, M., and Gutnick, M.J., in press, Effects of serotonin on extracellular potassium concentration in the rat hippocampal slice, Brain Res.

Skou, J.C., 1975, The $(Na^+ + K^+)$ activated enzyme system and its relationship to transport of sodium and potassium, O. Rev.Biophys., 7:401.

Somjen, G.G., 1969, Sustained evoked potential changes of the spinal cord, Brain Res., 12:268.

Somjen, G. G., 1970,Evoked sustained focal potentials and membrane potential of neurons and of unresponsive cells of the spinal cord, J. Neurophysiol., 33:562.

Somjen, G.G., 1973, Electrogenesis of sustained potentials, Progr. Neurobiol., 1:199.

Somjen, G.G., 1978a, Metabolic and electrical correlates of the clearing of excess potassium in cortex and in spinal cord, in: "Studies in Neurophysiology," R. Porter, ed., Cambridge University Press, Cambridge, p.181.

Somjen, G.G., 1978b, A comment on the effect of potassium on dorsal root potentials, in: "Iontophoresis and Transmitter Mechanisms in the Mammalian Central Nervous System", R.W. Ryall and J.S. Kelly, eds., Amsterdam, Elsevier, p. 282.

Somjen, G.G., 1979a, Extracellular potassium in the mammalian central nervous system, Ann. Rev. Physiol., 41:159.

Somjen, G.G., 1979g, Responses of extracellular calcium during afferent nerve stimulation and during seizures in the spinal cord of cats, Neuroscience Abstracts, 5:730.

Somjen, G.G., 1980, Influence of potassium and neuroglia in the generation of seizures and in their treatment, in: "Antiepileptic Drugs: Mechanisms of Action", G.H. Glaser, J.K. Penry, and D.M. Woodbury, eds., Raven Press, New York, p.155.

Somjen, G.G., in press (a), Stimulus-evoked and seizure-related responses of extracellular calcium activity in spinal cord compared to those in cerebral cortex, J. Neurophysiol.

Somjen, G.G., in press (b), The why and the how of measuring the activity of ions in extracellular fluid of the spinal cord and cerebral cortex, in: "The Application of Ion-selective Electrodes," T. Zeuthen, ed., Amsterdam, Elsevier.

Somjen, G.G., in press (c), Physiology of glial cells., Proc. 28th Internat'l Congr. Physiol.,Invited Lectures, Akadémiai Kiadó, Budapest.

Somjen, G.G., Connors, B., and Kinnes, C., in press, Calcium activity and seizure mechanisms in the spinal cord, in: "Physiology and Pharmacology of Epileptogenic Phenomena", M. Klee, ed., Raven Press, New York

Somjen, G.G., and Lothman, E.W., 1974, Potassium, sustained focal potential shifts, and dorsal root potentials of the mammalian spinal cord, Brain Res., 69:153.

Somjen, G.G., Lothman, E., Dunn, P., Dunaway, T., and Cordingley, G., 1978, Microphysiology of spinal seizures, in: "Abnormal Neuronal Discharges", N. Chalazonitis and M. Boisson, eds., Raven Press, New York, p.13.

Syková, E., Czéh, G., and Kříž, N., 1980, Potassium accumulation in the frog spinal cord induced by nociceptive stimulation of the skin, Neurosci. Lett., 18:253.

Syková, E., and Vyklický, L., 1977, Changes of extracellular potassium activity in isolated spinal cord of frog under high Mg^{2+} concentration, Neurosci. Lett., 4:161.

Vyklický, L., 1978, Transient changes in extracellular potassium and presynaptic inhibition, in: "Iontophoresis and Transmitter Mechanisms in the Mammalian Central Nervous System", Elsevier, Amsterdam, p. 284.

Vyklický, L., Syková, E., Kříž, N., and Ujec, E., 1972, Post-stimulation changes of extracellular potassium concentration in the spinal cord of the rat, Brain Res., 45:608.

Wong, R.K.S., and Prince, D.A., 1978, Participation of calcium spikes during intrinsic burst firing in hippocampal neurons, Brain Res., 159:385.

Yoshida, S., Matsuda, Y., and Samejima, A., 1978, Tetrodotoxin-resistant sodium and calcium components of action potentials in dorsal root ganglion cells of the adult mouse, J. Neurophysiol. 41:1096.

RELATIONS BETWEEN EXTRACELLULAR K^+ AND Ca^{++} ACTIVITIES AND LOCAL FIELD POTENTIALS IN THE SPINAL CORD OF THE RAT DURING FOCAL AND GENERALIZED SEIZURE DISCHARGES

J. Janus, E.-J. Speckmann and A. Lehmenkühler

Physiologisches Institut I der Universität

D - 44oo Münster, GFR

Focal interictal epileptiform discharges (FIED) as well as generalized cortical seizure activity are known to evoke spinal field potentials (SFP) (Elger and Speckmann, 1980). Origin and transmission of bioelectrical potentials are considered to be linked with changes of extracellular calcium and potassium activity. Several investigations revealed a transient increase of spinal extracellular potassium in the course of afferent nerve stimulation (c.f. Somjen, 1979). To analyze the mechanisms underlying SFP following efferent impulse transmission the reaction of potassium and calcium activity on epileptiform discharges within the cerebral cortex was measured in the lumbar spinal cord.

METHODS

Local application of penicillin to the motor cortex of anaesthetized, paralyzed, artificially ventilated and thermo-stabilized rats (weighing 300 to 500 g) was used to evoke FIED (Elger and Speckmann, 1980). Generalized seizure discharges were elicited by systemic administration of pentylenetetrazol (PTZ). EEG registrations out of the cortical epileptogenic focus and recordings within the lumbar spinal cord were made by double-barrelled ion-selective microelectrodes (c.f. Lehmenkühler, 1979; Oehme et al., 1976), stored on tape and analyzed by use of a PDP-12 computer program (Knoll et al., 1974). For identification of spinal registration sites alcian-blue was iontophoretically injected (c.f. Lee et al., 1969).

RESULTS

FIED within the motor cortex revealed a periodical pattern of cortical potential shifts consisting of a primary negative component of about 2 mV followed by a smaller positive deflection. Each potential transient lasting ca. 100 ms was accompanied by an SFP. At the dorsal surface of the lumbar spinal cord SFP showed a small and short negative shift prior to a steep positive one in total lasting about 150 ms. In the course of dorsoventral spinal penetration the positive SFP component changed polarity at a depth of ca. 500 μm. The primary negative portion of the signal disappeared slowly with depth. Below 1000 μm it changed into a positive going transient.

The baseline of the extracellular potassium activity (a_K^o) ranged from 3 to 4 mmol/l (c.f. Somjen, 1979). Increases of a_K^o could be observed concomitant with SFP in a depth of 500 to 1500 μm. The maximum accumulation in the order of 0.1 mmol/l was found at 8oo to 1000 μm of depth. Lasting between 500 and 1000 ms rises of a_K^o often were succeeded by a small undershoot (Fig.1, A1). Depending on the latency of the next interictal discharge the increases of a_K^o were superimposed. The baseline of extracellular calcium concentration (a_{Ca}^o) was about 0.8 mmol/l. Beginning in a depth of ca. 1000 μm below dorsal spinal surface transients of SFP were linked with increases of a_{Ca}^o the maximum of which was found at ca. 1500 μm. Disappearing at 2000 μm rises of a_{Ca}^o were in the order of up to 0.05 mmol/l and lasted between 100 and 150 ms. Succeedingly, an underswing in the range of 0.01 mmol/l was found for about 250 ms (Fig.1, A2). The pattern of the ionic reaction was bilaterally symmetrical, FIED, however, occurred strictly unilaterally.

Generalized cortical seizures indicated by negative DC potential shifts were accompanied by a persistent negative deflection of SFP. During ictal and interictal episodes a_K^o increased up to 1 mmol/l. This reaction was strictly found within the posterior grey matter. (Fig.1, B1). At the same time, a slow rise of a_{Ca}^o was observed within the anterior grey matter. After about 15 s accumulation of a_{Ca}^o reached a ceiling level of 0.1 mmol/l above resting activity. The returning of a_{Ca}^o to baseline outlasted the negative SFP shift by about 30 s (Fig.1, B2).

DISCUSSION

Experimental evidence points to neurons as the main source of rising a_K^o (c.f. Somjen, 1979). The overwhelming majority of motoneurons is located in the ventral horn of the lumbar spinal cord (Janzen et al., 1974). Changes of a_K^o, however, could only be detected in the posterior grey matter.The discrepancy might be explained by the fact that in addition to their endings at motoneurons the fibers of the corticospinal tracts simultaneously activate a large network of interneurons by means of axoncollaterals

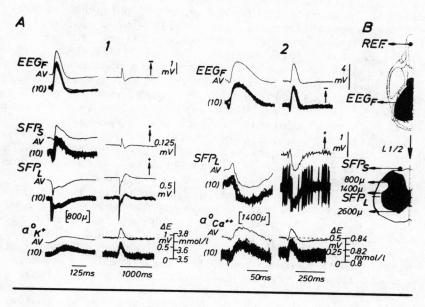

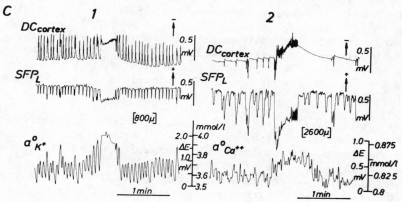

Fig. 1. Simultaneous recordings of local extracellular potassium (a^o_K+) and calcium ($a^o_{Ca}++$) activities, superficial and laminar spinal field potential (SFP_S, SFP_L) and cortical bioelectrical potential (EEG_F, DC_{cortex}) during focal (Part A) and generalized (Part C) seizure discharges. Scheme of registration in Part B. Calculated average potentials (AV) are drawn above 10 superimposed original recordings (10). Note different depths of spinal penetration and time scales.

(Erulkar and Soller, 1979). This idea is further supported by the finding that epicortical stimulation evoked polysynaptic EPSPs in lumbar motoneurons (Janzen et al., 1977).Calcium ions crossing neuronal membranes are thought to release transmitter substances at synaptic endings (c.f. Rahamimoff et al., 1976). This way of calcium movement is supported by the finding of decreasing extra-cellular calcium activity in the course of paroxysmal discharges (Heinemann et al., 1977). On the other hand, induced by PTZ abnormal discharges of isolated snail neurons revealed an initial marked decline of intracellular calcium activity (Zidek and Lehmenkühler, 1980). Additionally, showing an initial fast increase and a secondary prolonged decline a biphasic reaction of calcium could be demon-strated during interictal and ictal activity in the brain cortex of rats (Lehmenkühler et al., 1979). Since experiments using different techniques pointed into the same direction (Labeyrie and Koechlin, 1979) the pattern of calcium reaction in the spinal cord seems to be similar to that in the brain cortex. Under epileptiform activity enhanced oxygen consumption causes a large production of CO_2. (1) slow indirect CO_2 effects via pH changes and (2) rapid direct CO_2 reaction with macromolecules forming carbamic acids (c.f. Mitz, 1979) might liberate ionized calcium into the intracellular as well as the extracellular compartment. Investigations made in the cerebral cortex of rats pointed to exactly that action by CO_2 (Caspers et al. 1979). Increased concentrations of carbon dioxide in the inspiratory gas mixture caused an increase of tissue pCO_2 and led to an accumula-tion of extracellular calcium activity. Furthermore, varying complex-ation of calcium ions with oxoanions such as bicarbonate or phosphate might additionally to be taken into account for calcium transients entirely taking place within the extracellular space (Lehmenkühler et al., 1980).

In summary, the density of a large number of interposed small neurons activated by impulse transmission from centrifugal fibers is assumed to be responsible for increasing extracellular spinal potassium in the course of cortical seizure discharges. The rise of calcium activity in the extracellular space of the spinal cord is regarded to originate from binding sites of cellular membranes and/or of the extracellular space itself.

REFERENCES

Caspers, H., Speckmann, E.-J., and Lehmenkühler, A., 1979, Effects of CO_2 on cortical field potentials in relation to neuronal activity, in:"Origins of cerebral field potentials", E.-J.Speck-mann and H. Caspers, eds., Thieme, Stuttgart, pp. 151 - 163

Elger, C.E. and Speckmann, E.-J., 1980, Focal interictal epileptiform discharges (FIED) in the epicortical EEG and their relations to spinal field potentials in the rat, Electroenceph.clin.Neuro-physiol., 48: 447

Erulkar, S.D. and Soller, R.W., 1979, Neuronal interactions in a central nervous system model, in:"Origins of cerebral field potentials", E.-J. Speckmann and H. Caspers, eds., Thieme, Stuttgart, pp. 13 - 21

Heinemann, U., Lux, H.D. and Gutnick, M.J., 1977, Extracellular free calcium and potassium during paroxysmal activity in the cerebral cortex of the cat, Exp.Brain Res., 27: 237

Janzen, R.W.C., Speckmann, E.-J. and Caspers, H., 1974, Distribution of large ventral horn cells in the lumbar cord of the rat, Cell Tiss.Res., 151: 159

Janzen, R.W.C., Speckmann, E.-J., Caspers, H. and Elger, C.E., 1977, Cortico-spinal connections in the rat. II. Oligosynaptic and polysynaptic responses of lumbar motoneurons to epicortical stimulation, Exp.Brain Res., 28: 405

Knoll, O., Speckmann, E.-J. and Caspers, H., 1974, Ein Verfahren zur Korrelierung verschiedener bioelektrischer Vorgänge mit definierten Potentialmustern im EEG, Z.EEG EMG, 5: 200

Labeyrie, E. and Koechlin, Y., 1979, Photoelectrode with a very short time-constant for recording intracerebrally Ca^{++} transients at a cellular level, J.Neurosci.Methods, 1: 35

Lee, B.B., Mandl, G. and Stean, J.P.B., 1969, Micro-electrode tip position marking in nervous tissue: A new dye method, Electroenceph.clin.Neurophysiol., 27: 610

Lehmenkühler, A., 1979, Interrelationships between DC potentials, potassium activity, pO_2 and pCO_2 in the cerebral cortex of the rat, in:"Origins of cerebral field potentials", E.-J.Speckmann and H. Caspers, eds., Thieme, Stuttgart, pp. 49 - 59

Lehmenkühler, A., Lensing, J., Caspers, H. and Janus, J., 1979, Biphasic reaction of extracellular Ca^{++} activity during interictal discharges in the brain cortex, Pflügers Arch., 382: R42

Lehmenkühler, A., Zidek, W., Staschen, M. and Caspers, H., 1980, Cortical pH and pCa in relation to DC potential shifts during spreading depression and asphyxiation, this volume

Mitz, M.A., 1979, CO_2 Biodynamics: A new concept of cellular control, J.Theoretical Biology, in print

Somjen, G.G., 1979, Extracellular potassium in the mammalian central nervous system, Ann.Rev.Physiol., 41: 159

Oehme, M., Kessler, M. and Simon, W., 1976, Neutral carrier Ca^{++}-microelectrode, Chimia, 3o: 204

Rahamimoff,R., Erulkar,S.D., Alnaes,E., Meiri,H., Rotshenker,S. and Rahamimoff,H., 1976, Modulation of transmitter release by calcium ions and nerve impulses, in:"Cold spring harbour symposia on quant. Biol.", Vol. XL, The synapse, Cold spring harbour laboratory, New York, pp. 107 - 116

Zidek, W. and Lehmenkühler, A., 1980, Changes of intracellular Cl^- and Ca^{++} activities during abnormal discharges in snail neurons, Pflügers Arch., 384: R18

ION FLUXES ACROSS THE MEMBRANE OF MOTONEURONS DURING THE

ACTION OF GLUTAMATE

Ch. Ph. Bührle and U. Sonnhof

I. Physiologisches Institut, Universität Heidelberg
Im Neuenheimer Feld 326, 69 Heidelberg, F.R.G.

Continuous registration of ion activities in motoneurons (MNs) and in the extracellular space of the isolated frog spinal cord was performed to identify ion fluxes across the postsynaptic membrane during the depolarizing action of glutamate (GLUT).

When GLUT is applied in the superfusing solution of this preparation MNs as well as internuncial neurons are excited. Discharges of interneurons terminating at the membrane of the recorded neuron lead to uncontrolable permeability changes of this membrane and interfere with an exact analysis of the postsynaptic effects of GLUT.

Chemical synaptic transmission therefore had to be suppressed by Mn^{++} which causes a complete but reversible disappearance of synaptic events. Under these conditions the GLUT depolarization was found to develop without measurable changes of neuronal input resistance. A marked increase of extracellular K^+ activity (aK^+e) was always found to be part of the excitatory action of GLUT. As a GLUT induced efflux of K^+ from cells other than MNs and a consequent passive depolarization of the recorded MN by the diminution of the K^+ gradient across its membrane could not be excluded as cause of the excitatory action of GLUT, the sensitivity of the neuronal membrane to changes of aK^+e had to be determined.

MNs were depolarized to comparable levels by an experimental increase of aK^+e (substitution of NaCl against KCl in the superfusing medium) and by GLUT, while changes of aK^+e were measured with K^+ sensitive microelectrodes located in the immediate vicinity of the recorded cells. In close correspondence with the Nernst equation an experimental increase of aK^+e led to a depolarization of 56 mV/decade change of aK^+e while GLUT depolarized the MNs by

187

at least 80 mV/decade change of aK^+e. It is therefore evident that
GLUT depolarizes MNs by changing the relation between K^+ conductance
and other conductances. The excitatory action of GLUT has to be considered a postsynaptic effect.

A direct approach to detect ion fluxes arising from such shifts
of membrane permeability was chosen by simultaneously observing in-
tra- and extracellular ion activities. As membrane resistance is
virtually unchanged during the action of GLUT the depolarization was
assumed to be based on ion fluxes driven by a strong EMF and, therefore, requiring merely small conductance changes to considerably depolarize the membrane.

Measurements of the intra- and extracellular activities of K^+,
Na^+, Ca^{++} and Cl^- (aK^+i/e, aNa^+i/e, $aCa^{++}i/e$, aCl^-i/e) were performed
with conventional double barreled ion sensitive microelectrodes with
outer tip diameters of about 1 μm. Mean absolute ion activities ($a\bar{X}i$)
found in MNS and calculated respective equilibrium potentials (Ex)
are compiled in tab. 1:

Table 1

	n	$a\bar{X}i \pm SD$ (mmol/1)	$\overline{MP} \pm SD$ (mV)	Ex (mV)
Na^+	37	$53,1 \pm 13,8$	$-54,1 \pm 8,3$	$+ 22,1$
K^+	17	$87,8 \pm 34,1$	$-55,9 \pm 9,4$	$- 80,5$
Ca^{++}	57	$8,25 \times 10^{-2} \pm 6,25 \times 10^{-2}$	$-47,2 \pm 11,1$	$+ 36,5$
Cl^-	42	$34,4 \pm 9,9$	$-45,8 \pm 10,1$	$- 30,4$

Cross sensitivities of the respective ion exchangers to interfering inorganic or organic ions present in the MN generally lead to
overestimations of the measured ion activities. This especially
applies to aNa^+i and aK^+i in tab. 1 which are presumably overesti-
mated by 10 and 5 mmol/1 respectively. Due to the present ignorance
about the level of $aMg^{++}i$ no similar correction of $aCa^{++}i$ can be
made. For the determination of true aCl^-i interference by intracellular HCO^-_3 seems to be of some importance.

The EMF for the Na^+ (76,2 mV) and Ca^{++} (83,7 mV) batteries
seems to fulfill the criteria required for ionic mechanisms capable
to produce strong depolarizations at small changes of membrane conductance while the EMF for Cl^- is comparatively small.

Na^+: The GLUT depolarization was accompanied by an increase of
aNa^+i and a decrease of aNa^+e (Fig. 1). As with all other ion activities aNa^+i and aNa^+e monotonously returned to preexisting values
after termination of GLUT application. A depolarization during experimental elevation of aK^+e did not evoke changes of aNa^+i.

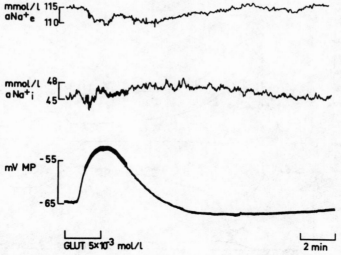

Fig. 1. Simultaneous registration of membrane potential (MP), aNa^+i and aNa^+e during the action of GLUT.

Ca^{++}: Potential dependent Ca^{++} influxes are known to exist in frog spinal MNs as well as in various other nerve cells. Passive depolarization of MNs by K^+ induced a marked decrease of $aCa^{++}e$ and an accompanying rise of $aCa^{++}i$. This potential dependent Ca^{++} influx was of threshold type and was activated at MP levels between $- 30$ mV and $- 25$ mV (Fig. 2). Ca^{++} influxes evoked by GLUT were already found when MP was far below the threshold (Fig. 2). Hence an activation of specific Ca^{++} channels in the MN membrane by GLUT has to be assumed.

Cl^-: As E_{Cl} deviates from MP by about 15 mV in the depolarizing direction, an increased Cl^- conductance could contribute to the GLUT depolarization. Due to the small EMF any significant Cl^- carried depolarization should be accompanied by a marked increase of membrane conductance. However, changes of aCl^-i during K^+ and GLUT depolarizations of comparable amplitude were nearly identical suggesting an essentially potential dependent displacement of Cl^- across the membrane and ruling out a Cl^- flux as specific part of the action of GLUT. Cl^- itself is not distributed passively between intra- and extracellular space as indicated by an E_{Cl} less negative than MP. An inwardly directed Cl^- transport providing an EMF of 15 mV has therefore to be postulated.

K^+: As K^+ conductance is thought to be the main constituent of membrane conductance in the resting state, changes of K^+ conductance should be reflected in variations of neuronal input resistance. As input resistance is not subject to detectable changes during the action of GLUT while aK^+i slightly de- and aK^+e markedly increases,

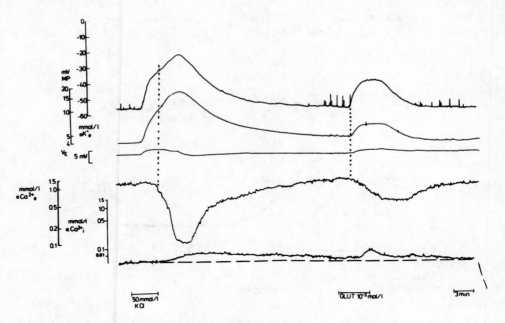

Fig. 2. Registration of MP, $aCa^{++}i$, $aCa^{++}e$ and aK^+e during experimental elevation of aK^+e as well as application of GLUT. Note threshold dependent Ca^{++} displacements during passive K^+ depolarization in opposition to instant changes of $aCa^{++}i$ and $aCa^{++}e$ evoked by GLUT.

a passive outward flux of K^+ without permeability changes of the membrane seems to explain sufficiently the accumulation of K^+ observed in the extracellular surroundings of the MNs. Calculations based on values of specific membrane resistance of cat MNs support the idea that the measured displacement of K^+ is in analogy to Cl^- - due to the shift of MP relative to the equilibrium potential during a depolarization mainly carried by an influx of Na^+ and Ca^{++}. However, an activation of K^+ conductance at remote dendritic sites can not be excluded at present, as such conductance changes may not necessarily be reflected in alterations of neuronal input resistance due to the electrotonic decrement between their point of origin and the recording electrode in the soma of the MN.

According to these results the GLUT depolarization can be attributed to a combined increase of membrane permeability for Ca^{++} and Na^+, while such effects are absent for Cl^- and at least unlikely for K^+.

THE IONIC BASIS OF THE IPSP IN SPINAL MOTONEURONS OF THE FROG

U. Sonnhof and Ch. Ph. Bührle

I. Physiologisches Institut, Universität Heidelberg

Im Neuenheimer Feld 326, 69 Heidelberg, F. R. G.

Although considerable effort has been dedicated to research into the constituents of the current that carries the hyperpolarizing IPSP in cat spinal motoneurons (Eccles, 1964), the results gained by ion injection experiments claiming a combined increase of membrane permeability for K^+ and Cl^- have not remained unopposed. An influx of Cl^- is by some workers (Lux, 1974; Llinás, Baker and Precht, 1974) supposed to be the main cause of the IPSP in this preparation.

As in spinal motoneurons (MNs) of the frog IPSPs are generally depolarizing (Katz and Miledi, 1963) a more direct analysis of their ionic basis by simultaneous measurements of intra- and extracellular K^+ and Cl^- activities (aK^+i/e, aCl^-i/e) with ion sensitive microelectrodes seemed worthwhile. Conventional double barreled micropipettes with an outer tip diameter of 1 μm were used in these experiments.

During the flow of the inhibitory current input resistance of the MN is reduced by 80% (Fig. 1 A,B). This change of membrane conductance and the reversal of this PSP at potential values 15 mV less negative than the resting MP discern the IPSP from the equally depolarizing EPSP which occurs without measurable changes of input resistance and the extrapolated reversal potential of which is assumed to be between + 10 mV and 0 mV.

Measurements of aK^+i and aK^+e revealed a transmembrane K^+ gradient corresponding to an E_K 15 - 20 mV more negative than the MP. An analogous determination of the Cl^- gradient indicated that Cl^- is also not passively distributed across the neuronal membrane.

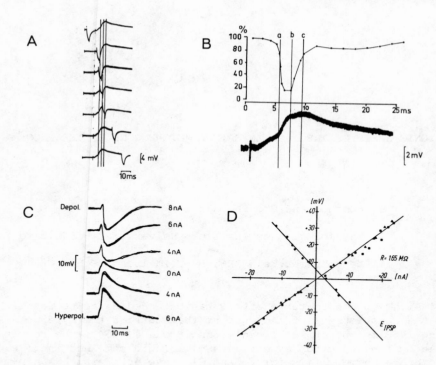

Fig. 1. A: Determination of input resistance during a depolari-
           zing postsynaptic potential following dorsal root
           stimulation
        B: During the IPSP a strong conductance increase is ob-
           served.
        C: The early component of the PSP (B, line a) is not re-
           versed by the depolarizing current injection while the
           late component is readily reversed.
        D: Reversal potential (E_{IPSP}) of a depolarizing IPSP
           (0 mV $\hat{=}$ resting MP)

The calculated E_{Cl} usually deviated little from the E_{IPSP} of the
respective cell, although E_{IPSP} was generally more negative.

An E_{Cl} less negative than MP calls for an inwardly directed
Cl^- transport along the activity gradient. The close correspondence between E_{Cl} and E_{IPSP} suggests an important role of a Cl^- efflux in the generation of the depolarizing IPSP. This idea was supported by the following observations:

During repetitive IPSPs aCl^-i decreased considerably accompanied by an increase of aCl^-e. During single IPSPs transient reductions of aCl^-i were observed (0,1 - 0,3 mmol/l). These signals,
however, being severely distorted due to the time constant of the
Cl^- sensitive electrode (80 - 100 ms) and of small amplitude (Fig. 2),

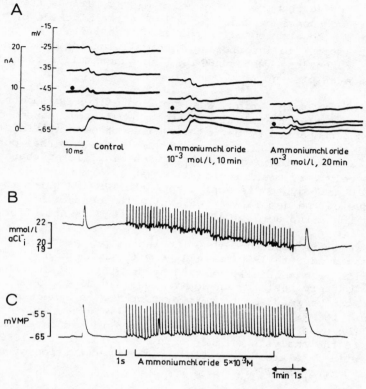

Fig. 2. A: Equilibration of E_{IPSP} with MP during application of NH_4^+
B: Registration of aCl^-i. During single IPSPs small transient reductions of aCl^-i are found. Upward deflection is due to incomplete subtraction of the signal of the reference barrel resulting from the great difference in time constants between both electrode barrels. NH_4^+ causes a continuous fall of aCl^-i.
C: MP and superimposed postsynaptic potentials

were suppressed when the IPSP was blocked by Strychnine. Reversal of the IPSP changed the transient decrease of aCl^-i to an increase.

Never were any transient changes of aK^+i observed during single IPSPs.

Application of NH_4^+ which is known to block Cl^- pumps (Lux et al., 1970) caused a reduction of aCl^-i and a parallel decrease of the amplitude of the IPSP. This blockade eventually led to a shift of E_{Cl} to values about 3 - 4 mV less negative than MP, i.e. a nearly passive distribution of Cl^- across the MN membrane and an equilibration of the E_{IPSP} with the MP, without affecting the increase of membrane conductance during single IPSPs.

The difference between E_{Cl} and E_{IPSP} as well as the incomplete correspondence between E_{Cl} and MP after blockade of the Cl^- transport may be attributed to the cross sensitivity of the Cl^- exchanger (Orion) to interfering intracellular ions such as HCO_3^-. For lack of knowledge about $aHCO_3^-$ i no quantitative correction can be made at present.

Inhibitory amino acids, when applied either iontophoretically or in the superfusing solution of the preparation, caused depolarizations accompanied by marked decreases of neuronal input resistance and a transient diminution of aCl^- i. The reversal potential of their action coincided with E_{IPSP}. No significant changes of aK^+ i and only very small increases of aK^+ e were found during their action. In analogy to its action upon the IPSP NH^+_4 led to a disappearance of the depolarization, while the conductance change induced by the amino acids (GABA, ß - Alanine) was not affected.

Hence it is concluded that the inhibitory postsynaptic current associated with IPSP as well as with the action of inhibitory amino acids is essentially carried by an efflux of Cl^-. The EMF of this Cl^- battery rests on an active inwardly directed Cl^- transport and can be reduced to zero by blocking this mechanism with NH^+_4. In frog MNs the great difference between the depolarizing E_{Cl} and the hyperpolarizing E_K must be considered an advantage in respect to the analysis of the ionic mechanism of the IPSP. The experimental data are incompatible with an activation of a K^+ conductance during the IPSP.

REFERENCES

Eccles, J.C., 1964, The physiology of synapses, Springer Verlag, Heidelberg, Germany.

Llinás, R., Baker, R., and Precht, W., 1974, Blockade of inhibition by ammonium acetate action on chloride pump in cat trochlear motoneurons, J. Neurophysiol., 37:522.

Lux, H.D., 1974, Fast recording ion specific microelectrodes Their use in pharmacological studies in the CNS, Neuropharmacology, 13:509.

Lux, H.D., Loracher, C., and Neher, E., 1970, The action of ammonium on postsynaptic inhibition of cat spinal motoneurons, Exp. Brain Res., 11:431.

EFFECTS OF INCREASED EXTRACELLULAR POTASSIUM ACTIVITY

IN THE FROG SPINAL CORD ON THE FLEXOR REFLEX

L. Vyklický and Eva Syková

Institute of Physiology
Czechoslovak Academy of Sciences
Vídeňská 1083, 142 20 Prague 4, Czechoslovakia

Neuronal activity causes potassium ions to accumulate in the extracellular space of the spinal cord. Their concentration may increase from the resting level of 2 or 3 mmol/l to as high as 9-10 mmol/l following tetanic stimulation of the dorsal roots or peripheral nerves (Vyklický et al., 1972; Krnjević and Morris, 1972; Kříž et al., 1974; Bruggencate et al., 1974; Somjen and Lothman, 1974; Kříž et al., 1975; Krnjević and Morris, 1975; Syková et al., 1976). Smaller increases, not exceeding 1 mmol/l are produced by adequate stimulation of the skin (Syková et al., 1980).

It has also been demonstrated that increased $[K^+]_e$ produces depolarization of primary afferent fibres in the spinal cord (Vyklický et al.,1976; Syková and Vyklický, 1978; Nicoll, 1979) which is considered to be the bases of presynaptic inhibition (Eccles, 1964). The findings that increased $[K^+]_e$ inhibits impulses transmission in the ganglion of the leech (Baylor and Nicholls, 1969) and decreases the efficacy of transmission in the giant synapse of the squid (Weight and Erulkar, 1976) supported this idea.

However, an increase in $[K^+]_e$ also depolarizes postsynaptic neurones (Syková and Orkand, 1980) and thereby increases their excitability (Nicoll, 1979). Furthermore, the increase in the spontaneous release of transmitters (Liley, 1956; Vizi and Vyskočil, 1979) and activation of ionic pumps (for review see Glynn and Carlish, 1975) make it difficult to predict the ultimate effects of increased $[K^+]_e$ on impulse transmission.

To elucidate this problem we dissected the spinal cord of the frog and cut it at the cervical level. The spinal cord was exposed and deprived of circulation. Innervation of both hind limbs was

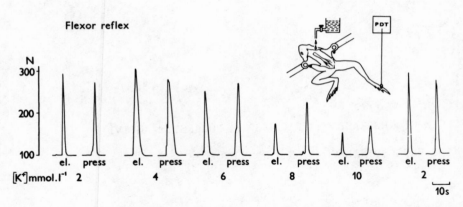

Fig. 1.   Flexor reflex responses in the frog during superfusion of
the spinal cord with various concentrations of extracellular
potassium
Diagram: The spinal cord was completely isolated, with the
exception of the ventral and dorsal roots IX and X which
remained connected with the periphery and perfused with
oxygenated Ringer solution. The flexor reflex was evoked
by pinching a toe of the foot with a forceps (press) or
with a series of electrical pulses (13 pulses at 100 Hz).
Concentration of K^+ in the Ringer solution was raised from
2 to 10 mmol/1 by substituting KC1 in the Ringer solution
for an equivalent amount of NaC1. Before testing, 30 min
were allowed for superfusion with Ringer solution containing
a higher concentration of K^+ and 60 min for recovery.

preserved. Immediately after the circulation had been arrested, the
spinal cord was superfused with oxygenated Ringer solution 95 % O_2
and 5 % CO_2 of the following composition: NaC1, 114.0 mmol/1;
KC1, 2.0 mmol/1; $NaHCO_3$, 2.0 mmol/1; $CaCl_2$, 1.8 mmol/1; glucose, 1g/1.
The flexor reflex was evoked either by pinching one of the toes with
a forceps or by stimulating the skin of the leg with a series of
rectangular, electrical pulses (7-13 pulses, 3.10^{-4} s, 10-40 V at
100 Hz) by means of a bipolar, platinum wire electrode placed on the
skin of the foot. Flexion was recorded by means of a photoelectric
displacement transducer (PDT in Fig. 1) the lever of which was fixed
to the foot by a thread sewn through the interdigital membrane.
Solutions, containing 4, 6, 8, 10 an 20 mmol/1 of K^+ were prepared
by substituting KC1 in the Ringer solution for an equivalent amount
of NaC1. Each test solution was superfused for 30 min at the rate
of 5-10 ml/min before testing started.

The effects of superfusing the spinal cord with solutions containing various concentrations of K^+ on flexor reflexes evoked by pinching a toe and by a series of electrical pulses (13 at 100 Hz) applied to the skin of the foot are shown in Fig. 1.

An increase in K^+ from 2 to 4 mmol/l enhanced and prolonged the flexion response of the hind limb. In 6 mmol/l K^+ the responses were shorter and somewhat weaker than when the solution contained 4 mmol/l; the duration, however, was still longer than that in the control Ringer solution containing 2 mmol/l of K^+. A further increase in K^+ to 8 or 10 mmol/l resulted in a pronounced decrease of the contraction tension. A full recovery of the flexor reflexes was observed when the normal Ringer solution was applied for one hour. When K^+ was raised to 20 mmol/l the effects were variable. Usually, fasciculations with a tendency to extension of the hind limbs were observed; sometimes, however, there was paralysis of the hind limbs or a residue of the flexor reflex in response to electrical stimulation or pinching.

Our results thus indicate two different actions of increased $[K^+]_e$ on impulse transmission in the spinal cord. Increases of up to 6 mmol/l which may be the maximum to be expected under physiological conditions facilitate the flexor reflex. Further increases in $[K^+]_e$, exceeding 6 mmol/l, which may occur only under extreme conditions inhibit impulse transmission. The apparent discrepancy between our results and those of Baylor and Nicholls (1969) and of Weight and Erulkar (1976) who exclusively observed inhibitory effects of increased $[K^+]_e$ can be explained by the fact that they used higher $[K^+]_e$ in control solutions which were 4 mmol/l and 9 mmol/l respectively, while we only used 2 mmol/l in our study.

Although the precise site at which the facilitatory effects of increased $[K^+]_e$ occur is still obscure, it is likely that the increased excitability of the second order neurones and motoneurones due to the depolarization, produced by raised $[K^+]_e$, and the increase of spontaneous transmitter release, more than compensate for the deficit in synaptic transmission that results from primary afferent depolarization.

REFERENCES

Baylor, D.A., and Nicholls, J.G., 1969, Changes in extracellular potassium concentration produced by neuronal activity in the central nervous system of the leech, J. Physiol., 203:555.
Bruggencate, G., ten, Lux, H.D., and Liebl, L., 1974, Possible relationship between extracellular potassium activity and presynaptic inhibition in the spinal cord of the cat, Pflügers Arch., 349:301.

Eccles, J.C., 1964, "The Physiology of Synapses", Springer Verlag, Berlin.

Glynn, I.M., and Carlish, S.J.D., 1975, The sodium pump, Physiol. Rev. 37:13.

Kříž, N., Syková, E., Ujec, E., and Vyklický, L., 1974, Changes of extracellular K^+ concentration induced by neuronal activity in the spinal cord of the cat, J. Physiol., 238:1.

Kříž, N., Syková, E., and Vyklický, L., 1975, Extracellular potassium changes in the spinal cord of the cat and their relation to slow potentials, active transport and impulse transmission, J. Physiol., 249:167.

Krnjevic, K., and Morris, M.E., 1972, Extracellular K^+ activity and slow potential changes in spinal cord and medulla, Can. J. Physiol. Pharmacol., 50:1214.

Krnjevic, K., and Morris, M.E., 1975, Factors determining the decay K^+ potentials in the central nervous system, Can. J. Physiol. Pharmacol., 53:923.

Liley, A.W., 1956, The effect of presynaptic polarization on the spontaneous activity at the mammalian neuromuscular junction, J. Physiol., 134:427.

Nicoll, R.A., 1979, Dorsal root potentials and changes in extracellular potassium in the spinal cord of the frog, J. Physiol., 290:113.

Somjen, G.G., and Lothman, E.W., 1974, Potassium sustained focal potentials of the mammalian spinal cord, Brain Res., 69:153.

Syková, E., Czéh, G., and Kříž, N., 1980, Potassium accumulation in the frog spinal cord induced by nociceptive stimulation of the skin, Neuroscience Lett., 17:253.

Syková, E., and Orkand, R.K., 1980, Extracellular potassium accumulation and transmission in frog spinal cord, Neuroscience, 5:1421.

Syková, E., Shirayev, B., Kříž, N., Vyklický, L., 1976, Accumulation of extracellular potassium in the spinal cord of frog, Brain Res., 106:413.

Syková, E., and Vyklický, L., 1978, Effects of picrotoxin on potassium accumulation and dorsal root potentials in the frog spinal cord, Neuroscience, 3:1061.

Vizi, E.,S., and Vyskočil, F., 1979, Changes in total and quantal release of acetylcholine in the mouse diaphragm during activation and inhibition of membrane ATPase, J. Physiol., 286:1.

Vyklický, L., and Syková, E., 1980, The effects of increased etracellular potassium in the isolated spinal cord on the flexor reflex of the frog, Neuroscience Lett., 19:203.

Vyklický, L., Syková, E., Kříž, N., and Ujec, E., 1972, Post-stimulation changes of extracellular potassium concentration in the spinal cord of the rat, Brain Res., 45:608.

Vyklický, L., Syková, E., and Mellerová, B., 1976, Depolarization of primary afferents in the frog spinal cord under high $Mg^{..}$ concentrations, Brain Res., 117:153.

Weight, F.F., and Erulkar, S.D., 1976, Modulation of synaptic transmitter release by repetitive postsynaptic action potentials, Science, 193:1023.

EXTRACELLULAR K^+ ACTIVITY DURING ELECTRICAL STIMULATION OF RAT SYMPATHETIC GANGLIA, VAGUS AND OPTIC NERVES IN VITRO

M. Galvan, J. Förstl and G. ten Bruggencate

Dept. of Physiology, University of Munich
Pettenkoferstr. 12, 8000 Munich 2, G.F.R.

INTRODUCTION AND METHODS

Measurements of extracellular K^+ (a_K) and Ca^{++} activities in the central nervous system indicate that, during electrical stimulation, ion concentrations are affected by fluxes in a variety of structural elements. In particular, presynaptic structures are believed to exert a major influence on extracellular ion levels. In order to quantify the changes in a_K that occur during activity in nerve fibres, we have measured the rises in a_K produced by electrical stimulation of 3 simple nervous preparations.
(a) The superior cervical ganglion.
(b) The vagus nerve.
(c) The optic nerve.

Experiments were performed in vitro on desheathed tissues obtained from urethane anaesthetized rats. Oxygenated Krebs' solution (vagus and ganglion: K=6, Ca=2.5; optic: K=3, Ca=1.5 mmol/l) was continuously superfused over the preparations at either 25 or 37 °C (Galvan et al., 1979). Stimulation and recording of summed potentials was effected by suction electrodes; extracellular K^+ activity was measured using double-barrelled liquid ion exchanger microelectrodes (Nicholson et al., 1978; Galvan et al., 1979).

RESULTS

Figure 1 summarizes the results of experiments on isolated vagus nerves, maintained at 25 °C. The left panel (an original recording) illustrates that repetitive stimulation of A and B-fibres led only to a very small change in a_K. However, when the stimulation voltage was increased so as to excite the unmyelinated C-fibres, stimulation at 16 Hz raised a_K from 6 to 8 mmol/l; a large ouabain-sensitive undershoot followed this period. The right panel of Fig. 1 shows data obtained from 6 nerves. It can be seen that activation of C-fibres resulted in frequency-dependent increases in a_K, however, even at fast stimulation rates, A and B-fibre activation did not greatly alter a_K.

When the temperature was raised to 37 ^OC, a_K increases resulting from C-fibre activity were slightly smaller than those measured at 25 ^OC. A and B-fibre activation now produced no significant change in a_K. Since the proportion of myelinated fibres in the vagus is low, we also measured a_K in the optic nerve, which is exclusively myelinated (Forrester and Peters, 1967). At 37 ^OC, stimulation of this nerve produced smaller increases in a_K than those seen during vagus C-fibre activation, however, changes of upto 2 mmol/l could be measured. These were followed by post-stimulus undershoots of upto 0.5 mmol/l.

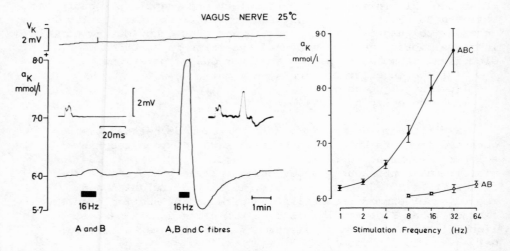

Fig. 1. The left panel shows a recording of extracellular K^+ activity (a_K) and reference potential (V_K) made from an isolated rat vagus nerve at 25 ^OC. The insets show averaged recordings of summed potentials (10 sweeps). The right panel illustrates the relationship between stimulatinn frequency and peak a_K achieved during stimulation. Means and SEMs are shown; n=6.

Previous experiments (Galvan et al., 1979) at 25 ^{O}C demonstrated that large rises in a_K and falls in Ca^{++} accompanied synaptic activity in sympathetic ganglia. We have now extended these experiments in an attempt to elucidate the role of synapses in K$^+$ release. Figure 2 shows a comparison of a_K rises produced by electrical stimulation of ganglia, vagi and optic nerves at 37 ^{O}C. Rises induced by vagus A and B-fibres at 25 ^{O}C are also included for comparison. For a given stimulation frequency, a_K rises were largest in ganglia and smallest in optic nerves. Antidromic stimulation of ganglia produced insignificant rises in a_K, suggesting that postsynaptic spiking probably does not contribute to rises seen during orthodromic stimulation.

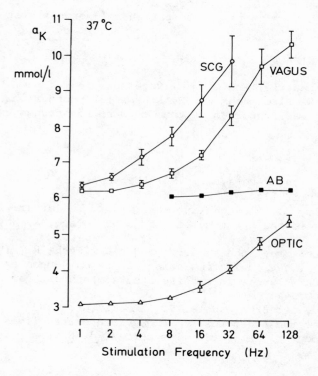

Fig. 2. The relationship between stimulus frequency and peak a_K produced by electrical stimulation of ganglia (o), vagus A, B and C-fibres (□), and optic nerves (Δ), all measured at 37 ^{O}C. The rises produced by activation of vagus A and B-fibres at 25 ^{O}C (■) are also included. Means and SEMs are shown; n ≤ 3. No error bars are drawn where they are less than the symbol size.

CONCLUSIONS

By using defined, in vitro preparations, we have been able
to investigate a_K changes due to nerve fibre activity more
quantitatively than is possible in the central nervous system.
Our experiments demonstrate that electrical stimulation of
unmyelinated nerve fibres leads to large rises in a_K. The presence
of nerve terminals (as in ganglia) probably contributes further
to observed a_K rises. Myelinated fibres release substantially
less K^+. The fact that large changes in a_K can be measured in
desheathed, superfused preparations confirms earlier suggestions
(Frankenhaeuser and Hodgkin, 1956) that significant diffusion
barriers exist in the extracellular space of nerve trunks.
Since synaptic function is highly dependent on the external K^+
concentration, we suggest that K^+ release from nerve fibres may
contribute to excitability changes and information processing
even within certain parts of the peripheral nervous system.

ACKNOWLEDGEMENTS

Miss E. Beuschel and Miss C. Vogel provided expert technical
assistance. We also thank Mr. H. Krauss for photographic work.
This research was supported by the Deutsche Forschungsgemeinschaft.

REFERENCES

Forrester, J., and Peters, A., 1967, Nerve fibres in optic nerve of
        rat, Nature, 214:245.
Frankenhaeuser, B., and Hodgkin, A.L., 1956, The after-effects of
        impulses in the giant nerve fibres of Loligo, J. Physiol.,
        131:341.
Galvan, M., ten Bruggencate, G., and Senekowitsch, R., 1979, The
        effects of neuronal stimulation and ouabain upon extracellular
        K^+ and Ca^{++} levels in rat isolated sympathetic ganglia, Brain
        Res., 160:544.
Nicholson, C., ten Bruggencate, G., Stöckle, H., and Steinberg, R.,
        1978, Calcium and potassium changes in extracellular micro-
        environment of cat cerebellar cortex, J. Neurophysiol., 41:1026.

EXTRACELLULAR POTASSIUM ACTIVITY AND AXON EXCITABILITY

Dean O. Smith

Department of Physiology
University of Wisconsin
Madison, Wisconsin 53706

INTRODUCTION

During repetitive action potential discharge, levels of extracellular K^+, $[K^+]e$, have been observed to increase. In experiments on squid nerves, Frankenhaeuser and Hodgkin (1956) showed that following nerve impulses K^+ accumulates in the periaxonal space between the axon and the surrounding Schwann cell. This was manifest as a progressive reduction in the undershoot of the action potential, which reflects a depolarizing shift of the potassium equilibrium potential.

Accumulation of extracellular K^+ may be expected to result in blockage of action potential propagation (Adelman and FitzHugh, 1975). Increased $[K^+]e$ in the region of axon conduction block has been inferred from voltage clamp records in the lobster (Grossman, et al., 1979). Indirect evidence has led to the conclusion that elevated $[K^+]e$ also underlies propagation failure in the crayfish (Smith, 1980). However, direct measurements describing such an accumulation have not been obtained. In this study, K^+-selective microelectrodes have been used in crayfish to measure changes in the activity of extracellular K^+, a_K, close to regions characterized by action potential propagation failure during prolonged repetitive stimulation. The kinetics of the K^+ buildup suggest that propagation block may be attributed to slow inactivation of the Na^+ conductance.

All experiments were performed on the excitor axon innervating the opener muscle of the first walking leg of the crayfish. A total of 22 animals were studied. The axon was stimulated with a suction electrode. Action potentials were recorded extracellularly at sites along the axon. Using a graduated reticle in the microscope eyepiece, the tip of the K^+-selective electrode was positioned between 10 and 50 μm from the axon.

POTASSIUM RESPONSE TO REPETITIVE NERVE STIMULATION

After the onset of repetitive stimulation of the excitor axon, the value of a_K in the vicinity of the nerve rose to a maximum and then either stayed at that level or decreased for the duration of the stimulation. Termination of the nerve stimulation resulted in a decay of a_K to values near those recorded prior to stimulation. Intermittent conduction failure at a site proximal to the recording site always led to a drop in a_K during the period of nerve stimulation. Conversely, increased rates of stimulation or addition of ouabain (10^{-3}M) to the bath resulted in a rise in a_K.

Values of a_K varied with not only time after the onset of nerve stimulation, but also distance, x, between the electrode tip and the axon. The maximum value of a_K was related inversely to the distance, x. This relationship could be described by the linear equation $\Delta a_K = 0.86 - 0.014x$. The kinetics of the change in a_K were slower as x increased. Thus, the time intervals between the onset of stimulation, the first detectable increase in a_K, and the attainment of steady-state maximum value were longer at larger distances. Using Fick's second law and the Einstein equation for free diffusion, two estimates of the diffusion coefficient for K^+ were calculated. The values obtained were 1.43×10^{-6} cm^2/s and 2.55×10^{-6} cm^2/s, respectively.

CONDUCTION FAILURE

In 5 experiments, axon conduction failure occurred at a location proximal to the site of the K^+-selective electrode tip. The exact point at which block occurred was not determined, but it was within 5 mm of the electrode tip in each preparation.

Failure occurred long after a_K had reached a maximum value in each case. The earliest time of block was 90s after stimulation (50 to 75 impulses/s) had begun; the average time was 169s. Values of a_K attained their maxima within less than 20s. The peak values of a_K were not significantly higher in these blocking preparations than those in which failure was not observed during the course of these experiments. Nor was there any consistent value of a_K at which propagation failed. From these data, however, the levels of a_K at the axon surface, within the periaxonal space, cannot be determined.

Experiments were performed in three animals to estimate the value of $[K^+]e$ at the axon surface when conduction fails. The concentration of K^+ in the physiologic saline was increased by 2 mM (initially, from 5.4 mM to 7.4 mM); in the absence of nerve stimulation, the preparation was allowed to rest for 15 min. Then, three stimuli were delivered to the axon at a rate of 1 impulse/s. If action potentials were evoked, the preparation was rinsed for 10 min in normal saline (i.e. $[K^+]e$ at 5.4 mM). The experiment was then repeated with an increment of an additional 2 mM, progressively increasing $[K^+]e$ in 2 mM steps until a level was reached at which action potentials were not conducted.

In each case, propagation failed only when $[K^+]e$ was raised to levels at least 18 mM above normal (from 5.4 mM to 23.4). There was no sign of failure at values lower than this. Furthermore, failure occurred only after at least 13 min in the 23.4 mM solution. To examine changes in the action potential during development of the block under these conditions, additional experiments were performed in which the axon was stimulated at a rate of one impulse every 30s after each 2 mM increment of $[K^+]e$. When $[K^+]e$ had been raised by less than 18 mM, there was no apparent change in action potential shape after 15 min. After raising $[K^+]e$ by 18 mM, the latency from the stimulus pulse to the action potential became progressively longer until conduction failed. The magnitude of the Na^+ inward current, which was manifest as the negative (downward) component of the extracellular record, also decreased. These results are similar to those observed during the development of a blocked state due to prolonged repetitive stimulation (Smith, 1980).

CONCLUSIONS

Accumulation of extracellular K^+ has been postulated to underlie the phenomenon of conduction failure in this (Smith, 1980) and other preparations (Grossman, et al., 1979). The results of this study are consistent with this hypothesis. However, the kinetics of the K^+ buildup indicate that mechanisms with slow time courses are involved.

At the ion-selective electrode tip, a_K reaches maximal values within less than 20s after the onset of axon stimulation. This is similar to kinetics reported for the mammalian central nervous system (Somjen, 1979). The time to reach this maximum decreases as the axon surface is approached. Thus, a_K in the periaxonal space must be maximal in less than 20s. This is well before any sign of conduction failure occurs (cf. Smith, 1980). Thus, if increased a_K is causing conduction block, it must do so by some process with a time constant of about 100 to 200s.

Slow inactivation of Na^+ channels is such a process (Rudy, 1978). It has been observed in axons from several different species to result from prolonged membrane depolarization. Inactivation of the Na^+ conductance is half-maximal when the membrane is depolarized by 30 to 50 mV (Rudy, 1978). When $[K^+]e$ was raised by 18 mM in this study, conduction block developed, presumably due to slow inactivation. This increase of 18 mmol/l corresponds to a drop in membrane potential of 29 mV, from -90 mV to -61 mV. Furthermore, as in slow inactivation, propagation can be restored by hyperpolarization of the axon membrane (Smith, 1980).

Although the temporal characteristics of conduction block and the rise in a_K during repetitive stimulation are similar to those of slow inactivation, the increases in a_K rcorded by the ion-selective electrode are not. Values of Δa_K less than 1 mmol/l were recorded. Such changes are expected to depolarize the axon membrane by only 2 to 3 mV. This is in marked contrast to the 18 mmol/l change in $[K^+]e$ found necessary to evoke failure.

These data do not rule out slow inactivation, however, for a_K in the periaxonal space was not measured with this technique; in fact, the space is too small (about 20 nm) to record from without destroying it. The increase in periaxonal a_K will be far higher than in the endoneurium and surrounding volume if the adaxonal glial layer represents a significant diffusion barrier (Frankenhaeuser and Hodgkin, 1956). Indeed, in squid axon Frankenhaeuser and Hodgkin (1956) inferred that $[K^+]e$ at the axon surface increased by about 17 mmol/l during stimulation at 125 impulses/s (cf. Adelman and FitzHugh, 1975). Thus, while there is no direct measurement of a_K in the periaxonal space during repetitive stimulation, it is possible that it rises to values high enough to cause conduction to fail due to slow inactivation of the Na^+ conductance.

ACKNOWLEDGEMENTS

This work was supported by NIH grants NS13600 and NS00380 (R.C.D.A.) and by the Alfred P. Sloan Foundation.

REFERENCES

Adelman, W.J., and FitzHugh, R., 1975, Solutions of the Hodgkin-Huxley equations modified for potassium accumulation in a periaxonal space, Fed. Proc., 34:1322.

Frankenhaeuser, B., and Hodgkin, A.L., 1956, The after-effects of impulses in the giant fibers of Loligo, J. Physiol. (Lond.), 131:341.

Grossman,Y.,Parnas, I., and Spira, M.E., 1979, Ionic mechanisms involved in differential conduction of action potentials at high frequency in a branching axon, J. Physiol. (Lond.), 295:307.

Rudy, B., 1978, Slow inactivation of the sodium conductance in squid giant axons. Pronase resistance, J. Physiol. (Lond.), 283:1.

Smith, D.O., 1980, Mechanisms of action potential propagation failure at sites of axon branching, J. Physiol. (Lond.), 301:243.

Somjen, G.G., 1979, Extracellular potassium in the mammalian central nervous system, Ann. Rev. Physiol., 41:159.

SESSION IV
IONIC ACTIVITY CHANGES IN THE BRAIN AND THEIR PHYSIOLOGICAL SIGNIFICANCE

EXTRACELLULAR POTASSIUM, CALCIUM AND VOLUME PROFILES

DURING SPREADING DEPRESSION

C. Nicholson, J.M. Phillips, C. Tobias and R.P. Kraig

Department of Physiology and Biophysics
New York University Medical Center
New York, N.Y. 10016

ABSTRACT

The characteristics and three hypotheses for the mechanism of spreading depression (SD) are outlined. The paper continues with a summary of some of our recent studies on the ion and potential profiles during SD in the cerebellum of the rat after conditioning with anion substitution. These experiments demonstrate that the characteristic negative potential of SD is accompanied by large increases in $[K^+]_0$ and decreases in $[Ca^{2+}]_0$. When the probe-ions tetramethylammonium (TMA^+) and α-naphthalene sulfonate (α-NS) were present, they concentrated during SD by a factor of about two indicating a decrease in extracellular volume. In many experiments the slow negative wave reversed to a positivity with depth; no ion changes accompanied the positive wave. It is concluded that SD is most likely generated at the site of presynaptic terminals and dendrites and may involve massive transmitter release.

INTRODUCTION

Phenomenology and Hypotheses of SD

SD was first clearly identified by Leão (1944) who noted the peculiar extinction of neuronal activity in the rabbit cerebrum. The loss of activity was only transient and had the remarkable characteristic of slowly propagating across the cortex with a speed of some 3 mm.min^{-1}. Other features of SD were soon discovered, including the fact that SD was usually accompanied by a slow negative potential in the brain tissue that could be 20 mV or more in amplitude.

211

Several hypotheses have been proposed to account for SD, three of which seem to embody concepts that remain useful, although the actual mechanism of SD is still obscure. The first significant concept was that of Grafstein (1956) who suggested that SD was caused by excessive firing of neurons leading to an increase in $[K^+]_0$. The rise in $[K^+]_0$ would lead to further neuronal depolarization and action potentials until the innactivation of sodium channels caused a cessation of neuronal firing, thus permitting recovery of the tissue. The slow propagation velocity was attributed, in part, to the rate of K^+ diffusion.

Changes in $[K^+]_0$ are undoubtedly very important in SD but the original hypotheses does not directly account for several features of the phenomenon, such as an apparent swelling of cellular elements and increases in tissue impedance. For these reasons, Van Harreveld (1959) proposed that the primary mechanism was the entry of NaCl into cells and that this was mediated by the release of endogenous glutamate from cells which then opened sodium channels in dendrites. Chloride would enter cells through the resting membrane permeability to maintain electroneutrality and water would follow to preserve osmolality. Although the NaCl movement is now confirmed it remains difficult to design conclusive experiments to demonstrate the pivotal role of glutamate.

The transmitter hypothesis has been advocated by several investiators (e.g. Somjen 1973; Mori et al 1976; Tuckwell and Miura 1978) and simply proposes that SD is caused by the massive simultaneous release of both excitatory and inhibitory transmitters. This would permit all mobile ions to move through subsynaptic channels down their electrochemical gradients.

One major question that is not resolved by any hypothesis is how the state of a brain region becomes susceptible to SD in the first place. The general phenomenology of SD is reviewed in detail in the monograph by Bureš et al.(1974). Since that book was written, studies with ISMs have further clarified the nature of SD.

Ionic Shifts During SD

The first direct measurements of $[K^+]_0$ with an ISM during SD (Vyskočil et al 1972) confirmed earlier indications that very large increases in $[K^+]_0$ occur during this event. Since then this observation has been repeated by numerous investigators in different brain regions and animal species. In addition it is now established that $[Ca^{2+}]_0$ falls precipitating during SD (Nicholson et al.1977, 1978; Kraig and Nicholson 1978) and that large decreases in $[Na^+]_0$ and $[Cl^-]_0$ also take place (Kraig and Nicholson 1978). These and other ISM studies on SD have been reviewed by Nicholson and Kraig (1980).

The ionic shifts that occur during SD appear to take place between extra- and intracellular compartments and to be mediated by transient increases in membrane permeability (Kraig and Nicholson, 1978; Phillips and Nicholson, 1979; Nicholson and Kraig, 1980). This raises the question of identifying the location of the ionic channels involved. For this problem the mammalian cerebellum is particularly favorable because of its laminar organization and relatively simple circuitry. We have used the rat cerebellum in the present work. SD was first demonstrated in this preparation by Fifková et al. (1961) and ISM data was later obtained by Nicholson et al. (1977) and Phillips and Nicholson (1979).

In the experiments described here we have correlated the changes in the slow extracellular potential that accompanies SD with the variations in $[K^+]_0$ and $[Ca^{2+}]_0$ as a function of depth. In addition we have monitored the spatial variations in extracellular volume using both cationic and anionic probe-ions (Phillips and Nicholson, 1979). These volume changes are caused by water movement induced by the loss of NaCl from the extracellular compartment (Kraig and Nicholson, 1978; Nicholson and Kraig, 1980). Our results show that, although the whole cerebellar cortex can support SD, it is often confined to the molecular layer and this evidence, when considered with other data, implicates presynaptic terminals and dendrites as the neuronal elements responsible for SD.

METHODS

Adult female Sprague-Dawley rats were anesthetized with urethane (160 mg/kg) and the cerebellum exposed. Warmed physiological saline (mM concentrations: Na^+: 160, K^+: 3.0, Ca^{2+}: 1.3, Mg^{2+}: 0.5, Cl^-: 145, HCO_3^-: 21, $H_2PO_4^-$: 0.5, gassed with 95% O_2 and 5% CO_2) flowed into a pool over the cerebellum and was continuously removed by suction. To condition (Nicholson and Kraig, 1980) the cerebellum for SD, 75% or more of the Cl^- in the saline was replaced by acetate, proprionate or benzoate. In those experiments where probe ions were used, 5 mM of either tetramethylammonium (TMA^+) chloride or sodium α-naphthalene sulfonate (α-NS^-) was added to this saline. SD was initiated in the conditioned cerebellum by local surface stimulation at 100 Hz for about 1 second at a stimulus strength that evoked normal field potentials when given as a single stimulus.

Recordings were made with double-barreled ISMs constructed from theta-glass (Nicholson and Kraig, 1980). For recording K^+ and TMA^+, Corning 477317 exchanger was used, for Ca^{2+}, ETH 1001 exchanger (Oehme et al., 1976) and for α-NS^-, crystal violet exchanger (Sĕnkýř and Petr, 1978; Phillips and Nicholson, 1979).

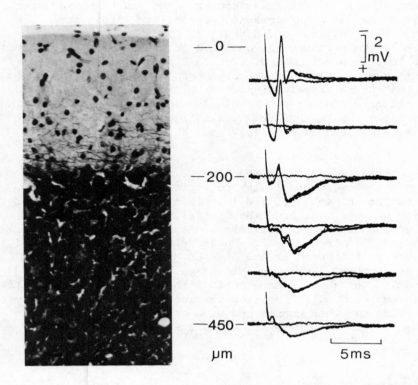

Fig. 1. Cerebellar cortex of the rat and laminar field potentials. Cortex consists of a molecular layer from 0-200 μm containing parallel fibers, Purkinje cell dendrites, stellate cells and Bergmann glia. The Purkinje cell layer, containing somata of those cells, extends from 200-230 μm. Below 230 μm is the granule cell layer. Photomicrograph is parasagittal section with reduced silver stain. Field potentials evoked by local surface stimulation. Near the surface they consist of a fast positive-negative wave generated by the compound action potential in the parallel fibers and a subsequent slower negativity reflecting the synaptically induced depolarization of the Purkinje cell dendrites. With depth the parallel fiber component is lost and the later negativity reverses to a positive wave which slowly attenuates with depth. Note the time scale for the field potentials shown here which is about 1000 times shorter than that for the slow potentials depicted in Figs. 2-5. Three sweeps have been photographically superimposed at each level.

RESULTS

Laminar Structure and Field Potentials of the Rat Cerebellum

In common with most other cerebellar cortices, that of the rat consists of three layers (Fig. 1), a molecular layer, a Purkinje cell layer and a granule cell layer. The molecular layer contains the axons of the granule cells, namely the parallel fibers and their postsynaptic elements, the dendrites of Purkinje cells and inhibitory interneurons. The Purkinje cell layer consists of a single layer of the cell bodies of the Purkinje cells and the granule cell layer is mainly populated by the cells of that name and their afferents, the mossy fibers. A second afferent system, the climbing fiber, makes direct contact with the dendrites of the Purkinje cells. Further anatomical details of the rat cerebellum are to be found in the monograph by Palay and Chan-Palay (1974).

The field potentials of the rat cerebellum, as evoked by local surface stimulation, are very characteristic of this laminar structure (Fig. 1). Near the surface an early fast negativity signifies the compound action potential of the parallel fibers while a second, slower negative wave corresponds to the synaptically induced depolarization of dendrites, mainly the Purkinje cells. In depth the parallel fiber volley is absent and the synaptic depolarization gives rise to a passive outflow of current from the vertically oriented core conductors that constitute the Purkinje cells; this outward current produces a positive extracellular potential. These field potentials are very similar to those seen in the cat cerebellum (Eccles et al., 1966). In that animal repetitive local surface stimulation also induces a laminar increase in $[K^+]_0$ and decrease in $[Ca^{2+}]_0$ that can be correlated with activity of the basic cerebellar circuit (Nicholson et al., 1978). Such ionic shifts are also seen in the rat under similar conditions (Nicholson et al., 1977).

Slow Potentials

During SD each set of ionic profiles is accompanied by the corresponding slow potentials recorded on the reference barrel of the ISM (records V in Figs. 2,3,4 and 5). It is seen that the potentials all show the characteristic negative wave form of some 15-30 mV amplitude near the cerebellar surface. In many experiments (illustrated here in Figures 2 and 3), the potential reverses to a positivity below the level of the Purkinje cell bodies. These characteristics are very similar to those seen in the postsynaptic wave of the field potentials evoked by local stimulation (Fig. 1).

In some instances, SD occurs at all depths in the cerebellar cortex (Figs. 3 and 4). Sometimes, as in Figure 3, the latency of the SD potential increases with depth. In other cases it appears

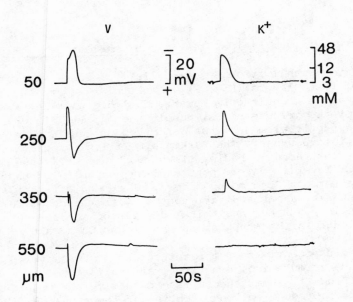

Fig. 2. $[K^+]_0$ profiles during SD. A slow negative potential, characteristic of SD, is seen at 50 µm (V). It appears to have two components and the second component reverses at 250 µm. By 550 µm the potential is wholly positive. A large $[K^+]_0$ increase is associated with the SD at 50 µm, but this becomes smaller and shorter at 250 and 350 µm. When the potential is all positive, no $[K^+]_0$ change is seen. Cerebellum conditioned with acetate.

that the potential of SD has two components both of which co-exist near the surface, but the earlier one also tends to persist in depth, sometimes with an increased latency relative to the surface (Fig. 2).

Potassium and Calcium Profiles

Figure 2 shows the $[K^+]_0$ signals associated with the slow potentials. It is clear that the large increases in $[K^+]_0$ are only seen in the region where the slow potential is negative. As the slow potential reverses to a positive potential, the $[K^+]_0$ signal rapidly diminishes and disappears. In the region where a large positive wave exists, no potassium change is seen. The small $[K^+]_0$ increase at 350 µm is apparently due to the persistance of the early component of SD at that level.

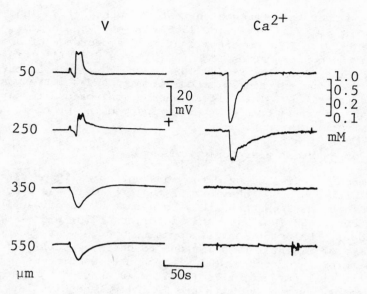

Fig. 3. $[Ca^{2+}]_0$ profile during SD. As in Figure 2, the slow potential (V) reverses with depth to a positivity. In this case $(Ca^{2+})_0$ shows a precipitous drop in concentration during SD, but again no ion changes are seen in the vicinity of the positive potentials. Cerebellum conditioned with benzoate.

The $[Ca^{2+}]_0$ profiles also show a sharp localization (Fig. 3). Here, however, the ionic change is a decrease in ion concentration. The changes in $[Ca^{2+}]_0$ take the ionic concentration down to levels as low as one tenth the resting value, but again they are only evident in the vicinity of the negative slow wave and are totally absent in vicinity of the positive potential. In this set of records neither negative potentials nor $[Ca^{2+}]_0$ changes occur in the granule cell layer.

As discussed elsewhere (Kraig and Nicholson, 1978; Nicholson and Kraig, 1980), the changes in $[K^+]_0$ and $[Ca^{2+}]_0$ are brought about by the movement of these ions down the electro-chemical gradients between the outside and inside of depolarized cells. This implies that K^+ leaves cells and Ca^{2+} enters.

Despite the impressive size of the shifts in $[K^+]_0$ and $[Ca^{2+}]_0$, relative to baseline, the amounts of these ions that move are quite small and will not affect the osmotic balance very much. Other studies, however, have suggested that movements of Na^+ and Cl^- also occur during SD (Van Harreveld, 1966; Kow and Van Harreveld, 1972). Measurements with ISMs have now confirmed a decrease of about 100 mM in the concentration of both $[Na^+]_o$ and $[Cl^-]_o$ (Kraig and Nicholson; Nicholson and Kraig, 1980). This will lead to the loss of water from the extracellular compartment and a corresponding reduction in volume. This effect can be monitored directly by looking at the concentration changes induced in "probe-ions" that remain extracellular during SD.

Profiles of Extracellular Ionic Probes

In these studies we used two ions not normally present in the brain as probes of the behaviour of the extracellular space. We chose TMA^+ and $\alpha-NS^-$ because they both remain predominantly extracellular during SD (Phillips and Nicholson, 1979; Nicholson and Kraig, 1980). By using ions of opposite charge we reduced the possibility of misinterpretation due to charge specific effects. The ions were introduced by allowing them to continuously diffuse in from the pial surface; this resulted in a standing gradient when the steady state was attained (Phillips and Nicholson, 1979). The diffusion characteristics of the extracellular space in the rat cerebellum for small cations and anions have been discussed elsewhere (Nicholson, 1980).

Figure 4A shows the distribution of TMA^+ changes during SD and Figure 5A shows those of $\alpha-NS^-$. Both ions behave very similarly in the experiments shown, where SD occurred at all levels. The probes concentrate during SD to about twice the baseline values. In other experiments, where SD was not seen in depth, as judged from the positive potentials (Figs. 4B and 5B), there was no change in TMA^+ or $\alpha-NS^-$. It is noteworthy that Figure 5A demonstrates that it is only when the positive phase of the potential gives way to negativity that an increase in $\alpha-NS^-$ occurs. These results are consistent with a decrease in the volume of the extracellular space within the region of the SD wave. This interpretation is supported by the finding that it is only cations and anions above a certain size that concentrate during SD; in fact, small ions fall in concentration during SD (Phillips and Nicholson, 1979; Nicholson and Kraig, 1980), apparently because they are able to enter cells.

DISCUSSION

Turning first to the slow potential profiles generated during SD we conclude that the reversal from a negative to positive wave with depth is reminiscent of the postsynaptic component of the fast field potentials (Fig. 1). This implicates a set of vertically oriented core conductors, such as the Purkinje cells or Bergmann glia, which are depolarized in the superficial region of the active

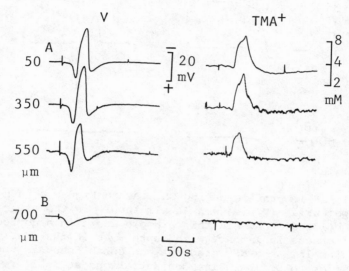

Fig. 4. $[TMA^+]_0$ profile during SD. In the first case (A) the SD potential (V) has the form of a positive-negative-positive wave at all depths. Prior to eliciting SD, the cerebellum was loaded with TMA^+ by superfusion and a standing gradient established (baseline values of $[TMA^+]_0$ were as follows: at 50 μm: 3.7 mM, at 350 μm: 3.2 mM, at 550 μm: 2.6 mM). During SD the TMA^+ concentrates. This concentration only occurs during the negative phase of the SD potential. In another experiment where the potential was wholly positive at 700 μm (B), no TMA^+ change is seen (baseline $[TMA^+]_0$: 2.2 mM). Cerebellum conditioned with benzoate.

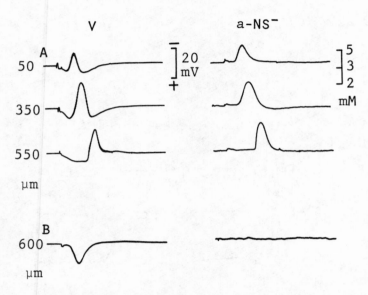

Fig. 5. $[\alpha\text{-NS}^-]_0$ profile during SD. As in Figure 4, a negative potential (V) is seen at all levels in the experiment depicted in A. In this example there is a noticeable increase in latency with depth. As in the TMA, for example, an $\alpha\text{-NS}^-$ gradient was established in the tissue prior to SD (baseline concentrations as follows: at 50 μm: 3.7 mM, at 350 μm: 3.0 mM, at 550 μm: 1.8 mM). During SD, the $\alpha\text{-NS}^-$ concentrates and the concentration is clearly related to the negative potential phase of SD. In another experiment (B) where only a positive potential was seen, no change in $[\alpha\text{-NS}^-]_0$ occurred (baseline $[\alpha\text{-NS}^-]_0$: 1.5 mM). Cerebellum conditioned with benzoate.

SD, thus forming there a current sink with respect to the extra-cellular space (Eccles et al., 1966; Nicholson and Llinás, 1971). The deeper positive wave would be generated by the current leaving the non-depolarized lower regions of the core conductors, thus forming a current source. It is likely, due to geometrical consider-ations and the physical nature of extracellular potential generation (Nicholson and Llinás, 1971) that the positivity would persist well below the level of the sources themselves. The large magnitude of the extracellular potentials during SD is likely due both to the high current densities established by the local depolarization of many cells and by the significantly increased resistance (Van Harreveld, 1966) of the extracellular medium due to ion depletion and decrease in size of the extracellular space.

In regard to the ionic measurements, our results show that the major changes in $[K^+]_0$ and $[Ca^{2+}]_0$ take place only in the region where there is a slow negative potential. In many of the present experiments, the slow negativity is confined to the molecular layer of the cerebellum, thus to the region of parallel fibers, presynaptic terminals, postsynaptic dendrites and Bergmann glial cells. Stellate cell somata also occur in the molecular layer, but the total membrane area is extremely small in comparison to the elements just listed. It is unlikely that the parallel fibers themselves are much involved in SD because they are axons and SD does not occur in regions in which axons predominate. Moreover, we have also demonstrated (Nicholson and Kraig, unpublished) that SD occurs in the tetrodotoxin treated rat cerebellum where all parallel fibers are inexcitable. There is no evidence that glia exhibit significant transient permeability increases to Ca^{2+}, Na^+ or Cl^- so that such elements cannot mediate these fluxes. This leaves the presynaptic terminals and Purkinje dendrites as the major locus of the ion changes.

Our studies with the probes TMA^+ and $\alpha-NS^-$ confirm our earlier studies (Phillips and Nicholson, 1979) and have also been substantiated by recent data obtained in the retina during SD using tetraethylammonium (TEA^+) and $\alpha-NS^-$ (do Carmo and Martins-Ferreira, 1980). The data presented here indicates that the volume of the extracellular space in the molecular layer decreases by a factor of about two, confirming other observations that a large amount of NaCl leaves the extracellular space. In other studies (Phillips and Nicholson, 1979) we have shown that an apparent anionic channel of well defined size opens during SD; since voltage-dependent anionic channels are rare this points to the involvement of one or more chemical mediators.

It seems from these data and other studies (Nicholson and Kraig, 1980) that the simplest hypothesis is that SD is brought about by a massive release of transmitter and the subsequent simultaneous opening of both cationic and anionic channels in dendrites. The effects may be augmented by voltage dependent Na^+ and Ca^{2+} channels in both pre- and postsynaptic membranes. K^+ is probably involved in the initial depolarization leading up to transmitter release and Ca^{2+} is obviously essential for the actual release.

In those instances where SD invades deep into the granule cell layer, presynaptic terminals and dendrites may still be the primary loci of the phenomenon, since the density of both these elements is very high, due to the enormous number of the tiny granule cells.

This sequence of events has elements in common with the K^+-hypothesis of Grafstein (1956) and the glutamate hypothesis of

Van Harreveld (1959, 1966) but is most in agreement with the
transmitter-release concepts advocated by Somjen (1973) and Mori
et al. (1976). Recently it has been shown that a simplified
model embodying these concepts can account for several features of
SD (Tuckwell & Miura, 1978) and Rodriguez and Martins-Ferreira
(1980) have produced direct evidence for the involvement of
transmitter release in retinal SD. It remains for the future,
however, to rigorously test these conjectures.

ACKNOWLEDGEMENT

The calcium exchanger was kindly provided by Prof. W. Simon,
Swiss Federal Institute of Technology, Zurich. Supported by
USPHS Grants NS-13742 and GM-07308 (J.M.P. and C.T.).

REFERENCES

Bureš, J., Burešová, O., and Křivánek, J., 1974, "The Mechanism
    and Applications of Leão's Spreading Depression of Electro-
    encephalographic Activity," Academic Press, New York.
Carmo, R.J.,do, and Martins-Ferreira, H., 1980, Na^+ activity and
    volume changes in the extracellular space during retinal
    spreading depression. An. Acad. brasil Cienc. Vol. 52
    (in press).
Eccles, J.C., Llinás, R., and Sasaki, K., 1966, Parallel fiber
    stimulation and the responses induced thereby in the Purkinje
    cells of the cerebellum. Exp. Brain Res. 1: 17-39.
Fifková, E., Bureš, J., Koshtoyants, O.Kh., Křivánek, J., and
    Weiss, T., 1961, Leão's spreading depression in the
    cerebellum of rat. Experientia 17: 572-573.
Grafstein, B., 1956, Mechanism of spreading cortical depression.
    J. Neurophysiol. 19: 154-171.
Kow, L.-M., and Van Harreveld, A., 1972, Ion and water movements
    in isolated chicken retinas during spreading depression.
    Neurobiol. 2: 61-69.
Kraig, R.P., and Nicholson, C., 1978, Extracellular ionic
    variations during spreading depression. Neurosci. 3:
    1045-1059.
Leão, A.A.P., 1944, Spreading depression of activity in the
    cerebral cortex. J. Neurophysiol. 7: 359-390.
Mori, S., Miller, W.H., and Tomita, T., 1976, Müller cell function
    during spreading depression in frog retina. Proc. Nat. Acad.
    Sci. 73: 1351-1354.
Nicholson, C., 1980, Dynamics of the brain cell microenvironment.
    Neurosci. Res. Prog. Bull. 18: 177-322.
Nicholson, C., ten Bruggencate, G., Steinberg, R., and Stöckle, H.,
    1977, Calcium modulation in brain extracellular microenviron-
    ment demonstrated with ion-selective micropipette. Proc.
    Nat. Acad. Sci. 74: 1287-1290.

Nicholson, C., ten Bruggencate, G., Stöckle, H., and Steinberg, R., 1978, Calcium and potassium changes in extracellular micro-environment of cat cerebellar cortex. J. Neurophysiol. 41: 1026-1039.

Nicholson, C., and Kraig, R.P., 1980, The behavior of extracellular ions during spreading depression, in: "The Application of Ion-Selective Electrodes," T. Zeuthen, ed., Elsevier/North-Holland, Amsterdam.

Nicholson, C., and Llinás, R., 1971, Field potentials in the alligator cerebellum and theory of their relationship to Purkinje cell dendritic spikes. J. Neurophysiol. 34: 509-531.

Oehme, M., Kessler, M., and Simon, W., 1976, Neutral carrier Ca^{2+}-microelectrode. Chimia 30: 204-206.

Palay, S.L., and Chan-Palay, V., 1974, "Cerebellar Cortex," Springer-Verlag, New York.

Phillips, J.M., and Nicholson, C., 1979, Anion permeability in spreading depression investigated with ion sensitive microelectrodes. Brain Res. 173: 567-571.

Rodriguez, P.S., and Martins-Ferreira, H., 1980, Cholinergic neurotransmission in retinal spreading depression. Exp. Brain Res. 38: 229-236.

Šenkýř, J., and Petr, J., 1978, Liquid ion-selective electrodes based on basic dyes, in: "Ion-Selective Electrodes," E. Pungor, ed., Elsevier, New York.

Somjen, G.G., 1973, Electrogeneis of sustained potentials. Prog. Neurobiol. 1: 201-257.

Tuckwell, H.C., and Miura, R.M., 1978, A mathematical model for spreading cortical depression. Biophys. J. 23: 257-276.

Van Harreveld, A., 1959, Compounds in brain extracts causing spreading depression of cerebral cortical activity and contraction of crustacean muscle. J. Neurochem. 3: 300-315.

Van Harreveld, A., 1966, "Brain Tissue Electrolytes," Butterworths, London.

Vyskočil, F., Kříž, N., and Bureš, J., 1972, Potassium-selective microelectrodes used for the extracellular brain potassium during spreading depression and anoxic depolarization in rats. Brain Res. 39: 255-259.

CORTICAL pH AND pCa IN RELATION TO DC POTENTIAL SHIFTS DURING SPREADING DEPRESSION AND ASPHYXIATION

A. Lehmenkühler, W. Zidek, M. Staschen and H. Caspers

Physiologisches Institut I der Universität

D - 4400 Münster, FRG

INTRODUCTION

Extracellular pCa in brain tissue increases considerably during spreading depression (SD) and terminal anoxia (Nicholson et al., 1977). The question arises as to whether this effect is attributable to transmembraneous Ca^{++} fluxes and/or to formation of Ca^{++} complexes resulting from an increase of extracellular oxoanions, e.g. of bicarbonate (Pedersen, 1971). Such a rise of oxoanion concentrations has been postulated by Kraig and Nicholson (1978) for reasons of electroneutrality in the extracellular space. To test this assumption tissue pH during SD and asphyxiation was measured since physiologically important oxoanions have more or less alkalizing properties. Indeed, pH shifts occurring on the surface of the cerebral cortex during SD have already been examined by several investigators. The results, however, are still controversial. Rapoport and Marshall (1964) described an acidic shift, whereas Tschirgi et al. (1957) found an alkalinization.

METHODS

The experiments were performed on the cerebral cortex of rats under urethane anaesthesia and artificial ventilation. SD was elicited by application of a small KCl crystal to the cortical surface remote from the recording site. Asphyxia was induced by ventilatory arrest after respiration with room air. Arterial pCO_2, pH and pO_2 were checked intermittently. For measuring pH and DC potentials a double-barrelled pH microelectrode of the antimony type was developed (Zidek et al., 1979). In the pH-sensitive barrel a dense column of metallic antimony was electrolytically precipitated from $SbCl_3$ dissolved in acetone using a current of 20 nA for 20 minutes. The

225

reference barrel contained 0.5 mol/l Na_2CO_3 solution in the tip during the electrolytic procedure. Then it was backfilled with 150 mmol/l NaCl. The slope of the electrode was ca. 55 mV/pH unit. The sensitivity to phosphates, proteins and oxygen in the physiological range was negligible. Measurements of Ca^{++} activity were also performed with double-barrelled microelectrodes. For construction borosilicate "theta"capillaries (Kuglstatter, D-8046 Garching, FRG) with a septum of the twofold thickness of the wall were preferred (Brown and Flaming, 1977). The tips were broken back to a diameter of two to three μm. The ion-selective channel was silanized by the hot vapour method (Coles and Tsacopoulos, 1977) and backfilled with 10 mmol/l $CaCl_2$. The tip contained a calcium-selective neutral carrier (Oehme et al., 1976). The electrodes were calibrated in different $CaCl_2$-NaCl solutions of constant ionic strength (0.16 mol/l). Standard reference solutions were made calculating individual activity coefficients as proposed by Moore and Ross (1965), Butler (1968) and Staples and Nuttall (1977). The microelectrodes were connected via Ag/AgCl wires to the symmetrical inputs of a high impedance buffer amplifier with capacitance neutralization of each electrode channel (Neher and Lux, 1973).

RESULTS AND DISCUSSION

Fig. 1A shows simultaneous recordings of the DC potential and of extracellular calcium activity ($a^°_{Ca}$) during SD. Resting $a^°_{Ca}$ was 0.3 $\pm$ 0.02 mmol/l. When the negative DC shift associated with SD had reached one third of its maximum amplitude $a^°_{Ca}$ began to fall by ca. one decade. The reincrease of $a^°_{Ca}$ showed first a rapid and then a slow time course (cf. Kraig and Nicholson, 1978). In Fig. 1B the changes of cortical tissue pH and of the DC potential during SD are displayed. The pH increased by ca. 0.3 units. The temporal relationship between the onsets of DC and pH changes was similar to that between DC and calcium activity shifts (Fig. 1A, 1B). The return of the pH to baseline level often started prior to the positive DC deflection. A transient decrease of pH was recorded after SD termination (Fig. 1B). During a train of SD waves these transient decreases summed up to a persistent depression of pH. Fig. 1C demonstrates changes of DC and of $a^°_{Ca}$ during asphyxia. Calcium activity initially increased during the primary positive DC shift (cf. Caspers and Speckmann, 1974) and then abruptly declined by more than one decade, when the terminal negative DC shift had passed DC baseline. The decrease of $a^°_{Ca}$ consisted of two phases with an initial rapid and a secondary slower one (cf. Nicholson et al., 1977). Fig. 1D shows the relation between DC potential and pH during asphyxia. After an initial acidic shift a transient increase of pH was recorded when the terminal negative DC shift had started. Thereafter a more or less pronounced reacidification was observed.

The alkalizing shift of pH during SD supported the hypothesis of Kraig and Nicholson (1978) who postulated an increase of an

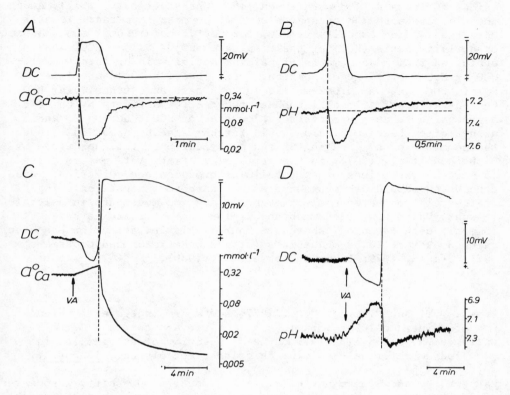

Fig. 1. Shifts of cortical DC potential (DC) in relation to changes
of extracellular calcium activity (a°_{Ca}) and tissue pH (pH)
during spreading depression (A, B) and asphyxiation (C, D).
VA: Start of ventilatory arrest.

unknown anion by 30 to 40 mmol/l during SD, since the measurements
of Na^+, K^+ and Cl^- revealed a deficit of anions with regard to extracellular electroneutrality. As derived from the Henderson–Hasselbalch
equation an increase in pH of 0.3 units would correspond to an increase of HCO_3^- by 40 mmol/l above an assumed resting value of 15
mmol/l (cf. Lübbers, 1972), provided that tissue pCO_2 does not fall
during SD below the systemic arterial value (Zidek et al., 1979).
Similar conclusions can be drawn as to phosphates, the efflux of
which from cellular stores is more likely, since the intracellular
phosphate concentration is known to be far higher than that of
bicarbonate.

When the changes of a°_{Ca} and pH are considered together, the
question arises as to what extent the decrease of a°_{Ca} may be caused
by the concomitant increase of alkalizing anions, because calcium
is known to form relatively stable complexes with a number of oxo-

anions (Greenwald, 1959; Pedersen, 1971;Christoffersen, 1975). Among these bicarbonate and phosphate seem to be most important. To estimate the binding capacity of HCO_3^- for Ca^{++}, the dissociation constant on activity basis (K_a) for the complex $CaHCO_3^+ \rightleftharpoons Ca^{++} + HCO_3^-$ was evaluated from measurements of calcium activity in different $CaCl_2$ - HCO_3^- - NaCl solutions of constant ionic strength (0.16 mol/l). K_a was in the range of 0.093 mol/l. In this case an extracellular HCO_3^- concentration of 15 mmol/l reduces the calcium activity by ca. 14% as compared to an equimolar solution free of HCO_3^-. During SD and asphyxiation calcium binding would further rise by about 35%. Thus, the decrease of a^o_{Ca} during SD and asphyxiation, first described by Nicholson et al. (1977) in the cerebellum of the rat, may be caused in part by variations of extracellular oxoanion concentration. This conclusion should be emphasized with regard to concepts existing on the relation between electrogenesis and ion movements in exitable tissues. Up to now, transmembraneous ion and water fluxes have commonly been favoured, whereas comparatively few attention has been paid on extracellular mechanisms (cf. also Katzmann and Grossmann, 1975; Somjen, 1979; Lehmenkühler et al., 1980).

REFERENCES

Brown, K.T. and Flaming, D.G., 1977, New microelectrode techniques for intracellular work in small cells, Neuroscience, 2: 813

Butler, J.N., 1968, The thermodynamic activity of calcium ion in sodium chloride - calcium chloride electrolytes, Biophys.J., 8: 1426

Caspers, H. and Speckmann, E.-J., 1974, Cortical DC shifts associated with changes of gas tensions in blood and tissue, in:"Handbook of Electroencephalography and Clinical Neurophysiology, Vol. 10 Part A", A. Remond, ed., Elsevier, Amsterdam, pp. 10 - 41

Christoffersen, G.R.J. and Skibsted, L.H., 1975, Calcium ion activity in physiological salt solutions: Influence of anions substituted for chloride, Comp.Biochem.Physiol., 52: 317

Coles, J.A. and Tsacopoulos, M., 1977, A method of making fine double-barrelled potassium-sensitive microelectrodes for intracellular recording, J.Physiol.(Lond.), 270: 12P

Greenwald, I., 1959, Complexes of bicarbonate with magnesium and calcium, J.phys.chem., 63: 1328

Katzmann, R. and Grossmann, R., 1975, Neuronal activity and potassium movement, in:"Brain Work", D.H. Ingvar and N.A. Lassen, eds., Munksgaard, Copenhagen, pp. 149 - 166

Kraig, R.P. and Nicholson, C., 1978, Extracellular ionic variations during spreading depression, Neuroscience, 3: 1045

Lehmenkühler, A., Zidek, W. and Caspers, H., 1980, Changes of extracellular Na^+ and Cl^- activity in the brain cortex during seizure discharges, IUPS Satellite Symposium on Physiology and Pharmacology of Epileptic Phenomena, Frankfurt

Lübbers, D.W., 1972, Physiologie der Gehirndurchblutung, in:"Der Hirnkreislauf", H. Gänshirt, ed., Thieme, Stuttgart, pp. 214-254

Moore, E.W. and Ross, J.W., 1965, NaCl and $CaCl_2$ activity coeffi-
     cients in mixed aqueous solutions, J.Appl.Physiol., 20: 1332
Neher, E. and Lux, H.D., 1973, Rapid changes of potassium concen-
     tration at the outer surface of exposed single neurons during
     membrane current flow, J.Gen.Physiol., 61: 385
Nicholson, C., tenBruggencate, G., Steinberg, R. and Stöckle, H.,
     1977, Calcium modulation in brain extracellular microenvironment
     demonstrated with ion-selective micropipette, Proc.natn.Acad.Sci.
     U.S.A., 74: 1287
Pedersen, K.O., 1971, On the presence of calcium complexes in aqueous
     bicarbonate solutions, Scand.J.clin.Lab.Invest., 27: 9
Oehme, M., Kessler, M. and Simon, W., 1976, Neutral carrier Ca^{++}-
     microelectrode, Chimia, 30: 204
Rapoport, J.L. and Marshall, W.H., 1964, Measurement of cortical pH
     in spreading depression, Am.J.Physiol., 206: 1177
Somjen, G.G., 1979, Extracellular potassium in the mammalian central
     nervous system, Ann.Rev.Physiol., 41: 159
Staples, B.R. and Nuttall, R.L., 1977, The activity and osmotic
     coefficients of aqeous calcium chloride at 298.15 K,
     J.Phys.Chem.Ref.Data, 6: 385
Tschirgi, R.D., Inanaga, K., Taylor, J.L., Walker, M. and Sonnen-
     schein, R.R., 1957, Changes in cortical pH and blood flow
     accompanying spreading cortical depression and convulsion,
     Am.J.Physiol., 190: 557
Zidek, W., Lehmenkühler, A. and Caspers, H., 1979, Extracellular pH
     transients in the rat cerebral cortex during spreading depression
     and asphyxiation, Pflügers Arch., 382: R43
Zidek, W., Lange-Asschenfeldt, H., Lehmenkühler, A. and Caspers, H.,
     1979, Relations between membrane potential and intracellular pH
     of snail neurons during CO_2 application in various buffer
     solutions, Pflügers Arch., 379: R39

CHANGES OF EXTRACELLULAR POTASSIUM IN RAT CEREBELLAR CORTEX INDICATE A REDUCED Na-K-PUMP ACTIVITY DURING ACUTE AND CHRONIC Li-APPLICATION

G. ten Bruggencate, A. Ullrich, P. Baierl

Dept. of Physiology, University of Munich
Pettenkoferstr. 12,
8000 Munich 2, G.F.R.

Although lithium salts (Li) are widely used in the treatment of mania and recurrent depression, their mechanism of action is still unclear (Schou, 1976). Since it seems possible that Li exerts direct or indirect actions on other ions, we investigated Li-effects upon extracellular potassium by means of ion selective microelectrodes (ISME) responding to Li^+ and K^+, respectively (Ullrich et al., 1980). The parallel fibre-Purkinje cell pathway of the cerebellar cortex was used as a convenient model of unmyelinated fibres with numerous synapses.

METHODS

Liquid ion exchanger electrodes of theta- or multibarrel-style were used. After exposure of the cerebellar cortex in urethane-anaesthetized rats, the parallel fibres were stimulated locally (see Nicholson et al., 1978) and the stimulus-induced changes in extracellular K^+ recorded within the parallel fibre beam. The potassium K-undershoot was taken as an indication of the activity of the Na-K-pump (Heinemann and Lux, 1975). Li-applications were given acutely by exchanging LiCl against NaCl in the artificial CSF with which the cerebellar cortex was continuously superfused (37^oC). The actual concentration within the cerebellar cortex was monitored using Li-ISMEs. In another set of experiments, rats were kept for 3 weeks to 3 months on a dry food-diet (Altromin), to which LiCl was added (groups receiving 30 and 100 mmol/l LiCl/kg dry food, respectively). The plasma levels of the Li-groups were about 0.5 and 1.0 mmol/l Li, respectively.

RESULTS

Figure 1 illustrates the main effects of acute (A) and chronic (B) Li administration upon the resting potassium (aK^+Cb), the stimulus induced peaks (ΔK^+p) and the poststimulus K-undershoots (ΔK^+u).

Acute application: In Fig. 1A, data were grouped (groups A-D) according to various Li-levels reached during Li-superfusion periods (a Li^+cb = extracellular level within cerebellar cortex, $mmol/1\pm SEM$. Clearly, there was a dose-dependent rise in the extracellular resting potassium reaching 200% (=7 mmol/1) at 20 mmol/1 Li (group D). As the high K-level in group D blocked excitation, no stimulus induced K-rise - and consequently no K-undershoots occurred in the highest Li-group. However, in the groups of rats which had average cerebellar Li-concentration of 5.3 and 7.4 mmol/1, respectively, stimulus-induced rises of K were increased. Despite the increased peak values, K-undershoots were reduced (groups B and C).

Chronic oral administration: Similar results were obtained in Li-treated rats (Fig. 1B). Control rats showed extracellular K-levels in cerebellar cortex of 3.5 ± 0.1 mmol/1. Group E (plasma Li-level 0.5 mmol/1) and F (plasma Li 1.0 mmol/1) had elevated resting K-levels (3.8 ± 0.1 and 4.2 ± 0.3 mmol/1, respectively). Simultaneously, poststimulus K-undershoots were reduced in these animals. Quantitatively, the reduction of K-undershoots seen in group F would correspond approximately to acute actions of about 6 mmol/1 Li.

Both an elevation of the extracellular resting potassium and the decrease of poststimulus K-undershoots agree with a Li-induced re - duction of the activity of the Na-K-pump.

Cardiac glycosides and conduction time: If Li interferes with the Na-K-pump, similar effects of other pump blockers can be expected. In fact, k-strophanthidin and other cardiac glycosides also increased K^+-levels and reduced K^+-undershoots. In addition, glycoside actions were more pronounced during acute or chronic Li-administration. An additional observation was a decrease in parallel fiber conduction time after prolonged stimulation under Li or k-strophanthidin. Such effects which also have been observed in vagus nerves (Ploeger, 1974) would be in accordance with a reduced sodium gradient across the axonal membrane.

DISCUSSION

The most likely interpretation of the results described is an inhibitory action of Li upon the activity of the Na-K-pump. Quantitatively, acutely applied Li at an extracellular concentration of 6-7 mmol/1 was about equipotent to a 1.3 mmol/1 Li-level in cerebellum in chronically treated rats. At both levels, the K^+-undershoots

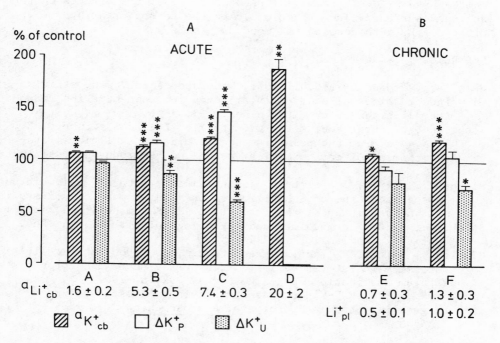

Fig. 1. Changes in extracellular potassium related to lithium
application.
A, effects of acute, B, of chronic oral Li-administration.
Bars represent changes in extracellular resting K$^+$ (aK$^+$cb)
stimulus-induced K$^+$-peaks (ΔK$^+$p) and poststimulus K$^+$-under-
shoots (ΔK$^+$u) with respect to control values (=100%). Groups
A-D represent rats which showed the indicated intracerebellar
Li-levels (aLi$^+$cb) during superfusion with various Li-con-
centrations. Groups E and F refer to chronic oral administration. Extracellular Li in cerebellar cortex was 0.7 and
1.3 mmol/1, respectively, in rats having 0.5 or 1.0 mmol/1
plasma Li.
x = P < 0.05, xx = P <0.01, xxx = P <0.001.

were reduced about 25-30%. The parameter identical in both situations
could be the intracellular Li-concentration.

An impairment of the transport capacity of the Na-K-pump ought
to mainly affect tiny neuronal elements having a relatively large
surface/volume ratio in addition to a lack of myelin. Thus, the parallel fiber-Purkinje cell pathway appears to be a very useful model
to study the general effects of pump blockade on the ionic microenvironment of neurons. Li-induced changes in transmitter release or
receptor sensitivity could well be secondary to its interference with

the Na-K-pump (see Vizi, 1978). A dependence of the effects on the neuronal surface/volume ratio could be the factor creating the specifity of Li with respect to "mood systems".

REFERENCES

Heinemann, U.,and Lux, H.D., 1975, Undershoots following stimulus-induced rises of extracellular potassium concentration in cerebral cortex of cat, Brain Res., 93:63-76.

Nicholson, C., Bruggencate ten G., Stöckle, H., and Steinberg, R., 1978, Calcium and potassium changes in extracellular microenvironment of cat cerebellar cortex, J. Neurophysiol.,41:1026-1039.

Ploeger, E., 1974, The effects of lithium on excitable cell membranes. On the mechanism of inhibition of the sodium pump of non-myelinated nerve fibres of the rat, Europ. J. Pharmacol., 25:316-321.

Schou, M., 1976, Pharmacology and toxicology of Lithium, Ann.Rev. Pharmacol. Toxicol. , 16:231-243.

Ullrich,., Baierl, P., and Bruggencate ten, G., 1980, Extracellular potassium in rat cerebellar cortex during acute and chronic lithium application. Brain Research, 192:287-290.

Vizi, E.S., 1978, Na^+-K^+-activated adenosinetriphosphatase as a trigger in transmitter release, Neuroscience, 3:367-384.

CHANGES IN EXTRACELLULAR FREE Ca^{2+} IN THE SENSORIMOTOR CORTEX OF CATS DURING ELECTRICAL STIMULATION AND IONTOPHORETIC APPLICATION OF AMINO-ACIDS

U. Heinemann and R. Pumain

Dept. of Neurophysiology
Max Planck Institute for Psychiatry
D-8000 München 40, F.R.G. and
Inserm U 97, Centre Paul Broca
F-75014 Paris, France

In the mammalian central nervous system extracellular free Ca^{2+} (a_{ca}) varies under a variety of conditions such as during repetitive electrical stimulation and seizures (Nicholson et al., 1977; Heinemann et al., 1977,1978). In order to gain insight into the mechanisms which are responsible for extracellular Ca^{2+} activity changes in cat neocortex, we measured a_{ca} changes with Ca^{2+} sensitive reference electrodes (Oehme et al., 1976) during iontophoretic application of excitatory and inhibitory amino acids and during repetitive electrical stimulation of the cortical surface and the thalamic ventrobasal complex. The effects of Ca^{2+} antagonists such as Co^{2+}, Mn^{2+} and La^{3+} and of the sodium channel blocker tetrodotoxin (TTX) on changes in a_{ca} were also investigated.

The baseline a_{ca} in the cat's cortex was found to vary between 1.1 and 1.4 mM. It was in average 1.2 mM. During repetitive stimulation of the cortical surface (CS) and the ventrobasal complex (VB) a_{ca} decreased by up to 0.45 mM. Reductions in a_{ca} (Δa_{ca}) were largest in depths of 100 to 300 μm below cortical surface. Below 700 μm usually only increases in a_{ca} were observed (Heinemann et al., 1979). This is particularly surprising in the case of VB stimulation, since thalamocortical fibers terminate predominantly in layer 3b, i.e. in depths of 600 to 900 μm. In fact, in these depths stimulus induced increases in extracellular potassium activity (a_k) are also largest (Heinemann and Lux, 1975) as expected if presynaptic K^+ release contributes strongly to increases in a_k (Nicholson et al., 1978). Therefore presynaptic Ca^{2+} entry is unlikely to be the major cause of reduction in a_{ca}. The increases in a_{ca} in deeper cortical layers are most likely due to reductions of extracellular space size, as suggested by recent measurements using nominally K^+ selective micropipettes to record concentration changes of marker substances for the extracellular space such as choline and tetramethylammonium (Dietzel et al., 1980).

The laminar distribution of stimulus induced Ca^{2+} signals points to the existence of postsynaptic Ca^{2+} conductances also in neocortical neurones. The existence of such Ca^{2+} conductances has been demonstrated already for a variety of neurones such as cat's motoneurones (Lux and Schubert, 1975), cerebellar Purkinje cells (Llinas and Hess, 1976) and hippocampal pyramidal cells (Schwartzkroin and Slawski, 1977). If neocortical Ca^{2+} conductances are voltage sensitive (for review see Lux and Heyer, 1979) iontophoretic application of excitatory aminoacids such as glutamate (Glu), aspartate (asp), and DL-homocysteic acid (DLH) should also result in reductions of a_{ca}. Therefore changes in a_{ca} were measured during iontophoretic application of these substances from a nearby phoresis electrode (tip intervals 20 to 80 µm). It was found that Glu, Asp and DLH usually evoked reductions of up to 1.2 mM in a_{ca} (see fig.1). Such Δa_{ca} were never seen in the white matter; it is therefore unlikely that the reductions in a_{ca} are caused by precipitation of Ca^{2+}. The largest reductions in a_{ca} were seen in upper cortical layers at depths of 100 to 300 µm, i.e. the same site at which also stimulus induced Δa_{ca} were largest (see fig.1C,D).

In principle such reductions in a_{ca} could be the result of Ca^{2+} movement through transmitter coupled channels (Takeuchi, 1963). However, in this case Ca^{2+} reductions should be unaffected by Ca^{2+} antagonists such as Co^{2+}, Mn^{2+} and La^{3+}, since Ca^{2+} displacement through glutamate activated channels is preserved in the presence of Mn^{2+} (Bührle et al., 1978). Therefore, we tested the effects of Co^{2+}, Mn^{2+} and La^{3+} on amino-acid induced reductions of a_{ca}. We found that all these substances could block amino-acid dependent Δa_{ca} (see fig.1B).

It may also be possible that these Δa_{ca} are due to Ca^{2+} entry in presynaptic endings as a result of local excitation of interneurones and recurrent collaterals and subsequent propagation of action potentials into presynaptic endings (Katz and Miledi, 1969). In order to block generation and propagation of action potentials and the resulting entry of Ca^{2+} into presynaptic endings we applied TTX to the cortical surface at a concentration of 10^{-5} M. After TTX stimulus induced Δa_{ca} were completely blocked and the accompanying slow negative field potentials were largely abolished or even reversed in polarity. Amino-acid induced Δa_{ca}, on the other hand, were only little affected by TTX and the average reduction of Δa_{ca} was less than 10%. Therefore we concluded, that reductions

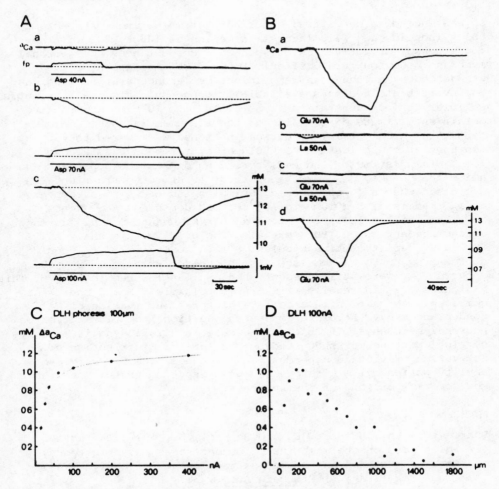

Fig. 1. Effects of iontophoretic application of excitatory amino-
acids on extracellular free Ca^{2+}. A: Iontophoretic application of Asp with varying current intensity induced dose
dependent changes in a_{ca} and negative shifts of the field
potentials (fp). B: Glutamate induced changes in a_{ca} are
blocked by La^{3+}. C: Dose response curve of DLH induced
Δa_{ca} obtained at a depth of 100 μm below cortical surface.
D: Plot of Δa_{ca} evoked by iontophoretic application of
Δa_{ca} versus recording depth below cortical surface.

in a_{ca} are probably mainly due to activation of voltage dependent
Ca^{2+} conductances in postsynaptic membrane. This interpretation is
supported by the observation that the inhibitory amino-acid GABA
reduced or even prevented the Δa_{ca} evoked by iontophoretic application of Glu, Asp or DLH. These Ca^{2+} conductances appear to be
particularly prominent in neuronal membranes of upper cortical

layers including dendrites, since both stimulus and iontophoretically induced Δa_{ca} were largest in depths of 100 to 300 μm. The
consequences of activation of such Ca^{2+} conductances on neuronal
membrane behaviour are difficult to predict. Among others they
are dependent on the transmembraneous Ca^{2+} concentration gradient.
In invertebrate neurones available evidence suggests that the intracellular Ca^{2+} concentration is below 10^{-7} to 10^{-8} M. In order to
obtain an estimate of the size of the transmembraneous Ca^{2+}-con-
centration gradient in neocortical neurones we lowered the a_{ca} by
iontophoretic application of HEDTA or citrate and examined at what
level of a_{ca} stimulus induced, spreading depression dependent and
amino-acid evoked Δa_{ca} were abolished. As expected transient Δa_{ca}
decreased when a_{ca} was lowered. Stimulus induced Δa_{ca} disappeared
at a_{ca} levels of 5 x 10^{-5} to 10^{-4} M. DLH dependent Δa_{ca} were
abolished at levels of 10^{-6} to 5 x 10^{-6} M. Changes in a_{ca} during
spreading depression (SD) were also included in this analysis. If
SD was evoked at resting baseline of 1.2 to 1.3 mM/l a_{ca} could
decrease by up to 1.2 mM (see also Nicholson et al., 1978). SD
induced Δ_{ca} were still present when a_{ca} was lowered to 10^{-6} M. This
indicates that intracellular Ca^{2+} is below 10^{-6} M and thus well
comparable to that in invertebrate neurones. Activation of Ca^{2+}
conductances may therefore impose an additional depolarization on
neuronal membranes. If this is the case in apical dendrites of neocortical neurones as suggested by the laminar distribution of Δa_{ca},
activation of voltage dependent Ca^{2+} conductances may serve to
amplify peripheral excitatory synaptic input so that it can reach
the somatic portions of the neurones.

REFERENCES

Bührle, Ch.,Ph., Buchert, B. and Sonnhof, U., 1978, The action of
    glutamate on the membrane of motoneurones investigated by
    measurements on intra- and extracellular ion activities
    (a_K^+, a_{Na}^+, $a_{Ca}2+$) Pflügers Arch., 377, R43.
Dietzel, J., Heinemann, U., Hofmeier, G. and Lux, H.D., 1980,
    Transient changes in the size of the extracellular space in
    the sensorimotor cortex of cats in relation to stimulus
    induced changes in potassium concentration. Exp.Brain Res.,
    in press.
Heinemann, U. and Lux, H.D., 1975, Undershoots following stimulus
    induced rises of extracellular potassium concentration in the
    cerebral cortex of cat. Brain Res., 93:63 .
Heinemann, U., Lux, H.D., and Gutnick, M.J., 1977, Extracellular
    free calcium and potassium during paroxysmal activity in the
    cerebral cortex of the cat. Exp.Brain Res., 27:237.
Heinemann, U., Lux, H.D., and Gutnick, M.J., 1978, Changes in
    extracellular free calcium and potassium activity in the
    somatosensory cortex of cats., in: Abnormal neuronal dis-
    charges, M.Chalazonitis and M. Boisson, eds., Raven Press,
    New York.

Heinemann, U., Lux, H.D., and Konnerth, A., 1979, Stimulus induced changes in extracellular Ca^{++} activity in the cerebral cortex of cats. Pflügers Arch. Suppl. 379, R46.

Katz, B., and Miledi, R., 1969, Tetrodotoxin - resistant electrical activity in presynaptic terminals. J.Physiol.,203:459 .

Llinas, R., and Hess, R., 1979, Tetrodotoxin - resistant dendritic spikes in avian Purkinje cells. Proc.nat.Acad.Sci.73:2520.

Lux, H.D., and Schubert, P., 1975, Some aspects of the electro-anatomy of dendrites, Advances in Neurol., Vol. 12.

Lux, H.D., and Heyer, C.B., 1979, A new electrogenic calcium-potassium system. in: The Neurosciences, Fourth Study Program, F.O.Schmitt and F.G.Worden, eds., MIT-Press, Cambridge.

Nicholson, C., Ten Bruggencate, G., Steinberg, R., and Stöckle, H., 1977, Calcium modulation in brain extracellular microenviron-ment demonstrated with ion-selective micropipette. Proc.nat. Acad. Sci., 74:1287.

Nicholson, C., Ten Bruggencate, G., Stöckle, H., and Steinberg, R., 1978, Calcium and potassium changes in extracellular micro-environment of cat cerebellar cortex. J.Neurophysiol.,41:1026

Oehme, M., Kessler, M., and Simon, W., 1976, Neutral carrier Ca^{++}-microelectrode. Chimia 30:204 .

Schwartzkroin, P.A., and Slawsky, M., 1977, Probable calcium spikes in hippocampal neurons. Brain Res., 135:157.

Takeuchi, N., 1963, Effects of calcium on the conductance change of the end-plate membrane during the action of transmitter. J.Physiol. 167:141 .

MEASUREMENTS OF ION ACTIVITY IN THE CNS:

EXTRACELLULAR K^+ AND CA^{2+} IN THE HIPPOCAMPUS

Mary E. Morris

Department of Pharmacology
University of Toronto
Toronto, Canada M5S 1A8

The highly stratified organization and well documented electro-physiology of the hippocampus (Green, 1964; Pribram and Isaacson, 1975), as well as the availability of techniques for localized measur-ements with ion-sensitive microelectrodes (Walker, 1971; Oeme et al., 1976), have encouraged recent studies (Benninger et al., 1980; Krnjević et al., 1980) of transmembrane ionic shifts which may be associated with the generation of consciousness and memory formation, and a marked susceptibility to seizure activation and anoxic damage.

Our experiments were carried out in vivo in stereotactically mounted rats, which were anaesthetized with either urethane or ket-amine. After exposure of the cerebral cortex stimulating electrodes were positioned in the fimbria, and evoked field potentials were re-corded from the reference side of ion-selective microelectrodes, in-serted vertically to varying depths in the CAI-CA3 region of the hippocampus. The micropipettes were prepared from theta-capillary tubing, with tips broken back to 2-4 μm diameter, according to methods described by Lux (1974). The reference channel was filled with 0.1 mol/1 NaCl or Li acetate, or 2% Pontamine Sky Blue dye in 0.5 mol/1 Na acetate. K^+-sensitive channels contained the Corning # 477317 exchanger or a neutral carrier (valinomycin)solution (Oeme and Lux, 1976) and 0.1 mol/1 KCl. For Ca^{2+} measurements a neutral ligand (Oeme et al., 1976) and 0.1 mol/1 $CaCl_2$ were used. To allow simultan-eous recordings of K^+ and Ca^{2+} activities electrodes were combined so that their shanks were nearly parallel and tips separated by $\leq$ 10 μm. The slopes for K^+ and Ca^{2+} electrodes, when calibrated in Ringer solutions, were respectively 38-46 mV and 21-29 mV.

Changes in the activities of $K^+(a_K)$ and $Ca^{2+}(a_{Ca})$ in response to repetitive stimulation of the fimbria were consistently greatest

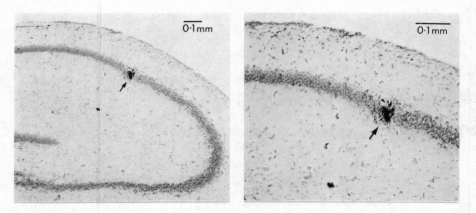

Fig. 1.   Localization with dye-marking shows the site of maximal
          evoked positive field, K^+, and Ca^{2+} potentials to be the
          pyramidal cell body layer.

in the pyramidal cell body layer, where the field potential recorded
at the same time, was maximally positive. This localization was confirmed by current ejection of Pontamine Sky Blue from the microelectrodes at the termination of experiments (Fig. 1). The observed ionic
shifts augmented rapidly over a narrow range of stimulation frequency
(3-8 Hz) and were considerably larger than those evoked by much higher
rates in most other central synaptic regions (Somjen, 1979; Nicholson
et al., 1978). In addition they frequently showed the unusual feature
of phasic fluctuations (at 30-60 s intervals) during prolonged application of the stimulus (Reiffenstein et al., 1980).

The evoked release and accumulation of K^+, from a resting level
of 2.5 - 3.0 mmol/l to as high as 12 mmol/l, was followed by an undershoot of the potential in the post-stimulus phase. With rates of stimulation $\leq$ 3-4 Hz the tendency for development of 'seizure activity'
(afterdischarge) and a more sustained elevation of the K^+ level was
increased. Relatively large changes were recorded over a considerable
depth of the hippocampal cortex. When simultaneous measurements of
the potential shifts were made with a microelectrode containing the
classical K^+ exchanger (which is more sensitive to ACh than to K^+)
and with one prepared with valinomycin (which has greater selectivity
for K^+ than for ACh), peak levels of responses were identical. A po-
tentially significant artefact, due to the activation of known cholinergic septal inputs, could therefore be ruled out.

Although the decrease in a_{Ca}, from initial levels of $\simeq$ 1.5 mmol/l
down to as low as 0.5 mmol/l, showed some degree of quantitative cor-

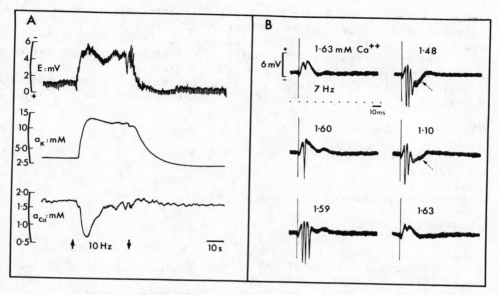

Fig. 2.   Recordings in stratum pyramidale at site of largest field potential. (A) DC focal, K^+, and Ca^{2+} potentials evoked by 10 Hz fimbrial stimulation; (B) oscilloscope traces of field potentials during 7 Hz stimulation. Spikes and negative after-potential (at arrow) develop and decline as $[Ca^{2+}]_o$ fell from 1.63 to 1.10 mmol/1 and recovered.

relation with the changes in a_K, they had a distinctly different time course (Fig. 2A) - being more transient and usually followed during the period of stimulation by an overshoot and/or secondary falls of varying degree and duration. They were more steeply related to the intensity and rate of stimulation than the changes in a_K, and much more localized in depth - large falls being limited to the pyramidal cell body layer.

The positive component of the field potential, which reflects the action of inhibitory synapses on the pyramidal cell bodies (Ben-Ari et al., 1979) also showed striking phasic changes in response to repetitive activation of the fimbria. Its depression was accompanied by the appearance of population spikes which increased in amplitude and number and were followed by a negative depolarizing after-potential - changes which show close correlation with both the localization and time course of the large transient falls in calcium (Fig.2B). The evidence therefore suggests that excitation is accompanied by not only a removal of inhibition, but also the activation of a large calcium inward current into the pyramidal cell bodies, rather than the dendrites, as previously hypothesized (Schwartzkroin and Slawsky,1977).

Although influx of Ca^{2+} into the inhibitory terminals located on the pyramidal cell bodies could contribute to the fall in $[Ca^{2+}]_o$, it is more likely that the lowered level of a_{Ca} would profoundly depress their release of transmitter. Finally, since there is recent evidence that the pyramidal cell bodies are coupled (MacVicar and Dudek, 1980), further significant functional contributions may arise from uncoupling effects of raised intracellular Ca^{2+}(Rose and Loewenstein, 1975).

ACKNOWLEDGEMENTS

This work was supported by the Medical Research Council of Canada and carried out in collaborative experiments in the Department of Anaesthesia Research, McGill University, Montreal, Canada. Professor W. Simon kindly donated the neutral carrier exchangers.

REFERENCES

Ben-Ari, Y., Krnjeviĉ, K., and Reinhardt, W., 1979, Hippocampal seizures and failure of inhibition, Can. J. Physiol. Pharmacol., 57:1462.

Benninger, C., Kadis, J., and Prince D.A., 1980, Extracellular calcium and potassium changes in hippocampal slices, Brain Res., 187:165.

Green, J.D., 1964, The Hippocampus, Physiol. Rev., 44:561.

Krnjeviĉ, K., Morris, M.E., and Reiffenstein, R.J., 1980, Changes in extracellular Ca^{2+} and K^+ activity accompanying hippocampal discharges, Can. J. Physiol. Pharmacol., 58:579.

Lux, H.D., 1974, Fast recording ion specific microelectrodes: their use in pharmacological studies in the CNS, Neuropharmacol., 13:509.

MacVicar, B.A., Dudek, F.E., 1980, Dye-coupling between CA3 pyramidal cells in slices of rat hippocampus, Brain Res., 196: in press.

Nicholson, C., ten Bruggencate, G., Stöckle,H.,and Steinberg, R., 1978, Calcium and potassium changes in extracellular microenvironment of cat cerebellar cortex, J. Neurophysiol., 41:1026.

Oehme, M., Kessler, M., and Simon W., 1976, Neutral carrier Ca^{2+} microelectrode, Chimia, 30:204.

Oehme, M., and Simon, W., 1976, Microelectrode for potassium ions based on a neutral carrier and comparison of its characteristics with a cation exchanger sensor, Anal. Chim. Acta, 86:21.

Pribram, K.H., and Isaacson, R.L., eds. ,1975,"Hippocampus: Structure and Development, Physiology and Behaviour", Vols. 1 and 2, Plenum Press, New York.

Reiffenstein, R.J., Krnjeviĉ, K., and Morris, M.E., 1980, Cyclic fluctuations in hippocampal firing and extracellular electrolytes during repetitive fimbrial stimulation, Proc. Can. Fed. Biol. Soc. , 23:154.

Rose, B., and Loewenstein, W.R., 1975, Permeability of cell junction depends on local cytoplasmic calcium activity, Nature, 254:250

Schwartzkroin, A., and Slawsky, M., 1977, Probable calcium spikes in hippocampal neurons, Brain Res., 135:157.

Somjen, G.G., 1979, Extracellular potassium in the mammalian central nervous system, Ann. Rev. Physiol., 41:159.

Walker, J.L., 1971, Ion specific liquid ion exchanger microelectrodes, Anal. Chem., 43:89A.

EVOKED IONIC ALTERATIONS IN BRAIN SLICES

D. A. Prince, C. Benninger, and J. Kadis

Department of Neurology
Stanford University School of Medicine
Stanford, CA 94305

INTRODUCTION

The use of ion sensitive microelectrodes (ISMs) has made it possible to obtain virtually real time measurements of extracellular ionic events in mammalian brain during a variety of experimental conditions (see Lux, 1974; Somjen, 1979 for reviews). Data emphasize that the concentrations of ionic species vary considerably during physiological and electrical stimulation, and that these changes have specific distributions which appear to depend on the anatomic organization of the structures studied (see also Moody et al., 1974; Nicholson et al., 1978, and others). Two important questions with respect to these ionic shifts relate to 1) their source in terms of the varieties and distributions of conductances in neuronal membranes and 2) their potential capacity to influence the excitability of stimulated, and nearby non-stimulated, neuronal elements.

We have used the hippocampal slice preparation to examine the changes in extracellular potassium ($[K^+]_o$) and calcium ($[Ca^{++}]_o$) concentrations during a variety of experimental maneuvers, under circumstances where the baseline ionic extracellular environment could be controlled. In another series of experiments we have studied the effects of iatrogenic alterations in ionic elements on neuronal activities in hippocampal and neocortical slices to attempt to determine whether changes in ionic microenvironment in the ranges measured following stimulation, can have potential effects on neuronal excitability.

247

METHODS

Techniques for preparation and maintenance of in vitro slices
were similar to those previously used (Schwartzkroin and Prince, 1977,
1980; Yamamoto, 1972). Standard techniques for manufacturing double-
barreled K^+ and Ca^{++} ISMs were employed (Lux and Neher, 1973). Some
other details of the experimental methods are described in an earlier
publication (Benninger et al., 1980). Experiments were done at 37 °C
in media containing (in mmol/1)NaCl 124; KCl 5; NaH_2PO_4 1.25; $MgSO_4$
2.0; $CaCl_2$ 2; $NaHCO_3$ 26; dextrose 10. Some studies were done in solutions containing higher (10 mmol/1) or lower (3 mmol/1) concentrations of K^+; and 1.2 mmol/1 Ca^{++}. Values obtained for activities of
Ca^{++} and K^+ from ISMs were converted to concentrations using the calibration curves for each electrode.

RESULTS

The baseline levels of $[K^+]_o$ and $[Ca^{++}]_o$ were those of the perfusion medium and therefore ranged from 3-10 mmol/1 for K^+ and 1.2-
2 mmol/1 for Ca^{++}. Maximal changes in ionic concentrations were elicited with 5-10 Hz stimulation in the stratum radiatum of the CA1
region. Recordings in stratum pyramidale of CA1 showed increases in
$[K^+]_o$ from baseline levels of 3 or 5 mmol/1 to peaks as high as 12
mmol/1 and decreases in $[Ca^{++}]_o$ from baseline levels of 2 mmol/1 to
as low as 1.4 mmol/1 (Fig. 1). No significant changes in $[Ca^{++}]_o$, and
rare small increases in $[K^+]_o$ were seen with 1 Hz stimulation. Significant undershoots in $[K^+]_o$ were regularly recorded following prolonged stimulus trains (e.g., second train of Fig. 1). When a

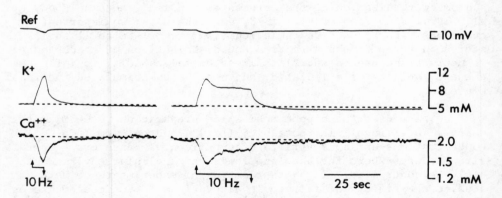

Fig. 1. Recordings from stratum pyramidale in one hippocampal slice
         during stratum radiatum stimulation. The effects of 5 sec
         (first segment) and 25 sec (second segment) trains of 10 Hz
         stimulation are shown. Dotted lines in K^+ and Ca^{2+} traces:
         baseline activity levels. Upper trace: low gain DC recording
         from K^+ reference micropipette. (From Benninger et al.1980).

laminar analysis of $\Delta[K^+]_o$ and $\Delta[Ca^{++}]_o$ was done at various sites (Fig. 2) it was found that maximal changes in these ionic species occurred in stratum pyramidale, with less striking alterations in stratum oriens and stratum radiatum, and still smaller changes in alveus and stratum lacunosum. The percent changes in K^+ and Ca^{++} mirrored each other precisely and the profile obtained was independent of the sequence of measurement sites. The laminar profile for $[K^+]_o$ was similar to that obtained in vivo when measurements were made of changes related to interictal epileptiform spikes in penicillin-treated hippocampus (Fisher et al., 1976).

The finding that maximal $[Ca^{++}]_o$ decrease occurs in stratum pyramidale was unexpected, since it has been shown that Ca^{++} spike electrogenesis in hippocampal pyramidal cells is prominent in dendrites (Wong and Prince, 1979). It is possible however that movement of Ca^{++} into presynaptic terminals or somata contributes to the observed pattern. At this point we are unable to control for the effect of neuronal packing density as a contributor to the laminar profiles seen. It is clear, however that K^+ and Ca^{++} changes are very closely coupled as might be expected from other results which show that voltage dependent increases in gK^+ and gCa^{++} are present in CA1 pyramidal neurons (Hotson et al., 1979),

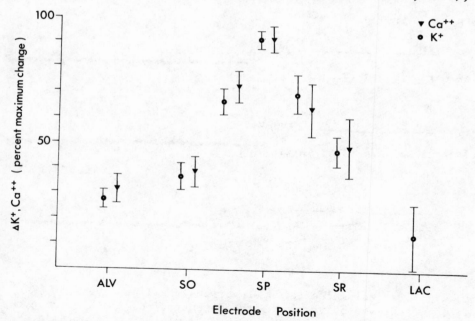

Fig. 2. Plot of maximum per cent change in $[K^+]_o$ and $[Ca^{2+}]$ against electrode position in the slice. Bars = $\pm$ 1 S.D. ALV, alveus LAC, stratum lacunosum. Each point represents average of measurements in 10 experiments. (From Benninger et al., 1980).

as are Ca^{++}-activated increases in gK^+ (Hotson and Prince, 1980).
The large and prolonged K^+ conductance changes activated by Ca^{++} entry
would presumably be a major factor in producing increases in $[K^+]_o$.
Slice Ca^{++} is thought to be rapidly bound at sites of entry, it appears
likely that $\Delta[K^+]_o$ due to Ca^{++} activated gK^+ will be maximal outside
neuronal elements with significant calcium conductances. The relatively small rises in $[K^+]_o$ produced in our experiments when synaptic
transmission was blocked and antidromic activation was produced by alveus stimulation (see below and Fig. 5B2), suggest that action potential generation in soma dendritic membrane does not make a large contribution to $\Delta[K^+]_o$. Results of studies in spinal cord tend to support this conslusion (see Somjen, 1979 for review.)On the other hand,
postsynaptic conductance increases for K^+ may significantly increase
$[K^+]_o$ (Nicholson et al., 1976; Segal and Gutnick, 1980).

We have conducted additional investigations of some of the factors which affect $\Delta[K^+]_o$. In earlier experiments in neocortex (Moody
et al., 1974) we found an inverse relationship between $\Delta[K^+]_o$ and
the baseline $[K^+]_o$, however these studies were done using K^+ release
during epileptogenesis as the mechanism for increasing baseline levels.
When baseline levels were adjusted by perfusion with solutions con-

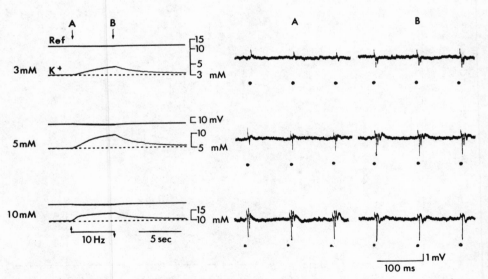

Fig. 3.   First column: effects of various baseline levels of $[K^+]_o$
          (achieved by varying bath concentrations) on K^+ rise evoked
          by stimulus train. Recordings from stratum pyramidale. Ref:
          reference trace recorded DC. A and B: representative field
          potential recordings from beginning (A) and end (B) of each
          stimulus train for each of the three baseline concentrations
          of $[K^+]_o$. (From Benninger et al., 1980).

taining different concentrations of K^+ (Fig. 3) it was found that the largest percent increases in $[K^+]_o$ occured from baseline of about 5 mmol/l, with lesser changes at 3 mmol/l and 10 mmol/l (compare evoked changes at different baseline $[K^+]_o$s in Fig. 3). A similar relationship between $\Delta[K^+]_o$ and baseline $[K^+]_o$ was found when $[K^+]_o$ was manipulated with iontophoretic K^+ pulses from a nearby micropipette. Very little stimulated rise could be obtained when iontophoresis raised the $[K^+]_o$ to levels between 15 and 20 mmol/l prior to the orthodromic stimulus. Field potential recordings also suggested that increments in the excitability of the population tended to occur when $[K^+]_o$ reached higher levels as judged by larger amplitude and multi-peaked population responses (see field potentials at baselines of 5 and 10 mmol/l $[K^+]_o$ in Fig. 3).

As mentioned above, undershoots in $[K^+]_o$ occured regularly following prolonged stimulus-induced rises. Previous studies in vivo have shown that there is an active uptake process for K^+ which is turned on by such stimuli (Heinemann and Lux, 1975). Results in the slice were also compatible with this interpretation. The envelope of $\Delta[K^+]_o$ usually showed an initial rise to peak followed by a sag toward baseline during prolonged stimuli. The amplitude of iontophoretic K^+ pulses increased during the early phases and close to the peak of an orthodromically induced K^+ rise (cf. Fig. 4A and B) and decreased in amplitude when pulses fell on the descending limb of the K^+ response or during the undershoot(Fig. 4D, E, and F). The larger responses at the peak of the orthodromic K^+ change suggest that the additional intophoretic K^+ application excites neurons and produces an additional $[K^+]_o$ release. Potassium undershoots were not seen following prolonged iontophoretically induced $[K^+]_o$ rises to levels as high as 15 mmol/l; i.e., iatrogenically increased $[K^+]_o$ in this range is not an adequate stimulus for active K^+ uptake.

Maneuvers which depressed synaptic activation of the CA1 region, such as use of perfusion solution containing 0.5 mmol/l Ca^{++} and 6 mmol/l Mg^{++}, markedly decreased $\Delta[K^+]_o$ produced by stratum radiatum stimulation as measured in stratum pyramidale (compare Figs. 5A1 and 5A2). During suprathreshold stimulation of the alveus significant rises in $[K^+]_o$ were also recorded in stratum pyramidale, presumably related to antidromic activation of CA1 neurons as well as synaptic activation due to current spread into stratum oriens (Fig. 5B1). After perfusion with 0.5 mmol/l Ca^{++} and 6 mmol/l Mg^{++}-containing solutions, the same alveus stimuli produced only small increments in $[K^+]_o$ in stratum pyramidale (Fig. 5B2). Similar effects were produced by perfusion with solutions containing 1-3 mmol/l Mn^{++}, a more effective calcium blocking agent, and were not reversed by increasing the stimulus intensity. These findings suggest that synaptic events are a major contributor to $[K^+]_o$ rises. The data do not allow separation of Ca^{++}-activated gK^+ in pre- and postsynaptic elements, versus transmitter-activated postsynaptic gK^+ as contributors to the $\Delta[K^+]_o$s recorded.

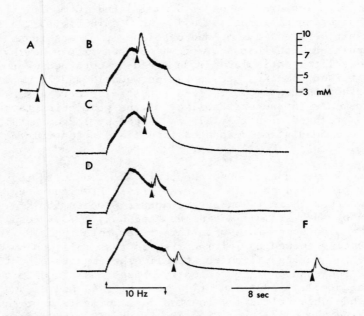

Fig. 4. Interactions between iontophoretically evoked $[K^+]_o$ increases and those produced by trains of orthodromic stimuli. A. iontophoretic K^+ pulse of 200 nA, 500 msec evokes a control $[K^+]_o$ increase of 2.0 mmol/1. Test pulse evokes larger changes in $[K^+]_o$ when it is delivered near the peak or early falling phase of the orthodromically evoked increase. (B: 2.8 mmol/1; C: 2.3 mmol/1). Iontophoretic pulses falling late during the orthodromically evoked rises (D: 1.4 mmol/1), or during the recovery phase (E: 1.5 mmol/1) or $[K^+]_o$ undershoot (F: 1.7 mmol/1) evoked $[K^+]_o$ increase which are smaller than control. Arrowheads: onset of 500 msec iontophoretic pulses. Calibration for K^+ ISM following segment (B) is for all traces. Baseline at the beginning of each segment except (F): 3 mmol/1. (From Benninger et al., 1980).

Since Ba^{++} is known to be an effective blocker of K^+ currents (Werman and Grundfest, 1961; Gorman and Hermann, 1979), we studied its effect on $\Delta[K^+]_o$ during spontaneous and evoked neuronal and field potential activities in slices. Barium (either 0.5 mmol/1 added to the normal perfusion medium containing 1.5 mmol/1 Ca^{++} or 2 mmol/1

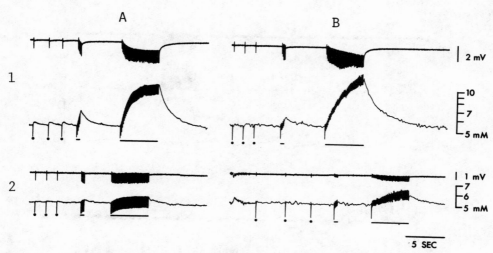

Fig. 5. The effects of stratum radiatum (A) and alveus (B) stimulation on $[K^+]_o$ levels measured in stratum pyramidale. Segments A1 and B1 were obtained from slices in normal bath solutions containing 2 mmol/1 Ca^{++} and 2 mmol/1 Mg^{++}. Segments A2 and B2 were obtained from the same slices as A1 and B1 after perfusion with solutions containing 0.5 mmol/1 Ca^{++} and 6 mmol/1 Mg^{++}. Dots under segments: single stimuli. Bars under segments: trains of stimuli delivered at 10 Hz. Upper lines: field potential recordings at site of ISM measurements. Lower traces: potassium signals. Time calibration in B1 for all segments. (From Benninger et al., unpublished).

substituted for Ca^{++}) regularly produced spike broadening, spontaneous bursts, and subsequent plateau potentials in CA1 pyramidal neurons (Fig. 6, 2 mmol/1 Ba^{++} 2) (see also Hotson and Prince, 1980, 1980 a). In 2 mmol/1 Ba^{++} -0 Ca^{++} solutions, it was possible to evoke multi-peaked field potential bursts associated with intracellular depolarizations and repetitive spiking. Although $[K^+]_o$ increases in control solutions following single stimuli were very small (Fig. 6 normal, 1st 5 stimuli), very significant increments were seen following single stimuli which evoked field potential bursts and intracellular depolarizations in Ba^{++} (Fig. 6, 2 mmol/1 Ba^{++}). Brief trains of stimuli in normal medium (Fig. 6 normal, middle of segment) evoked smaller rises in $[K^+]_o$ than single stimuli in Ba^{++}. Discharges of single neurons, even when characterized by prolonged plateaus and multiple bursts, did not produce detectable $\Delta[K^+]_o$s, presumably because of the position of the ISM relative to the impaled neuron (Fig. 6, 2 mmol/1 Ba^{++}). We presume that large stimulated releases of K^+ in Ba^{++} solutions reflect 1) incomplete block of voltage dependent and calcium activated gK^+ and enhancement of these residual K^+ currents during

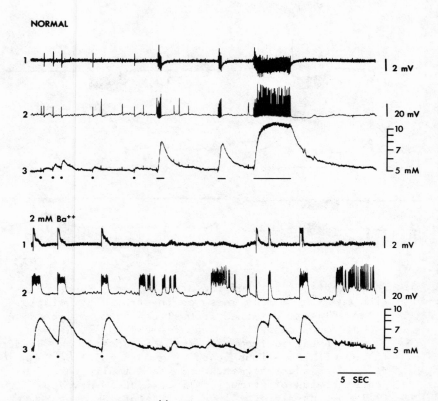

Fig. 6. The effects of Ba^{++} perfusion on orthodromically evoked $\Delta[K^+]_o$
Line 1: field potentials. Line 2: intracellular recording
near site of $[K^+]_o$ measurement. Line 3: K^+ signal. Upper
traces: stimuli in normal solution. Lower traces: stimuli in
solution containing 2 mmol/1 Ba^{++}. Dots and bars under line
3 represent single stimuli and trains at 10 Hz. Neuronal spikes are attenuated by penwriter recordings. Time calibration
in B for A-B. (From Benninger et al., unpublished).

prolonged depolarizations which may be associated with Ca^{++} entry; and
2) effective enhancement of transmitter release by Ba^{++} which may sub-
stitute Ca^{++} in this process (Fatt and Ginsborg, 1958). The latter
effect would cause added $\Delta[K^+]_o$ during synaptically activated K^+ conductances · (see also Nicholson et al., 1976 for discussion).

Prediction of the effects of measured ionic alterations on
activities of the neuronal elements which generated these changes

in the first place, or on neighboring neurons, is exceedingly difficult. Issues such as 1) the distribution of observed concentration gradients through the hippocampus in relation to neuronal elements located at various sites; and 2) the conductance and membrane potentials of elements which " see" the extracellular ionic changes, must be taken into account. Recent data indicate that hippocampal pyramidal neurons, dentate gyrus granule cells, and subtypes of neocortical neurons have marked heterogeneity in membrane properties and susceptibility to alterations in the ionic microenvironment (Connors, Fricke, Gutnick, Wong, and Prince, unpublished). For example, granule cells and neocortical neurons are much more resistant to burst generation produced by Ba^{++} or elevated $[K^+]_o$ than are CA1 pyramidal neurons.

As a first approach to these complex problems, we have studied the effects of changes in the ionic composition of the bathing medium on evoked activities in slices. When changes in $[Ca^{++}]_o$ and $[K^+]_o$ were produced, significant alterations in neuronal excitability occurred (Schwartzkroin and Prince, 1978; Prince and Schwartzkroin, 1978; Prince et al., 1978). In the case of K^+, increments to levels close to 10 mmol/l will produce spontaneous and evoked depolarization shifts and bursting in groups of CA1 neurons, as judged by intracellular recordings and the emergence of spontaneous and evoked multi-peaked field potentials (Fig. 7B; see also Ogata et al., 1976). Even small changes in $[K^+]_o$ produce a very significant alteration in the capacity of CA1 neurons to participate in penicillin induced epileptogenesis (Fig. 7A; Schwartzkroin and Prince, 1978). In bath solutions containing 3 mmol/l K^+ and penicillin orthodromic stimulation of CA1 cells usually evoke only EPSPs (Fig. 7A1-2). However, cells of such slices generate prominent depolarization shifts and bursts as soon as $[K^+]_o$ is increased to 5 mmol/l (Fig. 7A3-4).

The mechanisms by which increases in $[K^+]_o$ produce such changes are not clear. The small depolarizations of membrane potential expected to result from such increases in $[K^+]_o$ (Scholfield, 1978) might bring neurons close to burst threshold by depolarizing dendrites (Wong and Prince, 1979) or affecting synaptic events. Recent studies in neocortical slices (Wong and Prince, unpublished) show that neurons do not usually generate TTX-resistant (presumed) Ca^{++} spikes in normal medium (Fig. 8A), but may do so when $[K^+]_o$ is increased (Fig. 8C), or when agents which decrease gK^+ such as intracellular TEA, or extracellular Ba^{++} are applied (e.g., Fig. 8B). Increases in $[K^+]_o$ in the absence of significant alterations in membrane potential would produce positive shifts in the potassium equilibrium potential. Such shifts might in turn decrease repolarizing effects of voltage dependent and Ca^{++} activated potassium conductances and facilitate Ca^{++} mediated depolarization, which is critical for burst generation in hippocampal pyramidal cells (Wong and Prince, 1978, 1980).

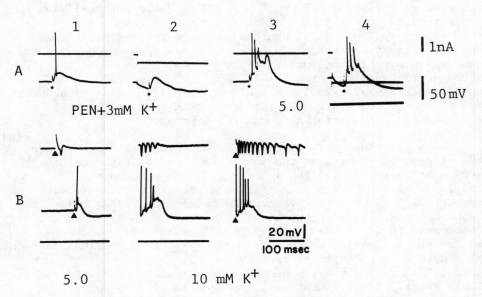

Fig. 7. Effects of increases in extracellular potassium concentration on activity in hippocampal slices. A: effects of $[K^+]_o$ on orthodromic responses in penicillin medium. Orthodromic stimuli to slice in solution containing penicillin + 3 mmol/1 K^+ evoke EPSPs (A1-A2) which may trigger single spikes (A1), or isolated EPSPs when hyperpolarizing current pulses are applied (A2). When $[K^+]_o$ is increased to 5 mmol/1 (A3-4) orthodromic stimuli evoke bursts riding on DSs in another CA1 neuron. Upper traces: current monitor; lower traces: intracellular recordings. B: Upper traces: representative field potentials; lower traces: intracellular recordings. Increases in $[K^+]_o$ from 5-10 mmol/1 changes the response to orthodromic stimulation from one of a single extracellular field spike and EPSP-IPSP sequence (B1) to one of DS generation with repetitive spike activity and multipeaked extracellular field potentials (B1-B3). Burst in B2 is spontaneous and in B3 evoked by stratum radiatum stimulation. Modified from Prince and Schwartzkroin (1978).

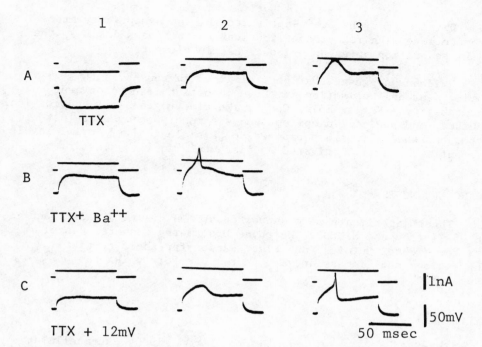

Fig. 8. TTX resistant spikes: A: Neuron which shows a depolarizing
"hump" which occurs at threshold (A3) during depolarizing
pulses delivered in TTX. B-C: TTX resistant spikes in 2
other cells. B: TTX resistant spike evoked at threshold (B2)
in the presence of 1 mmol/1 Ba^{++}. C: TTX resistant spike
(C3) evoked in medium containing 12 mmol/1 K^+. (From Wong
and Prince, unpublished).

SUMMARY AND CONCLUSIONS

1.   The use of ISMs in the <u>in vitro</u> hippocampal preparation has
provided additional information with respect to the size and
distribution in $\Delta[Ca^{++}]_o$ and $\Delta[K^+]_o$ produced by stimulation.

2.   Most of the features of ionic alterations found <u>in vivo</u> can be
reproduced in the slice, including evidence for active K^+ uptake,
and a laminar distribution of changes in Ca^{++} and K^+.

3. $\Delta[K^+]_o$ and $\Delta[Ca^{++}]_o$ are closely coupled at different sites in
the CA1 region during orthodromic activation with stratum radiatum
stimulation.

4.   The size of the $\Delta[K^+]_o$ is largest at baseline levels of 5-6 mmol/1
and decreases at higher levels.

5. Data suggest that Ca^{++}-activated gK^+ and synaptic events produce more significant contributions to increases in $[K^+]_o$ than spike generation in axons or postsynaptic elements.

6. Evidence suggests that physiological increases in $[K^+]_o$ during neuronal activation may have important effects on neuronal excitability. For example, Ca^{++} spike electrogenesis in neocortical neurons, and penicillin epileptogenesis in hippocampus are not prominent when slices are exposed to physiological (3 mmol/l levels of K^+, but are readily activated by increments in $[K^+]_o$ levels.

ACKNOWLEDGMENTS

These experiments were supported by NIH grants NS 12151 and NS 06477 from the NINCDS. We thank Drs. Barry Connors, Russell Fricke, Michael Gutnick, and Bruce Ransom for their critical suggestions and discussion, and Cheryl Joo for typing the manuscript.

REFERENCES

Benninger, C., Kadis, J., and Prince, D. A., 1980, Extracellular calcium and potassium changes in hippocampal slices, Brain Res., 187:165.

Fatt, P., and Ginsborg, B. L., 1958, The ionic requirements for the production of action potentials in crustacean muscle fibres, J. Physiol. (Lond.), 296:410.

Fisher, R. S., Pedley, T. A., Moody, W. J., Jr., and Prince, D. A., 1976, The role of extracellular potassium in hippocampal epilepsy, Arch. Neurol., 33:76.

Gorman, A. L. F., and Hermann A., 1979, Internal effects of divalent cations on potassium permeability in molluscan neurones, J. Physiol., 296:393.

Hotson, J. R., and Prince, D. A., 1980, A calcium-activated hyper-polarization follows repetitive firing in hippocampal neurons, J. Neurophysiol., 43:409.

Hotson, J. R., and Prince, D. A., 1980a, Penicillin and barium-induced epileptiform bursting in hippocampal neurons: actions on Ca^{++} and K^+ potentials, Ann. Neurol., in press.

Lux, H. D., 1974, Fast recording ion specific microelectrodes: their uses in pharmacological studies in the CNS, Neuropharmacol., 13:509.

Lux, H. D., and Neher, E., 1973, The equilibration time course of $[K^+]_o$ in cat cortex, Exp. Brain Res., 17:190.

Moody, W. J., Jr., Futamachi, K. J., and Prince, D. A., 1974, Extracellular potassium activity during epileptogenesis, Exp. Neurol., 42:248.

Nicholson, C., ten Bruggencate, G., and Senekowitsch, R., 1976, Large potassium signals and slow potentials evoked during aminopyridine or barium superfusion in cat cerebellum, Brain Res., 113:606.

Nicholson, C., ten Bruggencate, G., Stöckle, H., and Steinberg, R., 1978, Calcium and potassium changes in extracellular microenvironment of cat cerebellar cortex, J. Neurophysiol., 41:1026.

Ogata, N., 1976, The correlation between extracellular potassium concentration and hippocampal epileptic activity in vitro, Brain Res., 110:371.

Prince, D. A., Pedley, T. A., and Ransom, B. R., 1978, Fluctuations in ion concentrations during excitation and seizures, in: "Dynamic Properties of Glia Cells," G. Franck, L. Hertz, E. Schoffeniels, and D. B. Tower, eds., Pergamon Press

Prince, D. A. and Schwartzkroin, P. A., 1978, Nonsynaptic mechanisms in epileptogenesis, in: "Abnormal Neuronal Discharges," N. Chalazonitis, and M. Boisson, eds., Raven Press, New York.

Schwartzkroin, P. A. and Prince, D. A., 1977, Penicillin-induced epileptiform activity in the hippocampal in vitro preparation, Ann. Neurol., 1:463.

Schwartzkroin, P. A. and Prince, D. A., 1978, Cellular and field potential properties of epileptogenic hippocampal slices. Brain Res., 147:117.

Schwartzkroin, P. A., and Prince, D. A., 1980, Effects of TEA on hippocampal neurons, Brain Res., 185:169.

Scholfield, C. N., 1978, Electrical properties of neurones in the olfactory cortex slice in vitro, J. Physiol., 275:535.

Segal, M., and Gutnick, M. J., Effects of serotonin on extracellular potassium concentration in the rat hippocampal slice, Brain Res., in press.

Somjen, G. G., 1979, Extracellular potassium in the mammalian central nervous system, Ann. Rev. Physiol., 41:159.

Werman, R., and Grundfest, H., 1961, Graded and all or none electrogenesis in arthropod muscle II, J. Gen. Physiol., 44:997.

Wong, R. K. S., and Prince, D. A., 1978, Participation of calcium spikes during intrinsic burst firing in hippocampal neurons, Brain Res., 159:385.

Wong, R. K. S., and Prince, D. A., 1979, Intradendritic recordings from hippocampal neurons, Proc. Nat. Acad. Sci. USA, 76:986.

Wong, R. K. S., and Prince, D. A., 1980, Afterpotential generation in hippocampal pyramidal cells, J. Neurophysiol., in press.

Yamamoto, C., 1972, Intracellular study of seizure-like afterdischarges elicited in thin hippocampal sections in vitro, Exp. Neurol., 35:154.

SEROTONIN AND GABA-INDUCED FLUCTUATIONS IN EXTRACELLULAR

ION CONCENTRATION IN THE HIPPOCAMPAL SLICE

M. J. Gutnick and M. Segal

Faculty of Health Sciences, Ben Gurion University
Beersheva, Israel, and
Dept. of Isotopes, Weitzmann Institute
Rehovot, Israel

In central grey matter, activity-related release of K^+ from neurons can result in considerable K^+ accumulation in the extracellular space. It is likely that synaptic currents contribute to these rises in extracellular K^+ concentration ($[K^+]_o$). However, this contribution cannot be readily distinguished under conditions of neuronal excitation and associated high K^+ conductance. Increases in $[K^+]_o$ have been observed near medullary respiratory neurons during synaptic inhibition (Richter et al.,1978), and have also been noted following application of γ-aminobutyric acid (GABA) in cerebral cortex (Brinley et al., 1960) and spinal cord (Kudo and Fukuda, 1976). In the present investigation, we have studied the effects of two putative inhibitory neurotransmitters, serotonin (5HT) and GABA, on $[K^+]_o$ in the rat hippocampal slice preparation.

Experiments were performed on 350 μm thick slices of rat hippocampus, prepared and maintained in vitro as described elsewhere (Schwartzkroin, 1975; Segal and Gutnick, in press). Ion sensitive microelectrodes (ISMs) were manufactured from theta capillary tubing according to the techniques of Lux and Neher (1973). GABA and 5HT were prepared at a concentration of 0.5 mmol/l, and were focally applied by pressure ejection from a coarse micropipette.

The resting level of $[K^+]_o$ in the hippocampal slice was the same as that of the bathing medium; 5 mmol/l. Application of a droplet of 5HT to the pyramidal layer of area CA1 caused local $[K^+]_o$ to increase transiently by up to 0.8 mmol/l (Fig. 1-3). This $[K^+]_o$ rise reached a peak within 15 s and decayed to baseline with a halftime of about 75 s. Application of GABA produced a transient $[K^+]_o$ increase of up to 0.5 mmol/l within a similar time course (Fig. 1C,D). These $[K^+]_o$

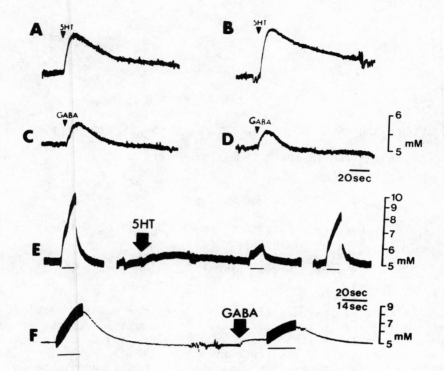

Fig. 1.   A–D. $[K^+]_o$ change following application of 5HT (A & B) or
GABA (C & D). Drugs applied and $[K^+]_o$ recorded in CA1
pyramidal layer in A & C and in CA1 lacunosum-moleculare
in B and D. E. $[K^+]_o$ increase evoked by 10 Hz stimulation
before, during and after 5HT-induced $[K^+]_o$ rise in CA1
pyramidal layer. F. $[K^+]_o$ increase evoked by 20 Hz stimulation before and during GABA-induced $[K^+]_o$ rise in CA1
pyramidal layer. In E and F, line indicates duration of
stimulus train. In this and subsequent figures, arrowhead
indicates droplet application of the drug.

changes were apparently mediated by specific receptors, since bathing
the slices in media which contained either the serotonin antagonist
methysergide (10^{-4} mol/l) or the GABA antagonist bicuculline
(10^{-5} mol/l) caused reversible attenuation of the K^+ response to
application of 5HT or GABA, respectively.

With both drugs, the $[K^+]_o$ increase was associated with an inhibitory process. Thus, whereas high frequency stimulation of the
Schaeffer collateral-commisural fiber system normally caused $[K^+]_o$
to rise by up to 4 mmol/l, stimulus-evoked responses were greatly
reduced when superimposed on drug-induced $[K^+]_o$ increases (Fig.1E.F).

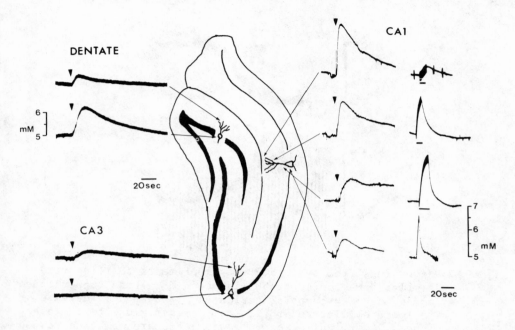

Fig. 2. Distribution of 5HT-induced $[K^+]_o$ rises in hippocampal slice. Recordings in CA1 from a different experiment than those in CA3 and dentate. In CA1, 5HT response at each electrode location followed by response to 10 Hz stimulation, indicated by line.

The regional distribution of $[K^+]_o$ responses to 5HT is shown in Fig. 2. In area CA1, responses were smallest in the pyramidal cell body layer and largest near the tips of the apical dendrites, in the vicinity of the hippocampal fissure. This was opposite to the laminar distribution of stimulus-evoked $[K^+]_o$ rises. In the dentate gyrus, 5HT-induced responses were greatest in the granular layer, and smaller in dendritic regions. In CA3, there was little or no response to 5HT. This distribution of responses is quite similar to the known distribution of 5HT-containing terminals in the hippocampus (Azmita and Segal, 1978).

These data demonstrate that activation of serotonergic receptors in the hippocampus produces an efflux of K^+ into the extracellular space. The $[K^+]_o$ increase my directly reflect activation of a synaptic K^+ conductance. Thus, in intracellular studies of CA1 pyramidal cells in rat hippocampal slices, Segal (in press) found that 5HT caused membrane hyperpolarization and increased conductance. When the drug was applied by pressure ejection, this effect, which was sensitive to changes in $[K^+]_o$ but was insensitive to changes in extra-

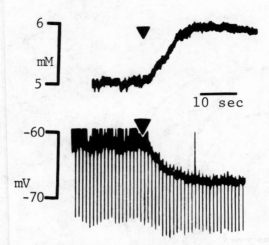

Fig. 3. Recordings from two different experiments to illustrate similar time-course of 5HT-induced $[K^+]_o$ rise (upper trace) and membrane hyperpolarization and conductance increase in intracellular recording from CA1 pyramidal cell (lower trace). Vertical lines in lower trace are membrane responses to 0.5 nA hyperpolarizing current pulses.

cellular chloride, had the same time course as does the 5HT-induced $[K^+]_o$ rise (Fig. 3).

Mechanisms underlying the GABA-induced $[K^+]_o$ increases are still unclear, since the ionic mechanisms underlying GABA's action on hippocampal neurons has yet to be resolved. It is not likely that GABA directly activates a significant K^+ conductance. However, since GABA can cause depolarization in these neurons (Alger and Nicoll, 1979), its application might indirectly lead to K^+ efflux due to secondary activation of voltage sensitive K^+ conductance. If the depolarization is mediated by chloride efflux, some passive outward movement of K^+ to preserve electroneutrality would also be expected (Deschenes and Feltz, 1976). Finally, the possibility that massive enhancement of chloride conductance results in neuronal swelling and shrinkage of the extracellular space cannot be ruled out.

Regardless of the precise mechanisms which give rise to these drug-induced $[K^+]_o$ elevations, it is clear that they are not secondary consequences of drug-induced enhancement of impulse generation, since both compounds inhibit hippocampal neurons. The use of ISMs in the in vitro preparation can thus be a useful approach to the study of the ionic consequences of transmitter action, and can provide important information regarding the regional distribution of these actions.

REFERENCES

Azmita, E.C., and Segal, M., 1978, An autoradiographic analysis of the differential ascending projections of the dorsal and medisn raphe nuclei in the rat, J. Comp. Neurol., 179:641.

Alger, B.E., and Nicoll, R.H., 1971, GABA-mediated biphasic inhibitory responses in hippocampus, Nature, 281:315.

Brinley, F.J., Kandel, E.R., and Marshall, W.H., 1960, Effect of gamma-aminobutyric acid (GABA) on K^{42} outflow from rabbit cortex. J. Neurophysiol., 23:237.

Deschenes, M., and Feltz, P., 1976, GABA-induced rise of extracellular potassium in dorsal root ganglia: an electrophysiological study in vivo, Brain Res., 118:494.

Kudo, Y., and Fukuda, H., 1976, Alteration of extracellular K^+ activity induced by amino-acids in the frog spinal cord, Jpn. J.Pharmacol., 26:385.

Lux, H.D., and Neher, E., 1973, The equilibration time course of $[K^+]_o$ in cat cortex, Exp. Brain Res., 17:190.

Richter, D.W., Camerer, H., and Sonnhof, V., 1978, Changes in extracellular potassium during the spontaneous activity of medullary respiratory neurones, Pflügers Arch., 376:139.

Schwartzkroin,P.A., 1975, Characteristics of CA1 neurons recorded intracellularly in the hippocampal slice, Brain Res., 85:423.

Segal, M., in press, Effects of 5HT on neurons in the hippocampal slice, J. Physiol.

Segal, M., and Gutnick, M.J., in press, Effects of serotonin on extracellular potassium concentration in the rat hippocampal slice, Brain Res.

THE SLOW COMPONENT OF THE DIRECT CORTICAL RESPONSE AND EXTRACELLULAR POTASSIUM

A.I. Roitbak[*], J. Machek, V. Pavlík, A.V. Bobrov[*], and I.V. Otcherashvili[*]

I.S. Beritashvili Institute of Physiology[*], Academy of Sciences, Georgian SSR, Tbilisi, and Institute of Physiology, Czechoslovak Academy of Sciences, Prague, Czechoslovakia

INTRODUCTION

Electrical impulses of definite intensity, when applied to the cortical surface under deep anaesthesia, elicit an electrical response, which consists of two negative components: 1. a dendritic potential which represents excitatory postsynaptic potentials (EPSPs) of apical dendrites, and/or 2. a slow negative potential (SNP) which has been suggested to result from additional postsynaptic depolarization of either apical dendrites (Goldring and O'Leary, 1960) or afferent fibres (Eccles, 1963). Alternative explanations of the nature of the latter component are hyperpolarization of the pyramidal cell somata in the depth (Li and Chou, 1962) or depolarization of glial cells due to increased extracellular potassium concentration $[K^+]_e$ following neuronal activity (Roitbak, 1963). The latter assumption was tested in the present study by comparing the time course of the SNP with the time course of $[K^+]_e$ transients elicited by single direct cortical stimuli.

METHODS

The experiments were performed on cats under Nembutal anaesthesia (60-80 mg/kg). All testing was made on the suprasylvian gyrus. The cortex was covered with a mixture of wax and vaseline. The temperature of the cortex was about 30 °C. Two stimulating silver electrodes insulated except for the tips, 0.2 mm in diameter, were placed 0.04 mm apart. The K^+ sensitive microelectrodes were manufactured by a modified procedure described by Walker (1971), Lux and Neher (1973), Kříž et al., (1974). The tips of the glass ion-selective

267

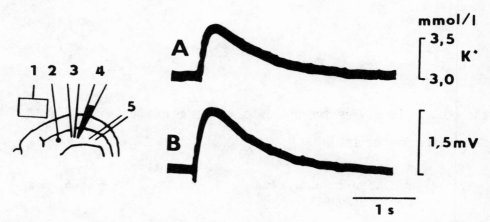

Fig. 1.   Extracellular K^+ change (A) and concurrent surface slow ne-
          gative potential (B) elicited by a single pulse to the cor-
          tical surface. Insert, scheme of electrode arrangement.
          1. Ag/AgCl common reference electrode in the neck muscles,
          2. AgCl silver ball electrode on the cortical surface,
          3. micropipette filled with NaCl, 4. ion-sensitive micro-
          pipette, 5. stimulating electrodes.

microelectrodes had a outer diameter of 3-4 μm. Each ion-selective
micropipette was first silanized and then filled with a liquid ion
exchanger (Corning 477317) and 0.5 mol/1 KCl. The second microelectrode with a diameter of less than 1 μm and resistance 10-30 MΩ which
served as reference for K^+ measurements and as the active electrode
for recording the field potential, was filled with a 1 mmol/1 NaCl
solution. The microelectrodes were fixed in a holder which made it
possible to maintain the inter-tip distance between 20-140 μm. The
distance between the recording and stimulating electrodes was 1 -
1.5 mm.

The $[K^+]_e$ was recorded simultaneously with the electrical cortical field potential using DC high impedance negative capacity input
preamplifiers (Kříž et al., 1974; Machek et al., 1975) and displayed
on two ink recorders KSP-4 or a double beam oscilloscope (Nihon
Kohden VC 8). The K^+ potential was correlated with the surface SNP
wave (Fig. 1), or with the field potential (Fig. 2).

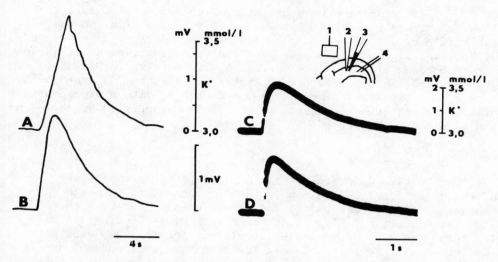

Fig. 2. Extracellular K$^+$ change (A,C) and concurrent field potential (B,D) elicited by a single pulse to the cortical surface. Insert, scheme of electrode arrangement. 1. Ag/AgCl common reference electrode in the neck muscles, 2. micropipette field with NaCl, 3. Ionsensitive micropipette, 4. stimulating electrode.

RESULTS

A single stimulus which elicited a SNP on the cortical surface resulted in an [K$^+$]$_e$ increase 0.5 - 1.5 mmol/l recorded at a depth of 300 μm in the cortex.

A K$^+$ transient of 0.6 mmol/l, photographed from the oscilloscope is presented in Fig. 1A; it demonstrates a slow time course with a rise time constant of about 45 ms and a decay time constant of 800 ms which means that it corresponds to the slow type of response (see Keller et al., in this volume). In Fig. 1B which was recorded simultaneously with A, a surface SNP is shown, with a rise time constant of 65 ms and a decay time constant of 800 ms.

Fig. 2 (A,B) demonstrates [K$^+$]$_e$ responses and field potentials. A very slow type (Keller et al., in this volume) is shown in the ink record (A,B). In A, the K$^+$ response exhibits a rise time constant

of 900 ms, a decay time constant of 1900 ms and total duration of
10 s. The field potential (B), which was recorded simultaneously
exhibits a rise time constant of 300 ms and a decay time constant
of 2300 ms. It can also be observed that the prestimulus levels were
not reached by either of the curves. A slow pattern (C,D) was photographed from the oscilloscope it lasted 3.7 s; the $[K^+]_e$ change (C)
rose with a time constant of 60 ms, and decayed with a time constant
of 1300 ms; the time constants of the field potential(D) were 100 ms
and 1300 ms, respectively.

DISCUSSION

Our results demonstrate that K^+ transients accompany the SNP
of the direct cortical response. The time course of both the $[K^+]_e$
changes and SNP correspond to the type two (slow)and type three
(very slow) cortical$[K^+]_e$ rises which were classified by analysing
the responses evoked by single stimuli applied to peripheral nerves
(Keller et al., in this volume). The rise time constants of hundreds
of milliseconds characteristic of the very slow K^+ transients in our
experiments were also found in intracellular records of glial depolarizations elicited by direct cortical stimulation (Roitbak and
Fanardjian,1979). The similarity in the time course of the three
phenomena very slow K^+ transients, SNPs and glial depolarizations
which all exhibited time constants of several hundreds of milliseconds, suggests that glial depolarization caused by excess K^+ released from active neurones is the main factor which produces the
SNP wave of the direct cortical response. This conclusion is in accord with previous experiments in which the SNP component of the
direct cortical response selectively disappeared after the selective
destruction of glial elements by X-irradiation (Roitbak et al., 1968;
Roitbak, 1970).

As the SNPs which exhibited the time constants of the rise of
50 - 60 ms do not correlate with the time course of glial depolarizations, it seems likely that other mechanisms are involved in the
onset of their generation such as a presynaptic $[K^+]_e$ dependent or
postsynaptic transmitter dependent depolarization of neural elements
(dendrites or fibres). In the patterns in which the SNP rises faster
than $[K^+]_e$, a transmitter dependent EPSPs may be suspected to contribute to the SNP.

The presence of a cortical response under deep barbiturate
anaesthesia deserves a comment on the possible sources of the K^+
transients (see Somjen, 1979). Since it has been repeatedly shown
(Stohr et al., 1963) that a direct cortical stimulus stopped unit
firing, neuronal action potentials are unlikely to be the main source
of the excess K^+. We were also unable to see any units in our experiments, despite the fact that our equipment was capable of recording them.

The present data do not allow valuable estimates which of the possible K^+ sources contributes most to K^+ emission from neuronal membranes activated by direct, orthodromic and antidromic excitation of axons or postsynaptic excitation and inhibition. From the post-synaptic processes, IPSPs would be a more potent and important K^+ source than EPSPs for the following reasons: 1. barbiturates potentiate the GABA-mediated inhibition in the central nervous system of vertebrates (Morris, 1978), 2. postsynaptic inhibitory potentials last many times longer than the EPSPs and thus provide more time for K^+ to escape from neurones (Coles and Tsacopoulos, 1979). But prolonged depolarization of apical dendrites and fibres as demonstrated during SNP by Roitbak (1970) could also contribute significantly to the K^+ transients.

CONCLUSION

Similarity in time course between glial depolarizations, the very slow type SNP, and concurrent K^+ transients is in accord with the presumption, that the main factor generating SNP is glial depolarization by excess K^+ released from active neurones.

Depolarization of neuronal structures probably participates in those SNPs the rise time constants of which are faster than those of glial depolarizations.

REFERENCES

Coles, J.A., and Tsacopoulos, M., 1979, K^+ activity in photoreceptors, glial cells and extracellular space in the drone retina: changes during photostimulation, J. Physiol., 290:525.

Eccles, J.C., 1963, Discussion, Progr. in Brain Res., 1:163.

Goldring, S., and O'Leary, J.L., 1960, Pharmacological dissolution of evoked cortical potentials, Feder. Proc., 19:612.

Kříž, N., Syková, E., Ujec, E., and Vyklický, L., 1974, Changes of extracellular potassium concentration induced by neuronal activity in the spinal cord of the cat, J. Physiol., 238:1.

Li, C.L., and Chou, S.N., 1962, Cortical intracellular synaptic potentials and direct cortical stimulation, J. Cell comp. Physiol., 60:1.

Lux, H.D., and Neher, E., 1973, The equilibrium time course of $[K^+]_o$ in cat cortex, Exp. Brain Res., 17:190.

Machek, J., Ujec, E., and Pavlík, V., 1975, Cortical extracellular potassium concentration during the development of the intra-hemispheric response into the selfsustained afterdischarge, Physiol. bohemoslov., 24:41.

Morris, M.E., 1978, The effect of anaesthesia on extracellular K^+ activity in the central nervous system, Arzneim.-Forsch. Drug Res., 28:875.

Roitbak, A.I., 1963,, On the nature of cortical inhibition (In Russian), Zh.vysh.nerv.Deyat., 13:859.

Roitbak, A.I., 1970, On negative components of the cortical direct
    response (In Russian), Neirophysiologya, 2:339.
Roitbak, A.I., and Fanardjian, V.V., 1979, Analysis of changes of
    the membrane potential of glial cells of the cortex at its elec-
    trical stimulation (In Russian), in: "Functions of Neuroglia",
    A.I. Roitbak, ed., Metsniereba, Tbilisi.
Roitbak, A.I., Nadareishvili, K.Sh., and Moiseienko, K.I., 1968,
    Analysis of electrical cortical p entials in the X-irradiated
    hemispheres of the brain (In Russian), in: Sovr. Probl. Deyat.
    Stroi. Nerv. Sist., Metsniereba, Tbilisi.
Somjen, G.G., 1979, Extracellular potassium in the mammalian central
    nervous system, Ann. Rev. Physiol., 41:159.
Stohr, P.E., Goldring, S., and O'Leary,J.L., 1963, Patterns of unit
    discharge associated with direct cortical response in monkey and
    cat, Electroenceph. clin. Neurophysiol., 15:882.
Walker, J.L.,Jr., 1971, Ion-specific liquid ion-exchanger micro-
    electrodes, Analyt. chem., 43:89A.

POTASSIUM CHANGES ELICITED IN THE FELINE SOMATOSENSORY CORTEX BY A SINGLE STIMULUS TO THE PERIPHERAL NERVE

O. Keller, E. Ujec, V. Pavlík and J. Machek

Institute of Physiology
Czechoslovak Academy of Sciences
Vídeňská 1083, 142 20 Prague 4, Czechoslovakia

INTRODUCTION

In previous studies we measured changes in extracellular potassium concentration ($[K^+]_e$) elicited by repetitive stimulation in the cerebral cortex. Cortical K^+ responses to single stimuli were buried in the noise to such a degree that they could not be differentiated for accurate measurements (Machek et al., 1975; 1976). This drawback of conventional double-barrel electrodes which were used in these studies was overcome by low-noise K^+ selective, coaxial, double-barrel microelectrodes (ISCM) (Ujec et al., 1979; 1980 and in this volume) which make it possible to measure very small and rapid changes in K^+ concentration.

The aim of this study was to classify various types of K^+ transients, evoked in the cortex by a single stimulus to a peripheral nerve, according to their time course.

METHODS

Cats anaesthetized with chloralose, immobilized by Flaxedil and artificially ventilated, were used in experiments in which blood pressure, pCO_2 in the expired air and rectal temperature were monitored and maintained within standard limits (more than 90 kPa, 3-4.5 CO_2, 38 $\pm$ 0.5 $^{\circ}C$, respectively). Trephine openings were made in the skull over the primary somatosensory region. The infraorbital and radial nerves contralateral to the recording site were stimulated by rectangular electrical pulses (0.1-0.3 ms, voltage less than 15 V, 0.1-6 Hz) applied via bipolar stainless steel electrodes inserted under the skin. The K^+ sensitive ion exchanger Corning Code Number

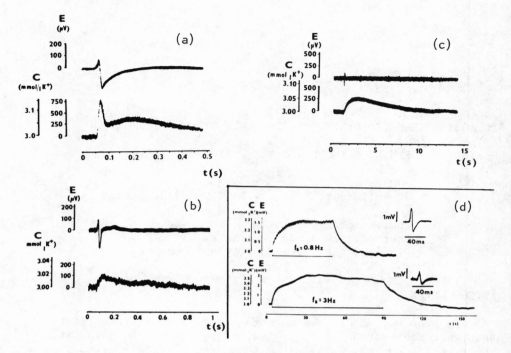

Fig. 1.   Types of single K^+ transients elicited in the somatosensory
          cortex by single electrical stimuli applied to the radial
          nerve (a,b,c). Small summated cortical K^+ changes elicited
          by repetitive stimulation of the infraorbital nerve (d).
          Upper traces in a,b,c, and insets in d, field potentials.
          Lower traces in a,b,c, K^+ transients. Note different time
          scales. C, calibration of K^+ concentration changes. E, ca-
          libration of electrical potential changes.

477317 was used in the sensitive channel of the ISCMs. The K^+ signal
was measured between the K^+ sensitive and reference channels of the
ISCM, and the field potential between the reference channel and an
Ag/AgCl electrode inserted in the neck muscles.

RESULTS

Classification of K^+ changes according to their time course

        The ISCMs enabled us to detect small changes in $[K^+]_e$ as small
as 10 μmol/1 (Ujec et al., 1979). In response to single peripheral

stimuli, we recorded K^+ transients of 20-200 μmol/l amplitude in the cortex of the cat. Three types of K^+ signals could be differentiated according to their time course: 1. The first type reaching 30-200 μmol/l K^+ was characterized by a short ascending phase with a time constant 4-6 ms (see Ujec et al., in this volume), and total duration of 40-50 ms. An example of this is shown in Fig. 1a, in which the lower trace demonstrates the K^+ transient and the upper trace the field potential. The fast K^+ signal is seen in front of the slower K^+ transient (which is classified as type two). In Fig. 2, left, the fast K^+ transient is shown alone. 2. The type two K^+ response lasted about one second or less. Its rise time constant was 20-60 ms and maximum increase 20-50 μmol/l. It appeared either in the wake of the type one K^+ transient (Fig. 1a, lower trace) or was solitary (Fig. 1b lower trace). 3. The type three K^+ response (Fig. 1c, lower trace) lasted several seconds, its maximum rise was 50-100 μmol/l and its time constant was 150-1000 ms.

Temporal summation of single K^+ responses

Only the type two and type three of K^+ transients summated at low frequency stimulation 0.8-3 Hz (Fig. 1d). The summation of accumulated K^+ reached 0.3-0.6 mmol/l and displayed characteristics similar to those observed following repetitive interhemispheric stimulation, i.e. an exponential rise, a more or less stabilized ceiling during stimulation followed by a poststimulation undershoot. In Fig. 1d, the upper trace represents a summated K^+ response to repetitive 0.8 Hz stimulation of the infraorbital nerve. After about 20 stimuli, K^+ activity reached its plateau exceeding the resting level by 300 μmol/l. Note that the response evoked by the first stimulus made up one third of the total K^+ elevation. A higher rate of stimulation - 3 Hz (Fig.1d, lower trace) - raised the K^+ level by 600 μmol/l. In this case, there was thus a twofold increase of $[K^+]_e$ for an approximately fourfold increase of stimulation frequency. Samples of the concurrent evoked phasic field potentials are seen in corresponding insets of Fig.1d. When repetitive stimulation of 0.8-6 Hz was applied in situations which a single stimulus evoked the K^+ transient of the first type, the K^+ signal progressively diminished with each subsequent stimulus of the train to give no response. The coinciding field potentials remained basically unchanged.

Localization of K^+ transients

Only the fast K^+ signals of the first type were sharply localized within several hundreds of micrometers in the cortex as is illustrated in Fig. 2 which demonstrates field potentials (upper traces) and K^+ signals (lower traces) recorded at various depths of the cortex. The records on the left side represent measurements at 1000 μm, the records in the middle at 1250 μm and those on the right hand side at 1500 μm. It can be seen that the increase of $[K^+]_e$ was only observed

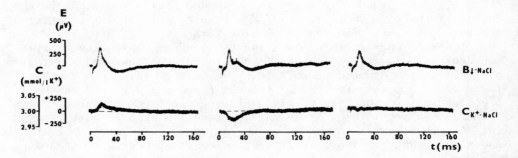

Fig. 2. Spatial distribution of the fast K^+ transients. Top traces, field potentials. Bottom traces, K^+ transients. Left, 1000 μm depth; middle, 1250 μm depth; right, 1750 μm depth. $B\downarrow$-NaCl, symbol indicating potential difference between the common Ag/AgCl reference electrode and the NaCl filled reference barrel of the ISCM. C_{K^+-NaCl}, potential difference between both barrels of the ISCM (see Ujec et al., this volume).

at the depth 1000 μm and that 250 μm deeper there was a transient decrease of $[K^+]_e$. At 1750 μm the K^+ response dissappeared completely. Similar patterns of responses were repeatedly observed at particular depths irrespectively of whether the electrode was moved in or out. The type two and type three K^+ transient gradually decreased within millimeter distances as the ISCMs were removed from the recording site of their maximum amplitude. A detailed analysis of their spatial distribution was not attempted.

DISCUSSION

We presume that the considerable differences in time parameters of K^+ changes reflect various types of processes responsible for K^+ movements in the extracellular space. We suggest that the fast type one K^+ transients reflect short distance space-independent K^+ exchange (Nicholson, 1980) between the intracellular and extracellular compartments, whereas the longlasting K^+ signals of the third type indicate the presence of a K^+ flux maintained over larger distances through brain tissue which is carried, at least partially, through cells, very probably of glial origin (Orkand et al., 1966; Somjen and Trachtenberg, 1979; Gardner-Medwin in Nicholson, 1980 and Coles and Tsacopoulos, in this volume).

The finding that a primary single stimulus transiently reduced $[K^+]_e$ may be relevant to that reported in the lateral geniculate body (Singer and Lux, 1975, Fig. 2G), where a primary K^+ decrease was detected by the averaging technique. This decrease was elicited by an electrical stimulus applied to the optic chiasm, lasted five seconds and exhibited a rise time constant of about 900 ms. In contrast to the fast K^+ decrease found by us, Singer and Lux's $[K^+]_e$ reduction was very slow and it is therefore not certain whether the same mechanisms are involved. Although no direct evidence in this respect can be presented, we can speculate that the fast "reflex" K^+ decreases may result from a synaptically induced transient arrest of ongoing K^+ releasing activities which maintain the $[K^+]_e$ resting level or a transient stepping up of K^+ pumping mechanisms responsible for the maintenance of the resting transmembrane K^+ concentration gradient.

CONCLUSIONS

1. K^+ sensitive, coaxial, double-barrel microelectrodes operating at a very low noise levels have made it possible to record and analyse single, very small K^+ transients in the cerebral cortex elicited by single stimuli to peripheral nerves.

2. Single K^+ signals of 20 to 200 $\mu mol/l$ were detected and classified according to their time course – as fast, slow and very slow.

3. It is being suggested that the single fast K^+ transients result from a direct K^+ exchange between the intracellular and extracellular compartments, whereas the very slow single K^+ changes probably reflect K^+ fluxes over longer distances carried by glial cells.

4. The single fast K^+ signals mirrored $[K^+]_e$ increases as well as $[K^+]_e$ reductions. They were sharply localized in the cortex at a distance of several hundreds of micrometers from each other.

REFERENCES

Machek, J., Ujec, E., and Pavlík V., 1975, Cortical extracellular potassium concentration during the development of the interhemispheric responses into the selfsustained afterdischarge, Physiol. bohemoslov., 24:41.

Machek, J., Ujec, E., and Pavlík, V., 1976, Extracellular potassium concentration and focal electrical potentials elicited in the cerebral cortex of rat by interhemispheric stimulation, Neuroscience Letters., 2:147.

Nicholson, Ch., 1980, Dynamics of the brain cell microenvironment, Neurosciences Res.Prog.Bull., 18:211.

Orkand, R.K., Nichols, J.G., and Kuffler, S.W., 1966, Effect of nerve impulses on the membrane potential of glial cells in the central nervous system of amphibia, J. Neurophysiol., 29:788.

Singer, W., and Lux, H.D., 1975, Extracellular potassium gradients and visual receptive fields in the cat striate cortex, Brain Research, 96:378.

Somjen, G.G., and Trachtenberg, M., 1979, Neuroglia as generator of extracellular current, in: "Origin of cerebral field potentials", E.-J. Speckmann and H. Caspers, eds., Georg Thieme Publishers, Stuttgart.

Ujec, E., Keller, O., Kříž, N., Pavlík, V., and Machek,J., 1980, Low-impedance, coaxial, ion-selective, double-barrel microelectrodes and their use in biological measurements, Bioelectrochemistry and bioenergetics, 7:363.

Ujec, E., Keller, O., Machek, J., and Pavlík, V., 1979, Low impedance coaxial K^+ selective electrodes, Pflügers Arch., 382:189.

THE MECHANISM AND INTEGRATIVE ROLE OF EXTRACELLULAR POTASSIUM

CLEARANCE IN THE RAT BRAIN

Jiří Křivánek, Jan Bureš, Vera I. Koroleva, Malla M.Reddy

Institute of Physiology
Czechoslovak Academy of Sciences
Prague, Czechoslovakia

INTRODUCTION

Both physiological and pathological forms of nervous activity are accompanied by K^+ release into the extracellular space (Somjen, 1979; Varon and Somjen, 1979). Various hypotheses atribute the $[K^+]e$ increase an important function in presynaptic inhibition (Kříž et al., 1975), neural plasticity (Roitbak, 1976) and epileptogenesis (Lux, 1974). The integrative role of K^+ accumulation in the extracellular space of brain neuropile is best demonstrated in the case of Leao's (1944) spreading depression (SD). A selfpropagating neurohumoral phenomenon mediated by a depolarizing substance, which is released from depolarized neurons in quantities sufficient to depolarize the adjacent nerve cells. Potassium ions are the most likely SD transmitter (Grafstein, 1956; Bureš et al., 1974). During the peak of SD wave$[K^+]e$ attains 40-70 mmol/l. Increase of $[K^+]e$ from the resting level of 3 mmol/l above the threshold value of 10 mmol/l is an essential prerequisite for induction and propagation of SD.

RESULTS

Blockade of SD by local brain stimulation

Whether $[K^+]e$ reaches the SD threshold or not depends on various influences affecting the steady state of $[K^+]e$ and modifying the susceptibility of the tissue toward SD-inducing agents (SD susceptibility). Intensity of the K^+-clearance from the extracellular space is such a factor. Under "basal" clearance intensity threshold depolarization of a critical volume of brain tissue elicits SD. However, when clearance is intensive enough to prevent $[K^+]e$ accumulation above the

279

level essential for SD propagation, the brain tissue becomes SD resistant.

Such a state can be induced by intensive electrical or chemical stimulation of the rat cerebral cortex (Fig. 1). Stimulation by electrical pulses (0.1 ms, 15 V, 6 Hz) or penicillin induced epileptic activity (spike frequency 3 Hz) block SD penetration into the stimulated area, in which $[K^+]e$ is raised to ceiling level of 10 mmol/1. The SD blockade, manifested by absence of the slow potential shift and of the $[K^+]e$ transient (above 40 mmol/1) persists for several minutes after cessation of stimulation, that is at a time when the $[K^+]e$ has returned to or below the resting level.

It is now widely accepted that under conditions of the above experiments, increased intensity of the extracellular $[K^+]$ clearance accounts for the ceiling of K^+ rise and for the undershoot of $[K^+]e$ after stimulation arrest. Blockade of SD propagation into the stimulated area is not due to K^+ depletion of the stimulated neurons and to diminished K^+ outflux, but rather to increased efficiency of the K^+ clearing mechanism which prevents $[K^+]e$ to rise to and above the SD-threshold value.

Role of vanadate in the activation of $(Na^+ + K^+)$ ATPase

The mechanism of the K^+-clearance, particularly the cellular aspects of the problem, have been intensively discussed (Hertz, 1978; Somjen, 1979; Walton and Sombjen, 1979; Orkand, 1980). It is generally agreed that clearance is accomplished by active metabolically supported pumping of K^+ mediated by the $(Na^+ + K^+)$ATPase, rather than by passive diffusion.

A possible mechanism of activation of the $(Na^+ + K^+)$ ATPase by intensive stimulation was revealed in our experiments in which activity of this enzyme was measured in the homogenates from the rat cerebral cortex stimulated at intensity leading to SD blockade. Increased activity of $(Na^+ + K^+)$ATPase was found when a Sigma-Grade ATP preparation, containing vanadate as a contaminant, was used as substrate with 20 mmol/1 $[K^+]$ in the assay medium. Vanadate is a potent inhibitor of $Na^+ + K^+$ ATPase in the presence of high potassium (20 mmol/1). With low $[K^+]$ in the medium, vanadate is inactive and preparations from both resting and stimulated cortex show the same activity approaching that found in the stimulated cortex. It seemed, therefore, that electrical stimulation induced disinhibition of the enzyme, probably by decreasing its suceptibility toward vanadate inhibition. This assumption was supported by the finding that vanadate $(2.5.10^{-7} mol/1)$ in the presence of 20 mmol/1 K^+ inhibits activity of the ATPase from the normal, but not from the stimulated cortex (Fig.1)

From the kinetic data, obtained in the studies into the mechanism of vanadate inhibition, Cantley et al. (1977) concluded, that

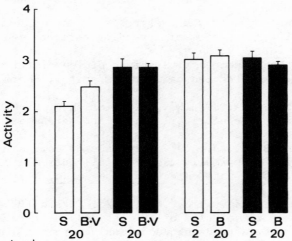

Fig. 1. (Na^++K^+)ATPase(μmol Pi/h/01 mg prot) of the rat cerebral cortex homogenates in the presence of the following ATP preparations: Sigma-Grade S contaminated with vanadate, Boehringer (B) without vanadate or with added $2.5.10^{-7}$M vanadate (B+V) . $[K^+]$: 2 or 20 mmol/1 . White and black columns: homogenates from control and electrically stimulated cortex, respectively.

under resting conditions, when vanadate is accessible to its binding site in the enzyme, at least 50% of (Na^++K^+)ATPase is inactive. Releasing vanadate from the binding site causes activation of the enzyme. The apparently diminished sensitivity of the enzyme toward the inhibitory action of vanadate (decreased affinity of the enzyme for vanadate) shown in our experiments may be interpreted as a manifestation of an active, disinhibited state of the enzyme, which is responsible for intensive clearing of potassium from the extracellular space.

CONCLUSION

The non-uniform spatial distribution of the active and inactive (Na^++K^+) ATPase may play the role of an integrative factor in the generation of reverberating SD, recurrent seizures and anomalous SD propagation (Koroleva and Bureš, 1979; 1980) and in other phenomena due to interaction between the resting, depressed and stimulated cortex.

REFERENCES

Bureš, J., Burešová , O.,and Křivánek, J., 1974, "The Mechanism and Application of Leao's Spreading Depression of Electroencephalographic Activity", Academia, Prague.
Cantley, L.C., Josephson, L., Warner, R., Yanagisawa, M., Lechene, C., and Guidotti, G., 1977, Vanadate is a potent (Na, K)-ATPase in-

hibitor found in ATP derived from muscle, J. Biol. Chem., 252:7421.

Grafstein, B., 1956, Mechanism of spreading cortical depression, J. Neurophysiol., 19:154.

Hertz, L., 1977, Drug-induced alterations of ion distribution at the cellular level of the central nervous system, Pharmacol.Rev., 29:35.

Koroleva, V.I.,and Bureš, J., 1979, Circulation of cortical spreading depression around electrically stimulated areas and epileptic foci in the neocortex of rats, Brain Res., 173:209.

Koroleva, V.I.,and Bureš, J., 1979, Blockade of cortical spreading depression in electrically and chemically stimulated areas of cerebral cortex in rats, Electroenceph. clin. Neurophysiol., 48:1.

Kříž, N., Syková, E.,and Vyklický, L., 1975, Extracellular potassium changes in the spinal cord of the cat and their relation to slow potentials, active transport and impulse transmission, J. Physiol. (London),248:167.

Leao, A.A.P., 1944, Spreading depression of activity in the cerebral cortex, J. Neurophysiol., 7:359.

Lux, H.D., 1974, The kinetics of extracellular potassium:relation to epileptogenesis, Epilepsia, 15:375.

Orkand, R.K., 1980, Extracellular potassium accumulation in the nervous sytem, Federation Proc., 39:1515.

Roitbak, A.I., 1976, "Function of Neuroglia", Metsniereba, Tbilisi.

Somjen, G.G., 1979, Extracellular potassium in the mammalian central nervous system, Ann. Rev. Physiol., 41:159.

Varon, S.,and Somjen, G.G., 1979, Neuron-glia interactions, Neurosci. Res. Prog.Bull., 17:1.

SESSION V
IONIC ACTIVITY CHANGES IN THE HEART AND SKELETAL MUSCLE

K^+ ACCUMULATION AND ITS PHYSIOLOGICAL REGULATORY ROLE IN HEART MUSCLE

M. Morad and G. Martin

Department of Physiology, School of Medicine
University of Pennsylvania, Philadelphia, PA 19104 U.S.A.

Electrophysiological as well as direct measurements of K^+ activity in heart muscle in the last decade suggest that ionic accumulation or depletion occurs under a variety of experimental conditions in the extracellular space (Niedergierke and Orkand, 1966; Kline and Morad, 1976; Kunze, 1977; Baumgarten and Isenberg, 1977; Martin and Morad, 1978; Morad, 1980). Although most of the quantitative data for ionic accumulation or depletion is obtained for K^+, direct and indirect experimental evidence is accumulating to suggest that significant intracellular accumulations of Na^+ and Ca^{2+} may also occur under a variety of experimental conditions (Deitmer and Ellis, 1978; Glitsch, 1972; Thomas, 1972; Langer, 1968). It is in fact, increasingly popular to suggest that intracellular or extracellular ionic accumulations play important local regulatory roles in controlling the electrical and mechanical events of the heart muscle under a variety of physiological and pharmacological interventions. For instance the ionotropic events associated with increased frequency of stimulations or exposure to cardiac glycosides, or variation in $[Na]_0$ or $[K]_0$ are suggested to be associated with alterations of $[Na]_i$ and $[Ca]_i$ which leads to the altered contractile state (Langer, 1973; Glitsch, Reuter and Scholz, 1970; Eisner and Lederer, 1979).

Although experimentally induced ionic accumulation or depletion occur for all of the physiologically important cations, in this communication we shall limit our discussion to directly measured accumulations or depletions of K^+ in the paracellular space of frog ventricular strips and consider their possible physiological or regulatory roles in controlling the excitable events in heart muscle.

MATERIALS AND METHODS

Double-barrel K^+ selective μ-electrode (2-4 μm in diameter) were prepared by placing a K^+ selective ion exchange resin (corning no. 474317) in one barrel and normal Ringers in the other (Kline and Morad, 1976). The output of the reference barrel was subtracted from that of Resin-containing barrel to eliminate possible artifacts due to local electrical fields. Only those electrodes were used which responded rapidly and to the same extent to changes of $[K^+]$, irrespective of whether the electrode was placed in the bath or in the extracellular space of the muscle (Kline and Morad, 1978). The selectivity of the K^+ electrode was found to be about 50/1 for K^+/Na^+ and 200/1 for K^+/Ca^{2+}. In some experiments K^+ activity was measured in frog ventricular strips which were voltage clamped using single sucrose gap voltage clamp technique (Cleemann and Morad, 1979a). Rabbit ventricular tissue, SA nodal strips, and frog ventricular tissue all essentially showed a similar K^+ accumulation or depletion profile in response to alterations of frequency.

TIME COURSE AND MAGNITUDE OF K^+ ACCUMULATION IN HEART MUSCLE

Figure 1 shows that K^+ activity increases continuously during the time course of a single action potential. $[K^+]$ decays back to resting level after the onset of rapid repolarization. On repetitive stimulation single beat accumulations seem to produce an increase in baseline K^+ concentrations which is often accompanied by depolarization of the resting membrane potential. The increase in paracellular K^+ activity accompanying a single action potential ranged between 0.5 to 1.0 mM. This amount of accumulation is equivalent to an efflux of 10-20 pmols. cm^{-2} sec^{-1} of K^+ (assuming a subenothelial accumulating space of 9%, and surface to volume ratio of 1.1; (Page and Niedergierke, 1972). Somewhat smaller single beat accumulations (0.05 to 0.1 mM) were measured in the rabbit SA nodal preparations (Maylie, Morad and Weiss, 1981). The increase in K^+ activity in the paracellular space ranging from 0.1 to 1.0 mM are sufficiently small as to be of little significance physiologically. However, it is important to remember that the magnitude of accumulation is directly related to the size and volume of accumulating space, which no doubt must be markedly distorted by a 2-4 μm electrode tip. Thus the electrode cannot directly sample the true increase in the smaller paracellular space or cellular clefts of 200-1000 Å. The actual changes in the activity of K^+ in these smaller and undistorted paracellular spaces has to be considerably larger, and may in fact exert a physiological role in controlling the electrical activity of the cardiac muscle.

Measurements of local changes in K^+ activity using K^+ electrode was made possible because of fairly high selectivity of the ion-exchanger resin to K^+ as compared to Na^+ (50-60 to 1). It is fair,

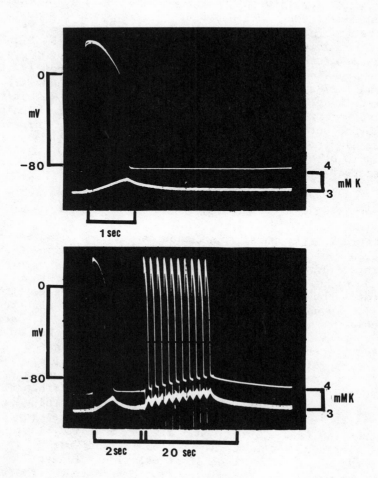

Fig. 1. Top panel: Simultaneous measurement of transmembrane potentil (upper trace) and K$^+$ activity (lower trace) during a
single action potential. A ground clamped double barrelled
K$^+$-selective electrode was used. Note the steady increase
in K$^+$ activity during the plateau phase of the action
potential. Bottom panel: As the stimulus frequency is
suddenly increased the interval between action potentials
decreases resulting in summation of the single accumulations
and membrane depolarization. Temperature, 22°C; [Ca^{2+}] =
0.2 mM (from Kline and Morad, unpublished records).

therefore, to suggest that in the presence of large and homogeneous changes in K^+ activity in the paracellular space, the resting membrane potential should also detect the transient changes in the K^+ concentration (because of its high selectivity for K^+ vs. Na^+). Detailed comparison between the profile of K^+ accumulation or depletion in the extracellular space as sensed by the resting ventricular membrane and K^+-selective μ-electrode were made recently (Cleemann and Morad, 1979a). It was concluded that both methods are equally sensitive in detecting changes in $[K]_0$. While, K^+-selective electrodes suffer from imposing a distortion on the paracellular space, the membrane potential as a "sensor" of K^+ activity suffers from possible electrogenic activity imposed on the membrane by $Na-K^+$ ATPase pump or other transporters activated during a physiological or pharmacological intervention.

K^+ ACCUMULATION AND K^+ REUPTAKE

Figure 1 lower panel shows that the rate-induced accumulation of K^+ decays back to resting levels after termination of short stimulus train. Time course of K^+ accumulation and its reuptake with longer duration "stimulus trains" are slightly different. Figure 2 illustrates the time course of K^+ accumulation in a ventricular strip in response to onset and termination of four different frequencies of stimulation. Note that in response to each stimulus frequency K^+ activity at first increases rapidly, then decays slowly to a steady state level. On termination of stimulation, K^+ activity decreases rapidly and undershoots below resting values. This actual paracellular depletion of K^+ below resting level suggests that reuptake process is active and that the process is sufficiently rapid as to overcome the equilibrating effects of higher bathing $[K]$, diffusing continuously into the paracellular space. Thus the slow diffusion of K^+ from the paracellular space allows for fairly large transient accumulation during the stimulation period and fairly large depletions of K^+ after termination of stimulation. Figure 2 also shows that the magnitude of K^+ depletion is related to the frequency of stimulation before the termination of "train". The accumulation profile, specifically the depletion of K^+ below bath concentration seems to be strongly attenuated by ionic or pharmacological interventions. For instance, increases in bathing $[K]$ increase the post stimulus depletion, while reducing bathing K concentration to about 1.5 mM strongly suppresses the depletion process. Figure 3 compares the effect of changing the bathing K concentrations on the accumulation and depletion profiles of K^+ in the paracellular space. Note that for any duration of stimulation, the bathing $[K]$ of 1.5 mM strongly suppresses while K^+ concentrations of 5.4 mM enchance the magnitude of paracellular depletion. Figure 3 also shows that although the bathing K^+ concentration alters the magnitude of depletion, the duration of "stimulus-train" seems to impose an even stronger influence on the magnitude of K^+ depletion. For instance,

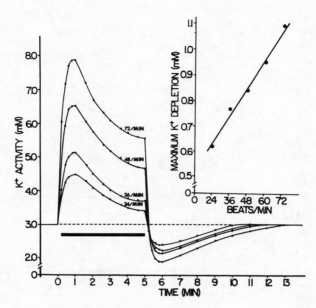

Figure 2.   Frequency dependence of K$^+$ accumulation and depletion.
            K$^+$ activity changes during and following stimulus trains
            of 24, 36, 48, and 72 beats/min ares shown. Inset
            (graph) shows the relation between the magnitude of
            maximum depletion and stimulus train frequency. Tem-
            perature, 23°C; [Ca^{2+}]$_0$ = 0.2 mM. (From Morad,1980).

note that in bathing K$^+$ concentrations of 3 or 5 mM termination of
stimulation within the first minute of the onset of stimulation does
not result in appreciable depletion of K$^+$ even though the paracellular concentrations of K$^+$ are very high 5.5 to 7.0 mM during this
time. With prolongation of stimulation period, even though paracellular K$^+$ concentration of K$^+$ are decreasing, post-stimulation
depletion continues to increase in magnitude. This finding suggests
that possible accumulation of Na$^+$ in an intracellular compartment
plays an important role in controlling the magnitude of post-stimulation depletion of K$^+$ from the paracellular space.

    Figure 4 compares the effect of frequency-induced accumulation
in the presence and absence of ouabain. Note that not only K$^+$ depletion below bath concentrations is completely suppressed but that
accumulation is no longer transient in nature. A similar change in
the profile of accumulation and depletion were observed when Li$^+$ was
replaced for Na in the bathing solutions. The finding that addition
of ouabain or replacement of 75% of [Na]$_0$ with Li$^+$, abolished the
post-stimulation depletion of K$^+$, supports the hypothesis that the
Na-pump plays a crucial role in accumulation and depletion processes.

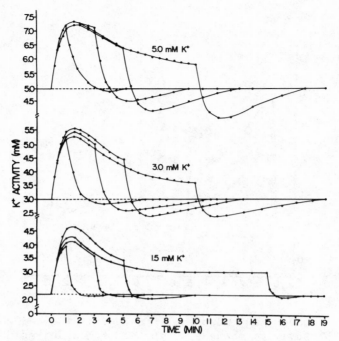

Figure 3. Effect of changes of bathing K^+ concentrations of K^+ accumulation and depletion. These curves represent linearization of original records. Muscles are stimulated for 1, 3, 5, and 10 min at 48/ min in solutions containing 1.5, 3.0 and 5.0 mM K^+. Note that increasing $[K^+]$ in the perfusate from 3.0 mM to 5.0 mM, increases the magnitude of K^+ depletion and decreasing $[K^+]$ in the perfusate from 3.0 mM to 1.5 mM decreases the magnitude of K^+ depletion. Temperature, $23°C$; $[Ca^{2+}]_0 = 0.2$ mM (from Morad, 1980).

These findings also suggest that Na^+-pump also influences the transient nature of accumulation profile, since in the presence of ouabain the accumulation profile changes markedly (Figure 4).

In experiments in which membrane potential was simultaneously monitored during the accumulation and depletion profiles, transient depolarization followed by steady state depolarization and finally a hyperpolarization at termination of stimulation could be consistantly recorded. On some occassion the transient depolarization was followed by return of the resting potential back to control level even though an increase in the extracellular K^+ was monitored. This finding supports the hypothesis that the $Na^+ - K^+$ ATPase system in heart muscle operates in an electrogenic manner.

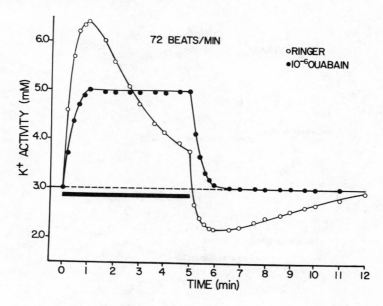

Figure 4.   Effect of ouabian on K^+ accumulation and depletion. Superimposed on a control stimulus train (0-0) at 72 shocks/min
is a stimulus train of the same frequency and duration
carried out after exposure of the preparation to 10^{-6} M
ouabain. Note the lack of K^+ redistribution during the
stimulus train and depleting phase following exposure of the
preparation to ouabain. Temperature, $23°C$; $[Ca]_0 = 0.2$ mM.

"PRIMING OF K^+-UPTAKE RPOCESS"

The transient increase in paracellular $[K]$ in response to high
frequency of stimulation, may be in part caused by a delay in activation of K^+ reuptake process. In order to test this hypothesis we
attempted to first prime the uptake of K^+ and then monitor the rate-
induced accumulation profile. Figure 5, illustrates K^+ accumulation
and depletion profiles in a ventricular strip in which the preparation
was first subjected to 5 min "conditioning" frequency of 60 shocks/
min, followed by "test" frequency applied with various delays (12
sec top panel; 36 sec middle panel; and 60 sec, bottom panel) after
termination of "conditioning" train. Note that the time course of
K^+ accumulation accompanying the "test" train is strongly affected
by the degree of activation of the reuptake process. If K^+ reuptake
process is sufficiently stimulated it may completely suppress or prevent the rate-induced accumulation of K^+. These results suggest that
K^+ reuptake process may be strongly enhanced in beating vs. quiescent
preparation. The results also suggest that the K^+ reuptake process
may be more sensitive to changes of $[Na]_i$ as compared to those
occuring in $[K]_0$.

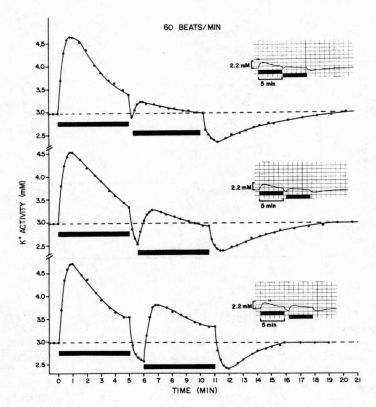

Figure 5.   "Pump priming" experiment. The tracings represent "lin-
            earizations" of the original records shown as insets.
            Stimulus trains of 60 shocks/min were initiated and
            maintained for 5 min after which time stimulation was
            terminated to allow for removal of K^+. Following three
            different periods, 12 sec top, 36 sec middle, and 1 min
            in bottom panel, a second stimulus train of 60 shocks/
            min was initiated and maintained for 5 min. Note that
            the earlier the second stimulus train is initiated in the
            reuptake of K^+ following the first train, the smaller
            the K^+ accumulation during the second train. Temperature,
            $23^\circ C$; $[Ca]_0 = 0.2$ mM.

VOLTAGE-DEPENDENCE OF K^+ ACCUMULATION

     Figure 6 shows the voltage dependence of accumulation and de-
pletion of K^+ in the paracellular space in response to clamp steps
of 5 seconds in duration. The change in K^+ activity in the paracellular space is monitored both with K^+-selective μ-electrode and
resting membrane potential. That is, the clamp pulse is terminated
and membrane is allowed to return to potential determined by E_K.
At the end of the clamp pulse membrane current, the post clamp after

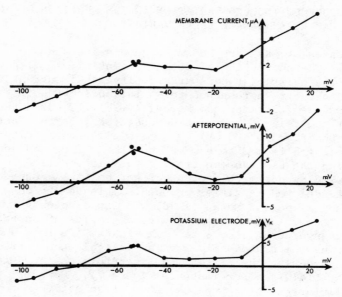

Figure 6. Simultaneous measurement membrane current, and K^+ electrode response versus the changed membrane potential. The duration of the clamp pulses was 5 sec. The membrane current is measured at the end of the clamp pulse. The after potential and K^+ electrode response were measured 0.5 sec after the termination of pulse. Note that the three curves are similar in shape with a maxima around -55 mV and minima around -20 mV (modified from Cleemann and Morad, 1979a).

potential, and the K^+ activity are measured. The voltage dependence of K^+ accumulation as sensed by the membrane or K^+-electrode are similar to the steady-state I-V relation. The N-shaped relation with respect to membrane potential is clearly apparent in all three parameters measured. These results suggest that the turnoff of K^+ current at potential around -20 mV is primarily responsible for the N-shaped nature of the steady state I-V relations. Investigations of the kinetics of activation of K^+ current and its differential blocking suggests that two distinct K^+ transport mechanisms are operating to generate the N-shaped I-V relation. At potentials negative to -20 mV, K^+ current is transported through an inwardly rectifying system which is time independent and is effectively blocked by Cs^+ or Ba^{+2}. At potentials positive to -10 mV a time-dependent K^+ current seems to be activated which is not significantly altered by blockers of the inward rectifier channel. As it will be discussed in subsequent sections, it is the interaction of these two channels during rest and activity which seems to control the duration of the action potential in a beating preparation.

ARE THE FREQUENCY-INDUCED VARIATION IN THE DURATION OF ACTION
POTENTIAL CAUSED BY PARACELLULAR VARIATIONS OF $[K^+]_0$?

Increases of $[K]_0$ are known to depolarize and shorten the action
potential. The shortening of action potential are likely to be secondary to the shift of the inward rectifying K^+ current experimentally
described to occur in response to variation in $[K]_0$ in the frog ventricular muscle (Cleemann and Morad, 1979b). These authors also
found that the delayed and time dependent K^+ current (activated at
potential positive to -20 mV) was not significantly altered when
$[K]_0$ was changed from 3 to 6 mM. Thus the efflux and accumulation
of K^+ during the plateau (in frog potentials positive to 0 mV, see
figure 1) would have little or no effect on the K^+ currents flowing
through the delayed rectifier channel. This assertion was further
confirmed by Kline and Morad (1978) who found no change in the
rate of K^+ accumulation, accompanying a single action potential, when
$[K]_0$ was changed from 3 to 6 to 3 mM. Thus K^+ efflux and its accumulation during the plateau may have an insignificant effect on the K^+
permeability during the plateau and therefore on the duration of the
action potential (see for instance figure 7). However, comparison
of paracellular $[K]$ prior to occurance of an action potential reveals
a direct relationship between the duration of subsequent action potential and the level of K^+ prior to occurence of the upstroke of the
action potential (figure 7). This finding suggests that accumulation
of K^+ does in fact alter the duration of action potential but that
the ionic mechanism controlling the duration of the plateau may be
brought about by the shift of inward rectifying K^+ system (shown by
a number of investigators to shift along the voltage axis as predicted
by the Nernst equation). The significant point to be emphasized is
that the concentration of K^+ in the paracellular space after fapid
repolarization phase will induce appropriate shifts in the inward
rectifying system as to produce more or less repolarizing currents
during the time course of the following action potential. Since it
is the turn off of the inward rectifying system which provides for
low conductance of the plateau, small voltage-dependent shifts in
this system will be highly effective in changing the plateau duration.
Thus local variations in K^+ concentration may serve as very effective
mechanisms for controlling the duration of action potential. In such
a scheme long action potentials will be followed by shorter action
potential, simply because of the level of K^+ accumulated prior to
onset of an action potential changes. Clearly other parameters such
as the reactivation of inactivated Na^+ or Ca^{2+} current will also
contribute to the overall changes in the action potential duration.

Other factors make the comparison of local K^+-accumulation and
duration of action potential more complicated. Among these is the
homogenity of K^+ accumulation profile across the depth of the muscle.
It has already been shown that the magnitude of K^+ accumulation is
directly related to the muscle diameter and/or the depth of sampled
area. That is, deeper areas of extracellular space produce larger

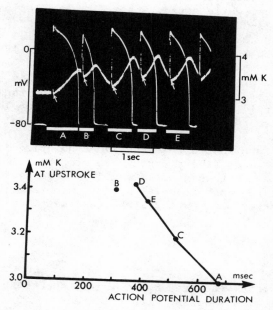

Figure 7. K$^+$ activity during a period of alternating action potential durations. Top panel: comparison of K$^+$ activity and membrane potential following a sudden change in frequency from zero to 90 shocks/min. In the graph above, K$^+$ activity at the start of each action potential (indicated by the arrows) is plotted vs. the action potential duration (indicated by time bars under each action potential). Note the close correlation between the [K]$_0$ prior to initiation of an action potential and its corresponding action potential duration. [Ca^{2+}]$_0$ = 50 μM; temperature, 22°C. (From Kline and Morad, 1978).

accumulations. Such a variation in K^+ accumulation profile would have a differential effect on resting and plateau potential, because of large differences of membrane resistance during rest and plateau. Thus the dependence of action potential duration on local paracellular K^+ concentration during the transition from a slow to a fast frequency may be complicated by the depth factor. In fact, it is often noticed that the action potential shortening is almost complete within the first three beats, while steady state K^+ accumulation values are not reached before 15-30 beats. The rapid shortening of action potential without any measureable change in resting potential seems to be inconsistent with the hypothesis that it is the shift in E_K (and therefore the inward rectifying current) which is responsible for determining the duration of action potential. This apparent inconsistency may be resolved when considering the radial K^+ accumulation profile within the fiber bundle in the trabeculum. For instance, it is probable that the large and more rapid accumulation at the core fibers would lead to early repolarization of these fibers, which could in turn induce regenerative repolarization of more superficially located fibers through an electrotonic process. The electrical influence thus exerted would be more pronounced at the plateau than at resting potential because membrane impedence differences at plateau and resting state (Weidmann, 1951, Goldman and Morad, 1977).

SUMMARY AND CONCLUSION

The experiments reported here clearly show that significant K^+ accumulation occurs during either increase of frequency of stimulation or under voltage clamp manipulations. The magnitude of accumulation per action potential suggests that K^+ efflux per beat is approximately 10-20 pmole/cm^2/sec. The accumulated K^+ is removed by an active reuptake process. That the reuptake process is strongly suppressed by ouabain, low $[K]_0$, and replacement of Na^+ by Li^+, strongly implies that the K^+ reuptake system has similar characteristics to the Na^+-K^+ ATPase. The voltage-dependence of accumulation provides evidence not only that the N-shaped I-V relation reflects the voltage dependence of K^+ current but also that there are two different types of K^+ channels. Our experiments suggest that local K^+ accumulation caused by efflux of K^+ during the plateau of the action potential alter the inward rectifying K^+ current such as to cause appropriate shortening or prolongation in the duration of action potential. It is, in fact, for this reason that there seems to be a direct relation between $[K^+]_0$ prior to occurence of an action potential and the duration of following action potential. We believe, therefore, that K^+ accumulation plays a physiological role in local control of the excitability in heart muscle.

REFERENCES

Baumgarten, C. M., and Isenberg, G., 1977, Depletion and accumulation of potassium in the extracellular clefts of cardiac Purkinje fibers during voltage clamp hyperpolarization and depolarization. Pflügers Arch., 368:19-31.

Cleemann, L., and Morad, M., 1979, Extracellular potassium accumulation in voltage-clamped frog ventricular muscle. J. Physiol. (London), 286:83-111.

Cleemann, L., and Morad, M., 1979b, Potassium currents in ventricular muscle: evidence from voltage clamp currents and extracellular K+ accumulation. J. Physiol. (London), 286:113-143.

Deitmer, J. W., and Ellis, D., 1978, Changes in intracellular sodium activity of sheep heart Purkinje fibres produced by calcium and other divalent cations. J. Physiol. (London), 277:437-453.

Eisner, D. A., and Lederer, W. J., 1979, The role of the sodium pump in the effects of potassium depleted solutions on mammalian cardiac muscle. J. Physiol. (London), 294:279-301.

Glitsch, H. G., Reuter, H., and Scholz, H., 1970, The effect of the internal sodium concentration on calcium fluxes in isolated guinea pig auricles. J. Physiol. (London), 209:25-43.

Glitsch, H. G., 1972, Activation of the electrogenic sodium pump in guinea-pig auricles by internal sodium ions. J. Physiol. (London), 220:565-582.

Goldman, Y., Morad, M., 1977, Ionic membrane conductance during the time course of the cardiac action potential. J. Physiol. (London), 268:655-695.

Kline, R., and Morad, M., 1976, Potassium efflux and accumulation in heart muscle: evidence from K+ electrode experiments. Biophys.J. 16:367-372.

Kline, R. P., and Morad, M., 1978, Potassium efflux in heart muscle during activity: extracellular accumulation and its implications. J. Physiol. (London), 280:537-558.

Kunze, D. L., 1977, Rate dependent changes in extracellular potassium in rabbit atrium. Circ. Res., 41 (1):122-127.

Langer, G. A., 1968, Ion fluxes in cardiac excitation and contraction and their relation to myocardial contractility. Physiol. Rev., 48:708-757.

Langer, G. A., 1973, Heart: excitation-contraction coupling 1089. Ann. Rev. Physiol., 35:55-86.

Martin, G., and Morad, M., 1978, K+ efflux and uptake in frog ventricular muscle. Biophys. J., 21:166.

Maylie, J., Morad, M., and Weiss, J., 1981, A study of pace-maker potential in rabbit sino-atrial node: measurement of potassium activity under voltage-clamp conditions (IN PRESS).

Morad, M., 1980, Physiological implications of K accumulation in heart muscle. Fed. Proc., 39:No.5.

Niedergerke, R., and Orkand, R. K., 1966, The dual effect of calcium
    on the action potential of frog's heart. J. Physiol. (London),
    184:291-331.
Page, S., and Niedergerke, R., 1972, Structures of physiological
    interest in the frog heart ventricle. J. Cell. Science, 11:
    179-203.
Thomas, R. C., 1972, Electrogenic sodium pump in nerve and muscle
    cells. Physiol. Rev., 53 (3):563-594.
Weidmann, S., 1951, Effect of current flow on the membrane potential
    of cardiac muscle. J. Physiol. (London), 115:227-236.

MEASUREMENT OF INTRACELLULAR IONIC CALCIUM CONCENTRATION IN GUINEA PIG PAPILLARY MUSCLE

Adolf Coray and John A.S. McGuigan

Institute of Physiology, University of Berne
Bühlplatz 5
3012 Berne, Switzerland

The measurement of intracellular calcium has been greatly facilitated by the introduction of calcium-sensitive ligands. In this study we have used microelectrodes filled with a resin containing the Ca-sensitive neutral ligand ETH 1001 (Simon et al., 1978) to measure intracellular calcium concentration in guinea pig ventricular muscle.

The microelectrodes were pulled on a vertical puller and then bevelled, to yield a tip diameter of less than 1 μm. Silanization of the electrodes was done according to the technique of Coles and Tsacopoulos (1977) with dimethylchlorosilane for 3 minutes at 200° C. The tip of the microelectrode was filled with the ligand by injection with a syringe. The shank of the microelectrode was then filled with calibrating solution with a calcium concentration of 4 x 10^{-8} mol/l.

Calibration of the calcium electrodes was carried out in a cation solution chosen to resemble the internal cation concentration of heart muscle (KCl 120 mmol/l; NaCl 7 mmol/l; $MgCl_2$ 1 mmol/l; buffered to pH 7.2 with either Tris or HEPES). Ionic calcium was buffered with either EGTA or nitrilotriacetic acid. The apparent stability constant for EGTA was calculated and also determined in the calibrating solution using the pH method of Miller and Moisescu (1976).

The result from an experiment to measure the resting calcium concentration in papillary muscle is shown in Fig. 1. In this experiment the difference between the calcium electrode signal and the resting potential was 132 mV, which corresponds to an internal calcium concentration of 2 x 10^{-7} mol/l. The mean value ± S.E. for 10 such experiments was 2.7 x 10^{-7} mol/l ± 0.8 x 10^{-7} mol/l. These values

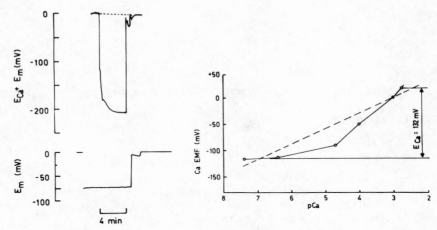

Fig. 1.   Resting calcium concentration in guinea pig papillary muscle.
          Upper left, signal measured by the calcium electrode (-207 mV)
          Lower left, resting potential (-75 mV). The calibrating curve
          is shown on the right. The dotted line is the Nernstian
          relationship. Temperature 22 °C; $[Ca]_o$ 1.8 mmol/l. Log of
          the apparent stability constant used in calculation of pCa
          was 6.80.

are similar to those found in ventricular muscle of sheep (Coray et
al., 1980) and ferrit ventricle (Marban et al., 1980). However, we
regard this value as the upper limit for the free calcium since im-
perfect impalements might lead to increased calcium levels.

     Contracures elicited in these papillary muscles (diameter 0.6 to
0.8 mm) by Na removal reach about twitch height. During such contract-
ures the internal ionic calcium intreased roughly ten times from the
resting value. During a contracture the calcium concentration was
maintained.

     Tests carried out on the relative sensitivity of the electrodes
to H^+, Mg^{2+} and Na^+ showed little or no interference from either H^+
and Mg^{2+} and only minimal interference from Na^+.

     In conclusion it appears that these electrodes are capable of
measuring not only the resting calcium levels, but also slow changes
in internal calcium concentration such as produced by Na-free contract-
ures.

ACKNOWLEDGEMENTS

We wish to acknowledge the help of Drs Fry and Miller with the initial experiments. The work was supported by the Swiss National Science Foundation, grant number 2.071-0.76. Dr Fry's stay in Berne was made possible by a stipend from the Roche Research Foundation. The ligand was a gift from Dr Ammann, Zürich.

REFERENCES

Coles, J.A., and Tsacopoulos, M., 1977, A method of making fine double-barrelled potassium-sensitive micro-electrodes for intracellular recording. J. Physiol., 270:12P.

Coray, A., Fry, C.H., Hess, P., McGuigan, J.A.S., and Weingart, R., 1980, Resting calcium in sheep cardiac tissue and in frog skeletal muscle measured with ion-selective microelectrodes, J. Physiol., in the Press (abstract).

Marban, E., Rink, T.J., Tsien, R.W., and Tsien, R.Y., 1980, Free calcium in ferrit ventricular muscle measured with an ion-sensitive microelectrode. J. Physiol., in the Press (abstract).

Miller, D.J., and Moisescu, D.G., 1976, The effects of very low external calcium and sodium concentrations on cardiac contractile strength and calcium-sodium antagonism, J. Physiol., 259:283.

Simon, W., Ammann, D., Oehme, M., and Morf, W.E., 1978, Calcium-sensitive electrodes, Ann. N.Y. Acad. Science, 307:52.

INTRACELLULAR Na ACTIVITY DURING K OR Rb ACTIVATED RESPONSE IN SHEEP PURKINJE FIBRES--CORRELATION WITH CHANGES IN MEMBRANE POTENTIAL

H. G. Glitsch, W. Kampmann and H. Pusch

Dept. of Cell Physiology and SFB 114
Ruhr University
D-4630 Bochum, West Germany

Cardiac Purkinje fibres hyperpolarize transiently in Tyrode solution containing KCl after superfusion with a K free medium. There are strong reasons to suppose that this K activated response is caused by enhanced electrogenic Na pumping (Hiraoka and Hecht, 1973; Deitmer and Ellis, 1978; Gadsby and Cranefield, 1979). However, it has been demonstrated only recently that changes in the intracellular Na activity (a^iNa) are in fact correlated with changes in membrane potential during the K activated response (Glitsch and Pusch, 1980). Similarly, Eisner, Lederer and Vaughan-Jones (1980) have recently shown that both, the current underlying the transient hyperpolarization and a^iNa decline with much the same time constant (τ) during a Rb activated response in voltage clamped sheep Purkinje fibres. We report here that the correlation between changes in membrane potential and a^iNa persists after variation of the external K (K_O) or Rb (Rb_O) concentration while the time course of decline in a^iNa and membrane potential varies according to the K_O or Rb_O concentration.

Sheep Purkinje fibres were pinned down to the bottom of a chamber (volume c. 1.5 ml) through which the bathing media run at 4 ml/min. The fibres were equilibrated for at least 40 min in normal Tyrode solution bubbled with 95% O_2 and 5% CO_2 at 35°C (pH 7.2) and stimulated at 0.8 shocks/s. Afterwards stimulation was stopped and the preparations were impaled with a Na^+ sensitive microelectrode (Thomas, 1970). The Na^+ electrode was filled with a standard solution containing (mM) 150 NaCl, 5 KCl and 10 TRIS, pH 7.2. Additionally the fibres were impaled with a conventional microelectrode as near as possible (distance between the electrodes ~ 100 μ) to the Na^+ electrode. This was done for the following reason: The Na^+ electrode measures the sum of the membrane potential and a potential (V_{Na}) which represents $a^i Na$. In order to obtain V_{Na} it is necessary to subtract the membrane potential from the total potential measured by the Na^+ electrode. The internal Na^+ activity is then calculated from V_{Na} by calibrating the electrode in test solutions with various Na concentrations.

After both electrodes had been impaled and steady-state values of the membrane potential and $a^i Na$ in normal Tyrode solution had been obtained, the bathing fluid was switched to a K(Rb) free medium for 10 to 25 min. Finally, solutions with 2.2 to 10.8 mM K or Rb were applied.

The upper part of Fig. 1 shows the total potential measured by the Na^+ electrode (lower envelope curve), the membrane potential (vertical bars) and V_{Na}, which represents $a^i Na$ (upper envelope curve) in a sheep Purkinje fibre before, during and after super-fusion with a K free solution. Application of a medium without K causes an increase in the potentials towards more positive values. The membrane potential depolarizes first and repolarizes slowly afterwards while V_{Na} depolarizes continuously. Switching back to Tyrode solution (5.4 mM KCl) induces a shift of all potentials to more negative levels. A closer inspection reveals that the membrane potential (vertical bars) hyperpolarizes transiently. The time course of $a^i Na$ (●) and membrane potential (o) is graphed in the lower part of the figure. The internal Na activity of the fibre in Tyrode solution amounts to 7 mM. The membrane potential is measured to be -67 mV. $a^i Na$ increases continuously in the K free solution and reaches about 15 mM after 25 min in OK. The membrane potential depolarizes upon application of the K free medium to about -40 mV and repolarizes later on by a few millivolts. Note that depolarization is complete 5 min after solution change. The intracellular Na^+ activity declines continuously after a certain delay towards its steady-state value if Tyrode solution (5.4 mM KCl) is again applied. The cell membrane hyperpolarizes during the $a^i Na$ decline (K activated response). This hyperpolarization is probably not due to K depletion at the cell membrane because a re-duction in K_O causes depolarization, not hyperpolarization (at the beginning of the OK period). Afterwards the membrane potential reaches the resting value with a time course similar to that of the $a^i Na$ diminution. For each experiment the increase of $a^i Na$ ($\Delta a^i Na$) above its steady-state value and the hyperpolarization (ΔV) of the cell membrane during the K(Rb) activated response were normalized with respect to their maximum values and plotted semilogarithmically. Such a plot is shown in Fig. 2. As can be seen from the figure the time constants of decline in $a^i Na$ and membrane potential are in fact very similar during a K(Rb) activated re-sponse. A strong correlation between changes in membrane potential and $a^i Na$ is present regardless whether 2.2 mM Rb_O or 10.8 mM K_O are used to activate the response. However, the time constants of these changes are quite different. The time constant is about

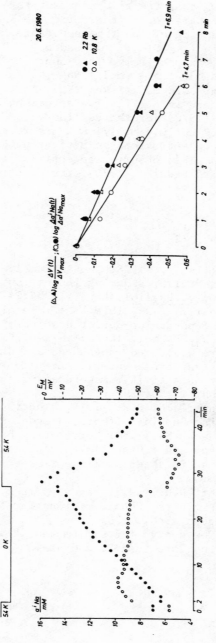

Fig. 1. Upper part: Total potential measured by a Na$^+$ sensitive microelectrode (lower envelope curve), membrane potential (vertical bars) and V$_{Na}$ representing a^{i}Na (upper envelope curve) of a sheep Purkinje fibre in Tyrode solution with and without 5.4 mmol/1 KCl. Lower part: a^{i}Na (left hand ordinate) and membrane potential (right hand ordinate) of the same fibre.

Fig. 2. Correlation between changes in membrane potential ($\Delta V(t)\triangle,\triangle$) and a^{i}Na(t) $\triangle,\triangle$) during a K(Rb) activated response in sheep Purkinje fibre. ΔV_{max} and a^{i}Na$_{max}$ are the values of $\Delta V(t)$ and Δa^{i}Na(t) at t=5 min (2.2 mmol/1 Rb$_o$) and t=6 min (10.8 mmol/1 K$_o$) after the change to the K(Rb) containing solution. Variations in K$_o$(Rb$_o$) due to the solution change had ceased at this time.

1.5 times larger at 2.2 mmol/l Rb_o than at 10.8 mmol/l K_o. A detailed investigation shows that the time constant is the same at corresponding Rb or K concentrations. Increasing the Rb_o or K_o concentration causes a reduction of the time constants. For example, is about 6.7 $\pm$ 1.5 min ($\bar{x}$ $\pm$ S.D.; n=3) and 5.6 $\pm$ 0.8 min, n=6 at 2.2 mmol/l Rb_o or K_o, respectively. It amounts to 4.1 $\pm$ 0.6 min, n=5 (3.9 $\pm$ 1.0 min, n=8) at 5.4 mmol/l Rb_o (K_o) and to 3.9 $\pm$ 0.5 min, n=2 (3.8 $\pm$ 0,8 n=3) at 10.8 mmol/l Rb_o (K_o). As to the K activated response the results are in qualitative agreement with data reported by Deitmer and Ellis (1978) for the decline in a^iNa. Furthermore, the findings show that 2.2 to 10.8 mmol/l Rb_o are roughly as effective as corresponding K_o concentrations in activating Na extrusion from sheep Purkinje fibres. This observation confirms an earlier conclusion drawn by Eisner and Lederer (1979) from electrophysiological experiments.

REFERENCES

Deitmer, J.W., and Ellis, D., 1978, The intracellular sodium activity of cardiac Purkinje fibres during inhibition and re-activation of the Na-K pump, J. Physiol.(Lond.), 284:241.

Eisner, D.A., and Lederer, W.J., 1979, The role of the sodium pump in the effects of potassium-depleted solutions on mammalian cardiac muscle. J. Physiol. (Lond.), 294:279.

Eisner, D.A., Lederer, W.J., and Vaughan-Jones, R.D., 1980, Electrogenic Na pumping in cardiac muscle: simultaneous measurement of intracellular Na activity, membrane current and tension, J. Physiol. (Lond.), 300:42P.

Gadsby, D.C., and Cranefield, P.F., 1979, Electrogenic sodium extrusion in cardiac Purkinje fibers, J. gen. Physiol.,73:819.

Glitsch, H.G., and Pusch, H., 1980, Correlation between changes in membrane potential and intracellular sodium activity during K activated response in sheep Purkinje fibres. Pflügers Arch., 384-189.

Hiraoka, M., and Hecht, H.H., 1973, Recovery from hypothermia in cardiac Purkinje fibers: Considerations for an electrogenic mechanism. Pflügers Arch., 339:25.

Thomas, R.C., 1970, New design for sodium-sensitive glass microelectrodes. J. Physiol.(Lond.), 210:82P.

INTERACTION BETWEEN pH_i and pCa_i IN CARDIAC TISSUE

Robert Weingart and Peter Hess

Dept. of Physiology, University of Berne
Bühlplatz 5
3012 Berne, Switzerland

It was Gaskell (1880) who originally made the observation that pH can have remarkable effects on cardiac contractility. Subsequently, although both the negative inotropic effect of acidosis and the positive inotropic effect of alkalosis on heart muscle have been well documented, we still do not fully understand the underlying mechanisms. There are several ways whereby protons might regulate resting and twitch tension. For example, the free sarcoplasmic Ca level could be changed, or the response of the contractile proteins to Ca might be altered. The latter possibility, namely a decrease of Ca sensitivity of the contractile proteins in acidosis, has been demonstrated by a number of workers in skinned preparations (e.g. Fabiato and Fabiato, 1978) as well as in isolated myofibrils from cardiac muscle (e.g. Schädler, 1967).

The aim of our study was to investigate the effect of pH_i on the intracellular calcium level of sheep cardiac Purkinje fibres at rest. The experiments were carried out at room temperature. The pH of all solutions was 7.3. Ca activity was kept constant by adjusting all solutions to that measured with a Ca-sensitive macroelectrode in Tris-buffered Tyrode solution containing 1.8 mmol/l $CaCl_2$. pH_i was measured using recessed-tip pH-sensitive glass microelectrodes as described by Thomas (1978), and pCa_i was monitored with Ca-sensitive microelectrodes. Their fabrication was as follows: Micropipettes were pulled from borosilicate glass and bevelled on an air-driven rotating disc (Stähli AG, Pieterlen, Switzerland). Optical examination revealed tip diameters ranging from about 0.5 μm to 1.4 μm. Subsequently the microelectrodes were siliconized according to one of the following methods: a) Nitrogen gas saturated with dimethylchlorosilane was blown through the electrode from the back at 4 atm. pressure, while the tip was heated to 200 °C by a heating

307

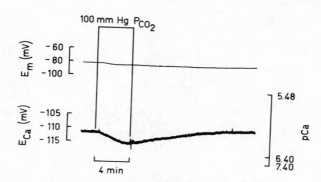

Fig. 1. Effect of pH_i on the intracellular Ca level. Top: Membrane
         potential (E_m) recorded with a 3 mol/1 KCl reference micro-
         electrode; bottom: Signal of the difference between the
         electromotive force seen by a Ca-sensitive and the reference
         microelectrode. A 4 min exposure to 100 mm Hg P_{CO_2} revealed
         a reversible decrease in $[Ca]_i$ from $8.7 \cdot 10^{-7}$ mol/1 to
         $5.3 \cdot 10^{-7}$ mol/1. Sheep Purkinje fibre, 22 $^\circ$C. P24-1.

filament (Coles and Tsacopoulos, 1977). b) A series of bevelled electrodes, kept in a petri dish, was first preheated to 200 $^\circ$C in an
oven, before a droplet of N,N-dimethyltrimethylsilylamine was added.
The neutral Ca ligand ETH 1001 (Simon et al., 1978) was then introduced into the tip of the electrodes from the back. Calibration of the
Ca electrodes was performed using a set of solutions which contained
the following "intracellular background": KCl 120 mmol/1, NaCl 7
mmol/1, $MgCl_2$ 1 mmol/1, Tris 24 mmol 1 or HEPES 10 mmol/1 to give a
pH of 7.2. [Ca] was varied between 10 mmol/1 and 40 nmol/1 by buffering the solutions either with NTA, HEDTA or EGTA. The resulting calibration curves showed typical Nernstian slopes for [Ca] between
10 and 0.1 mmol/1, hyper-Nernstian slopes between 0.1 mmol/1 and
1 μmol/1 and progressive flattening below 1 μmol/1. Calibration of
the Ca electrodes at different pH values showed no interference of
protons with the Ca measurements. Ca electrodes prepared and calibrated in this way can be successfully used to measure the intracellular
free calcium level and slowly changing calcium signals in cardiac
tissue (Coray et al., 1980; Coray and McGuigan, this volume).

    Intracellular acidosis was produced in sheep Purkinje fibres by
a sudden increase of P_{CO_2} from 0 to 100 mm Hg. Extracellular pH was
kept constant at pH 7.3 by buffering the solutions either with Tris
or with bicarbonate. 5 min exposure to the high P_{CO_2} resulted in a
reversible intracellular acidification ranging from 0.5 to 0.9 pH
units. Very similar intracellular acidosis resulted from short exposure (3-5 min) to solutions in which NaCl had been replaced by the
sodium salt of a weak organic acid, such as propionic acid. Measurements with Ca electrodes under both of these experimental conditions
revealed a decrease of the intracellular Ca level by a factor of 2-3

(Fig. 1). Separate experiments showed that this decrease in the cellular Ca was parallelled by a decrease in resting tension.

In order to obtain intracellular pH shifts in the alkaline direction, 15 mmol/l of NH_4Cl were added to the normal Tris-buffered Tyrode solution. The resulting intracellular alkalosis was rather moderate. During a 15 min exposure to the NH_4Cl, pH_i typically showed a transient increase of 0.2 to 0.3 pH units. In parallel sets of experiments, it was found that this pH intervention not only led to a roughly twofold increase in the cellular free Ca concentration, but also to an increase in resting tension.

It is concluded that with the relatively short-lasting alterations of pH_i studied, intracellular free calcium decreases with decreasing pH_i and increases as pH_i increases. It therefore seems reasonable to assume that in cardiac tissue at least part of the observed changes in contractility under conditions of intracellular acidosis or alkalosis are due to these changes in intracellular free calcium.

The ligand was a gift from Dr. D. Ammann. The work was supported by the Swiss National Science Foundation (3.565-0.79).

REFERENCES

Coles, J.A. and Tsacopoulos, M., 1977, A method of making fine double-barrelled potassium-sensitive micro-electrodes for intracellular recording, J. Physiol. (London), 270:12P.

Coray, A., Fry, C.H., Hess, P., McGuigan, J.A.S. and Weingart, R., 1980, Resting calcium in sheep cardiac tissue and in frog skeletal muscle measured with ion-sensitive microelectrodes, J. Physiol. (London), (London Meeting April 1980, in press).

Coray, A. and McGuigan, J.A.S., 1980, Measurement of intracellular ionic calcium concentration in guinea pig papillary muscle (this volume).

Fabiato, A. and Fabiato, F., 1978, Effects of pH on the myofilaments and the sarcoplasmic reticulum of skinned cells from cardiac and skeletal muscles, J. Physiol. (London), 276:233.

Gaskell, W.H., 1880, On the tonicity of the heart and blood vessels, J. Physiol. (London), 3:48.

Schädler, M., 1967, Proportionale Aktivierung von ATPase-Aktivität und Kontraktionsspannung durch Calciumionen in isolierten contractilen Strukturen verschiedener Muskelarten, Pflügers Arch., 296:70

Simon, W., Ammann, D., Oehme, M. and Morf, W.E., 1978, Calcium-selective electrodes, in:"Calcium Transport and Cell Function", A. Scarpa and E. Carafoli, eds., Ann.N.Y. Acad. Sci., 307:52.

Thomas, R.C., 1978, "Ion-sensitive Intracellular Microelectrodes", Academic Press, London.

THE USE OF ISMs IN WORKING SKELETAL MUSCLES AND

VENOUS EFFLUENT BLOOD

P. Hník, F. Vyskočil, N. Kříž, E. Ujec, O. Keller

Institute of Physiology
Czechoslovak Academy of Sciences
Vídeňská 1083
142 20 Prague 4, Czechoslovakia

INTRODUCTION

Even before the introduction of ion-selective microelectrodes (ISMs), it was known that K^+ is released from contracting muscles. Loss of muscle K^+ during contraction was described by Fenn (1936), and increased levels of K^+ were subsequently demonstrated in the venous effluent blood by a number of authors (e.g. Kjellmer, 1965; Lind et al., 1966). Hinke (1959, 1961) was the first to employ ion-selective glass electrodes for measuring Na^+ and K^+ activities in muscle fibres. Since the tips of these electrodes were rather large, only giant muscle fibres could be impaled. Sorokina in 1964 succeeded in making microelectrodes selective for Na^+ and K^+ with tip diameters below 0.5 μm. It was not until 1972, however, that Gebert (1972) used K^+ and Na^+ ion-selective glass electrodes and our group (Hník, Vyskočil, Kříž and Holas 1972) used the liquid ion-exchanger potassium ISMs to measure the time course and the extent of potassium accumulation in the contracting muscles and to assess potassium losses into venous effluent blood. In 1977, Hirche reported results on K^+ changes and Friedman (1973) and Hirche (1977) have also measured pH changes in contracting muscles with microelectrodes.

The aim of our work published in extenso in 1976 (Hník et al., 1976) was a/ to investigate the time course of K_e^+ accumulation in mammalian muscles induced by muscle activity, b/ to ascertain the time course of the changes in K^+ concentration in venous blood from working muscles, c/ to assess the losses of K^+ accompanying muscle activity of various durations and performed either under isometric or isotonic conditions, and d/ to attempt direct measurements of K_e^+ released from superficial fibres of the frog sartorius muscle in vitro.

311

RESULTS

K_e^+ measurements in contracting muscle

The problem of measuring K_e^+ using ISMs in contracting muscles was solved by the introduction of ISMs with a side-pore (Vyskočil and Kříž, 1972). The insertion of this semimicroelectrode (tip diameter 50-100 μm) damages some muscle fibres and consequently causes a transient rise in K_e^+ (Hník et al.,1972). Indirect muscle stimulation (0.3 ms pulses, 50 Hz, supramaximal intensity) caused K^+ accumulation in both rabbit and cat gastrocnemius muscles. For example, a 20-second isometric tetanus increased K_e^+ from around 5 to 8-10 mmol/1 K^+. Control experiments showed that it is highly unlikely that this work-induced K_e^+ accumulation was due to further damage of muscle fibres. The longer the period of stimulation, the higher the K_e^+ levels (Fig. 1). The K_e^+ increase was not dependent upon the type of muscle contraction(isometric or isotonic).

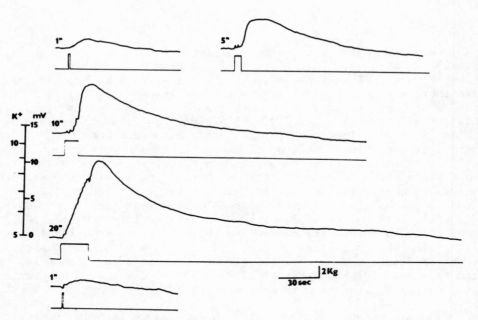

Fig. 1.   Changes of extracellular K^+ in cat gastrocnemius muscle during and after isometric tetanic contractions induced by nerve stimulation lasting 1,5,10 and 20 s respectively. The myographic curves are given below each record. Calibration for K^+ concentrations (in mmol/1) is given in scale on the left, calibration of myograph is given below (Hník et al., 1976).

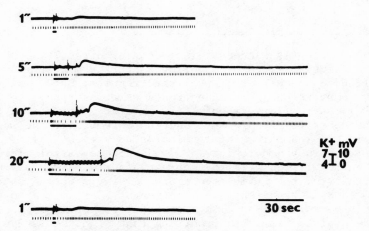

Fig. 2.   Changes of K$^+$ concentration in venous effluent blood
          (upper records) and blood flow (lower records from drop-
          counter) after isometric tetani of cat gastrocnemius. Sti-
          mulation indicated by thick horizontal bars below drop-
          counter record. Numerals on the left indicate duration
          of isometric tetani in seconds. Scale for K$^+$ concentration
          changes is given on the right (Hník et al., 1976).

K$^+_{ven}$ measurements in venous effluent blood

These side-pore electrodes were also employed for measuring K$^+$
in venous effluent blood (K$^+_{ven}$) from contracting muscles (Hník et
al., 1976)(Fig. 2).
It was possible to assess the loss of K$^+$ from the contracting cat
gastrocnemius muscle from the K$^+_{ven}$ changes and the blood flow.
This muscle lost about 0.5 % of its total K$^+$ content after contracting isometrically for 20 s (with 50 Hz tetanic stimulation). This
corresponds to a loss of 0.3 nmol/g per impulse from the cat gastrocnemius muscle. The value is very similar to that obtained by flame
photometry from the dog by Mohrman and Sparks (1974).

An interesting aspect of the K$^+$ changes occurring in the contracting muscle is the finding that the uptake of the lost K$^+$ by the
muscle fibres was relatively slow. Arteriovenous occlusion was used
to prevent the loss of K$^+$ from muscles during stimulation and recovery period of variable duration. The measurements of K$^+_{ven}$ after
release of the occlusion at various times after a 10-second tetanus
showed that the occlusion must last for at least 45-60 s if it was
to prevent the loss into venous blood of most of K$^+$ released into
the interstitial space.

K_e^+ released from single frog muscle fibres

We have recently succeeded in recording directly the K_e^+ released from single fibres of the frog sartorius muscle in vitro (Vyskočil, Ujec and Keller, unpublished results; Hník and Vyskočil, 1980). Two conventional microelectrodes were inserted into the same superficial muscle fibre, about 10-20 mm apart. One served for stimulation, the other for recording of action potentials. The muscles were immersed in hyperosmotic Ringer solution to prevent them from contracting (Hodgkin and Horowicz, 1957). A double-barrel microelectrode with one barrel filled with the ion-exchanger was brought into the close vicinity of the stimulated fibre. A single action potential was followed by a transient accumulation of K^+ from 2.5 to 4-5 mmol/l K^+. Repetitive stimulation with 2 or 6 pulses caused an increase to even higher values. It is thus obvious that K^+ accumulation in the muscle depends upon electrical and not mechanical activity of the muscle.

CONCLUSIONS

The use of ISMs has thus confirmed earlier reports that K^+ accumulates in the extracellular space during muscle work and that K^+ is released into venous blood. In addition, ISMs have provided more exact quantitative data about the actual concentrations, their time course and the amount of K^+ lost into venous effluent blood. It is being suggested, on the basis of these results, that the work-induced K^+ accumulation in skeletal muscles may affect excitable tissue elements present in skeletal muscles (Hník and Vyskočil, 1980), namely: a/ presynaptic nerve terminals, b/ muscle fibres themselves (membrane enzymes, contractile properties, muscle metabolism), c/ smooth muscles of blood vessels, d/ afferent muscle nerve terminals (both proprioceptive and non-proprioceptive).

It is thus obvious that ISMs have provided some basic information about ionic changes in contracting muscles, just as they have in other excitable tissues. It may be expected that even more pertinent data will be obtained when ISMs for other ions are employed for studying ionic movements in skeletal muscles under various physiological and pathophysiological conditions.

REFERENCES

Fenn, W.O., 1936, Electrolytes in muscle, Physiol. Rev., 16:450.
Gebert, G., 1972, Messung der K^+- und Na^+-Aktivität mit Mikro-Glaselektroden im Extracellulärraum des Kaninchenskeletmuskels bei Muskelarbeit, Pflügers Arch.,331:204.
Gebert, G., and Friedman, S.M., 1973, An implantable glass electrode used for pH measurement in working skeletal muscle, J. appl. Physiol., 34:122.

Hinke, J.A.M., 1959, Glass micro-electrodes for measuring intra-cellular activities of sodium and potassium, Nature, 184:1257.

Hinke, J.A.M., 1961, The measurement of sodium and potassium activities in the squid axon by means of cations-selective glass micro-electrodes, J. Physiol. (Lond.), 156:314.

Hirche, Hj., 1977, Changes of ion-activities in heart and skeletal muscle during exercise and ischemia, in: IUPS Satellite Symposium on "Theory and Application of Ion-selective Electrodes in Physiology and Medicine", Dortmund, p.26.

Hník, P., and Vyskočil, F., 1980, Ion-selective microelectrodes - A new tool for studying ionic movements in working muscles, in: "The Application of Ion Selective Microelectrodes", T. Zeuthen, ed., Elsevier, Amsterdam, in press.

Hník, P., Vyskočil, F., Kříž, N., and Holas, M., 1972, Work-induced increase of extracellular potassium concentration in muscle measured by ion-specific electrodes, Brain Res., 40:559.

Hník, P., Kříž, N., Vyskočil, F., Smieško, V., Mejsnar, J., Ujec, E., and Holas, M., 1973, Work-induced potassium changes in muscle venous effluent blood measured by ion-specific electrodes, Pflügers Arch., 338:177.

Hník, P., Holas, M., Krekule, I., Kříž, N., Mejsnar, J., Smieško, V., Ujec, E., and Vyskočil, F., 1976, Work-induced potassium changes in skeletal muscle and effluent venous blood assessed by liquid ion-exchanger microelectrodes, Pflügers Arch., 362:85.

Hodgkin, A.L., and Horowicz, P., 1957, The differential action of hypertonic solutions on the twitch and action potential of a muscle fibre, J. Physiol. (Lond.), 136:17P.

Kjellmer, I., 1965, The potassium ion as a vasodilator during muscular exercise, Acta physiol. scand., 63:460.

Lind, A.R., McNicol, G.W., and Donald, K.W., 1966, Circulatory adjustments to sustained static muscular activity, in: Proc. of the Beitostölen Symposium on Physical Activity in Health and Disease, K. Evang and K.L. Andersen, eds., Williams and Wilkins Co., Baltimore, p.38.

Mohrman, D.E., and Sparks, H.V., 1974, Role of potassium ions in the vascular response to a brief tetanus, Circ. Res., 35:384.

Sorokina, Z.A., 1964, Aktivnost ionov kaliya i natriya v protoplazme poperechnopolosatykh myshechnykh volokon lyagushki, Byul. eksper. Biol. Med., 58:(12)17.

Vyskočil, F., and Kříž, N., 1972, Modifications of single and double-barrel potassium-specific microelectrodes for various physiological experiments, Pflügers Arch., 337:265.

CHARACTERISTICS OF Ca^{2+}-SELECTIVE MICROELECTRODES AND THEIR APPLICATION TO CARDIAC MUSCLE CELLS

Chin O. Lee and Dae Y. Uhm

Department of Physiology and Biophysics
Cornell University Medical College
New York, N.Y. 10021

INTRODUCTION

The direct measurements of cytosolic Ca^{2+} activities are important for the study of roles of the ion in the regulation of cellular functions. One of the methods for such measurements is to use Ca^{2+}-selective microelectrodes. It appears that activities of cytosolic Ca^{2+} are much lower than those of other cytosolic ions such as K^+, Na^+ and Mg^{2+}. Therefore, Ca^{2+}-selective microelectrodes must have sufficient selectivities for Ca^{2+} over the interfering ions, i.e., K^+, Na^+ and Mg^{2+} so that the influence of the interfering ions on the microelectrodes could not produce errors. In this study, Ca^{2+}-selective microelectrodes were made and some of their properties were investigated to measure sarcoplasmic Ca^{2+} activities in cardiac muscle cells.

CONSTRUCTION OF Ca^{2+}-SELECTIVE MICROELECTRODES

Ca^{2+}-selective microelectrodes were made using the neutral ligand ETH 1001 as a sensor (Simon et al., 1978). Glass micropipettes with tip diameters of 1 µm or less were pulled from borosilicate glass capillaries (Corning Glass Works, Code 7740). Before pulling the micropipettes, the glass capillaries were cleaned with alcohol and boiled in deionized water, and dried completely. The inner surface of the micropipettes was silanized by exposure to dichlorodimethylsilane gas under pressure of nitrogen at room temperature. The shank and shoulder of the micropipettes were first filled with 100 mmol/l $CaCl_2$ solution using a syringe and the solution was driven by pressure to the end of the tip. Subsequently the Ca^{2+}-selective liquid was drawn up to 300 - 1500 µm from the tip by suction.

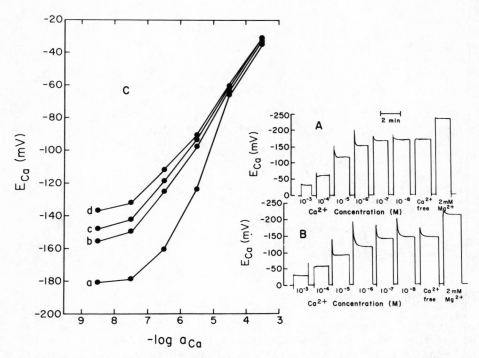

Fig. 1. Potential changes of a representative Ca^{2+}-selective microelectrode with time. Potential recordings A and B were
measured about 10 min and 1 h respectively after the microelectrode was made. Ion concentrations of the calibration
solutions are shown below each recording. Note that at Ca^{2+}
concentrations $\geq 10^{-4}$ mol/l the potentials in A are similar
to the corresponding potentials in B, while at the Ca^{2+}
concentrations $\leq 10^{-5}$ mol/l the potentials in A are about
30 mV more negative than the corresponding potentials in B.
In C, the curves a and b represent the plots of the potential recordings A and B respectively, c and d were obtained
about 2-6 h respectively after the microelectrode was made.

POTENTIAL RESPONSE OF THE MICROELECTRODES

The electrochemical system used for measurements of the Ca^{2+}-
selective microelectrode potentials was similar to that used in our
previous study (Lee, 1979). Fig. 1 A and B show potential recordings
measured with a representative microelectrode about 10 min and 1 h
respectively after it was made. The potentials were measured with
solutions containing Ca^{2+} concentrations of 10^{-3} to 10^{-8} mol/l and
a Ca^{2+} free solution. These solutions contained 150 mmol/l K^{+},

1 mmol/l Mg^{2+} and had a pH of 7.0. The solution containing 2 mmol/l Mg^{2+} had no Ca^{2+} and no K$^+$. The Ca^{2+} in the solutions was controlled by EGTH except for 10^{-3} and 10^{-4} mol/l Ca^{2+} solutions. The potentials in Fig. 1 A are different from those in Fig. 1 B particularly at Ca^{2+} concentrations lower than 10^{-4} mol/l. The difference indicates that the microelectrode potentials change with time after construction of the microelectrodes. The microelectrode potentials measured with time were plotted against $-\log a_{Ca}$ as shown in Fig. 1 C. After about 10 min (Fig. 1 C a), the potential changes (slopes) for a 10 fold change in Ca^{2+} activities between 0.32 x 10^{-4} and 0.32 x 10^{-6} mol/l were greater than those predicted by the Nernst equation (29.6 mV at 25 $^{\circ}$C). At Ca^{2+} activities greater than 0.32 x 10^{-4} mol/l, the potential changes were linear with a slope of about 30 mV. At Ca^{2+} activities lower than 0.32 x 10^{-6} mol/l, the slopes were less than those predicted by the Nernst equation. After about 1 h (Fig. 1 C b), the potentials became more positive and the slopes at Ca^{2+} activities greater than 0.32 x 10^{-6} mol/l were similar to those predicted by the Nernst equation. The slopes at Ca^{2+} activities lower than 0.32 x 10^{-6} mol/l remained the same or sometimes were improved. At Ca^{2+} activities between 0.32 x 10^{-6} and 0.32 x 10^{-7} mol/l, the slopes varied from one electrode to another, i.e., from 10 to 25 mV. At Ca^{2+} activities between 0.32 x 10^{-7} and 0.32 x 10^{-8} mol/l, the slopes varied from 5 to 10 mV, and rarely to 15 mV. With more time (Fig. 1 C c and d) the microelectrode potentials became more positive, and eventually the slopes at Ca^{2+} activities lower than 0.32 x 10^{-6} mol/l decreased. It was observed that the rate of the potential changes depended on the filling length of the Ca^{2+}-selective liquid. The microelectrode used in Fig. 1 had a filling length of about 550 μm. As the filling length of the Ca^{2+}-selective liquid was increased, the rate slowed. Although the reason for the potential changes is not known, one possible reason may be the nature of the solvent in the Ca^{2+}-selective liquid. When the microelectrodes filled to a proper length are aged for certain periods, they can be used to measure cytosolic Ca^{2+} activities.

With the microelectrode potentials measured with the solutions containing an interfering ion only, selectivity coefficients of the microelectrodes can be determined by an equation (Lee, 1981). To determine the selectivity coefficients (k_{CaK} and k_{CaMg}), the microelectrode potentials were measured with the solution containing 150 mmol/l K$^+$ and that containing 2 mmol/l Mg^{2+} (no Ca^{2+}) as shown in Fig. 1 A and B. With the potentials measured in Fig. 1 B, the calculated values of k_{CaK} and k_{CaMg} were 2.1 x 10^{-6} and 0.9 x 10^{-7} respectively. The k_{Cak} and k_{CaMg} values of the Ca^{2+}-selective microelectrodes were usually in the ranges of 7 x 10^{-6} to 1 x 10^{-6} and 5 x 10^{-7} to 0.7 x 10^{-7} respectively. These values are satisfactory for measurements of cytosolic Ca^{2+} activities. To express the results as Ca^{2+} activities rather than Ca^{2+} concentrations, the microelectrode potentials were plotted against Ca^{2+} activities (Fig. 1 C). To determine Ca^{2+} activities in the calibration solutions, an activity coefficient of 0.32 for Ca^{2+} was calculated by the extended Debye-

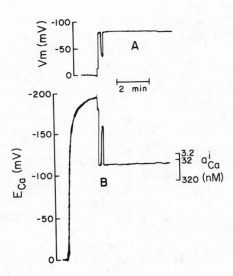

Fig. 2.   A and B represent the potential recordings with a conventional
          microelectrode and a Ca^{2+}-selective microelectrode respect-
          ively. In B the microelectrode potential in Tyrode's solution
          (1.8 mmol/1 Ca^{2+} concentration) was arbitrarily set to zero.
          The a^i_{Ca} values displayed on the right side of the trace were
          determined from the calibration curve of the microelectrode.
          Papillary muscles of rabbit ventricles were perfused with
          Tyrode's solution. Preparation of the muscle and solutions
          were described (Fozzard and Lee, 1976). All experiments were
          done at 35 °C - 36 °C.

Huckel equation (Robinson and Stokes, 1965). The results were presented as Ca^{2+} activities rather than Ca^{2+} concentrations, because: 1) many electrophysiological processes of cells respond to ion activities,
2) the microelectrodes measure potentials related to ion activities,
3) expressing the results as ion concentrations rests on the assumption that the activity coefficient of Ca^{2+} in the cytosol is equal to
that of Ca^{2+} in the calibration solutions, 4) other ions in cells such
as K^+, Na^+ and Cl^- have been expressed as their activities. Assuming
that the activity coefficients of the ions in cytosol is equal to those in calibration solutions, however, the results can be expressed
as ion concentrations.

SARCOPLASMIC Ca^{2+} ACTIVITY

    Fig. 2 illustrates the measurement of sarcoplasmic Ca^{2+} activity
(a^i_{Ca}) in a cell of rabbit ventricular muscle. A muscle cell was first
impaled with a Ca^{2+}-selective microelectrode (Fig. 2B). When the potential had reached a stable value, a second cell of the muscle was
impaled with a conventional microelectrode to measure a cell membrane
potential, V_m (Fig. 2A). Upon this impalement, the potential recorded

by the Ca^{2+}-selective microelectrode, E_{Ca}, fell by an amount equal to the cell membrane potential, and then reached another stable value. The rapid change in E_{Ca} represents the electronic subtraction of V_m from E_{Ca}. The E_{Ca} following the subtraction represents the sarcoplasmic Ca^{2+} activity. In ten successful measurements, the sarcoplasmic Ca^{2+} activity of the cells averaged 38 ± 17 nmol/1 (mean $\pm$ S.D.). Assuming that the activity coefficient for Ca^{2+} in sarcoplasm is the same as that (0.3), calculated for extracellular fluid, the Ca^{2+} activity of 38 nmol/1 is equivalent to a sarcoplasmic free Ca^{2+} concentration of 127 nmol/1. This assumption can be justified provided the sarcoplasmic ionic strength is not too different from that of extracellular fluid.

ACKNOWLEDGEMENTS

This work was supported by NIH Grant HL - 21136. We are grateful to Dr. W. Simon for providing the neutral Calcium Ligand, D.Y. Uhm was on leave from the Department of Physiology, Chungang University College of Medicine, Seoul, Korea, under the support of the Korean Ministry of Education. C.O. Lee was an Established Investigator of AHA.

REFERENCES

Fozzard, H.A., Lee, C.O., 1976, Influence of changes in external potassium and chloride ions on membrane potential an intracellular potassium ion activity in rabbit ventricular muscle, J.Physiol., 256:663.

Lee, C.O.,1979, Electrochemical properties of Na^+- and K^+-selective microelectrodes, Biophysical J., 27:209.

Lee, C.O., 1981, Determination of selectivity coefficients of ion-selective microelectrodes, in: this issue.

Robinson, R.A., and Stokes, R.M., 1965, The theoretical interpretation of chemical potentials (Chapter 9), in: Electrolyte Solutions, Butterworth and Co., Ltd., London.

Simon, W., Ammann, D., Oehme, M., and Morf, W.E., 1978, Calcium-Selective Electrodes, in: Calcium Transport and Cell Function, A. Scarpa and E. Carafoli, eds., Ann. N.Y. Acad. Sci.

SESSION VI
OTHER TECHNIQUES FOR THE STUDY OF IONIC ACTIVITY CHANGES IN BRAIN RESEARCH

ION-SELECTIVE PROPERTIES OF THE NERVE CELL MEMBRANE

P.G. Kostyuk

A.A. Bogomoletz Institute of Physiology
Academy of Sciences of the Ukrainian SSR
Kiev 24, 252601 GSP, U.S.S.R.

The development of methods for precise control of the ionic content of the intra- and extracellular media, combined with effective membrane potential clamping for transmembrane current measurements, formed the technical basis for the recent studies of the ionic-selective properties of the cellular membrane. The main conclusion from these studies states that the transmembrane ionic currents which appear during active cellular reaction are based on parallel membrane conductances each of which is capable of passing selectively a flux of a certain type of ions.

Recently a way was found for continuous perfusion of isolated nerve cells, enabling the extension of these analytical possibilities to the somatic nervous membrane (Kostyuk et al., 1975a). Already the first results obtained in this respect were of considerable interest because they also described, apart from the already known sodium and potassium conducting systems, the presence of a well developed system of calcium conductance in this membrane. Thus the somatic membrane may in fact act as a sodium, potassium or calcium electrode depending on the type of membrane structures activated by the external signal (change in transmembrane electric field).

An extensive series of experiments made it possible to describe in detail all these electrode properties, which appear to be quite similar in both invertebrate and vertebrate neurones (cf. Kostyuk and Krishtal,1977; Fedulova and Veselovsky, 1980).

To determine the microstructure of the conducting systems, recording of the corresponding specific currents were made from a small patch of somatic membrane ($10-20\ \mu m^2$) sucked into a small pore of a

325

plastic membrane. Very effective electric insulation of this patch from the rest of the membrane was achieved. Under such recording conditions stochastic fluctuations of sodium and calcium currents of the order of 10^{-11} A were observed. Statistical analysis of these fluctuations has shown that they are produced by discrete conducting units ("ionic channels") which switch from the nonconducting to the conducting state due to changes in the intramembrane electric field. The conductance of a single sodium channel is about 7 pS at zero membrane potential, and the conductance of a single calcium channel - about 0.5 pS. The density of channels in the membrane is only few hundreds per μm^2 (Kostyuk et al., 1980).

The ionic channels are highly selective for the given type of ions. For the sodium channel the sequence of relative permeabilities (determined from the shifts in reversal potential) is $P_{Na} : P_{Li} : P_{NH_4} : P_K = 1.0 : 0.9 : 0.4 : 0.01$. For the calcium channel the corresponding current-voltage characteristic is not linear; it approaches the potential axis exponentially with high depolarizing potential shifts and no reversal of the calcium current can be obtained even when the intracellular free calcium concentration is increased artificially. On the contrary, already a small increase in the intracellular calcium (up to 10^{-7} mol/l) blocks the calcium conductance (Doroshenko et al., 1978). For these reasons the selectivity of the calcium channel could be estimated only from the maximum current values; it follows the sequence $P_{Ba} > P_{Sr} > P_{Ca} > P_{Mg}$, the relative permeabilities for these ions being 2.8 : 2.6 : 1.0 : 0.2.

The measurements of the concentration and potential-dependence of the ionic currents carried through these channels by different permeable ions provide a basis for certain suggestions about the nature of their selective properties and for the construction of appropriate energy profiles of the ion in the channel.

A characteristic feature of the functioning of calcium channels in the presence of effective binding of the penetrating ions in the region of both the external and internal channel mouth; the apparent dissociation constants for the external binding site are: $K_{Ca} = 5.4$ mmol/l; $K_{Sr} = 10$ mmol/l; $K_{Ba} = 15$ mmol/l (Valeyev, 1979). The presence of binding is the reason for effective competitive blocking of the calcium current by other divalent cations. The dissociation constants for the blocking cations (measured in the presence of 4 mmol/l Sr) are: $K_{Ni} = K_{Co} = 0.74$ mmol/l; $K_{Mn} = 0.36$ mmol/l and $K_{Cd} = 0.07$ mmol/l (Krishtal, 1976; Ponomaryov et al., 1979). Effective binding of the penetrating ions on both sides of the channel indicates that the energy profile of the ion inside the channel can be approximated by two energy wells separated by an energy barrier; the penetrating ions have to fill up these wells in succession. The free-energy levels at different points of the calcium channel profile have been computed by Kostyuk and Mironov (1980) using a diagrammatic technique (Fig. 1).

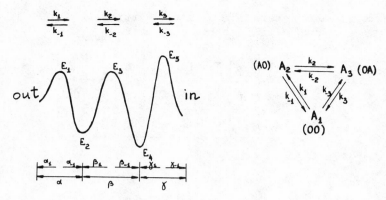

Fig. 1. Schematic description of three-barrier model for calcium channel and the diagramme of ion-channel states used for the calculations.

The parameters of this model are presented in Table 1. Because of the deepness of the internal energy well, the calcium channel in fact can pass ions only in the inward direction and in the virtual absence of internal calcium ions. Even a small increase in intracellular calcium fills up this well and blocks the channel (Kostyuk et al., 1980).

Contrary to the calcium channel, in the sodium channel there is no appreciable decrease in the energy of the passing ion, and the latter is stabilized in a partly dehydrated state by a negatively charged group inside the channel (cf. Hille, 1972). A peculiar feature of the sodium channels in vertebrate neurones is the separation of the produced current into two components – the fast (I_{Na}^f) and slow (I_{Na}^s). Both currents can be reversibly eliminated by replacement of the Na^+ ions in the external solution with Tris or tetramethylammonium (TMA), but only I_{Na}^f can be completely blocked by tetrodoxin (TTX) in a concentration of 5×10^{-8} g/ml. I_{Na}^s is not affected by increases in TTX concentration by 1-2 orders of magnitude. On the other hand, it can be effectively blocked by agents which normally block calcium channels (Co^{2+}, Mn^{2+}, Cd^{2+}, D-600 and its analogues). All these agents have no definite depressive action on the TTX-sensitive I_{Na}^f (Veselovsky et al., 1980).

The selectivity of the two sets of sodium channels does not markedly differ; it should be noted that the TTX-resistant inward current switched-off by the elimination of Na^+ ions from the external solution cannot be restored here by increasing the concentration of Ca^{2+} or introduction of other divalent cations. Moreover, the maximal

Table 1.   Parameters of the three-barrier model for calcium
channel. E_i given in RT units.

	E_1	E_2	E_3	E_4	E_5	α	β	γ
Ca^{2+}	4,2	-4,6	3,5	-6,0	7,5	0,3	0,4	0,3
Ba^{2+}	5,3	-2,4	4,0	-6,5	7,5	0,3	0,4	0,3

amplitude of the TTX-resistant sodium current is somewhat depressed
in this case by elevation of extracellular Ca^{2+} together with the
shift of its current-voltage characteristics in the depolarizing
direction.

A characteristic property of the outward (potassium) current in
the somatic membrane is also its separation into a fast and a delayed
component (I_K^f and I_K^s) differing in their activation and inactivation
kinetics. These components have been studied in detail in non-per-
fused molluscan neurones (Neher, 1971; Connor and Stevens, 1971;
Kostyuk et al., 1975) and now also in perfused mammalian neurones
(Tsyndrenko, 1979), An important functional characteristic of I_K^f is
a strong steady-state inactivation already at resting potential level
and its removal by hyperpolarization; due to this property the corresponding channels play an important role in the generation of auto-
rhythmic membrane potential waves.

The measurements of equilibrium potentials for both potassium
currents indicate that their channel selectivity is similar; if the
potassium gradient is switched-off by replacement of Tris ions for
K^+, these currents disappear completely. At the same time a potential-
dependent outward current still remains after such replacement due to
a flux of replacing ions through less-specific ionic channels (I_{ns}).
It differs from the fast and delayed potassium currents in its activation kinetics, absence of inactivation and resistance to the
action of tetraethylammonium (TEA). An increase in intracellular Ca^{2+}
concentration potentiates this current. All its characteristics are
similar to those of the TEA-resistant component of potassium currents,
which is also potentiated by intracellular Ca^{2+} (Heyer and Lux, 1976;
Thompson, 1977) and produced by less selective ionic channels (Doroshenko et al., 1979). These channels probably form the basis for the
activation of potassium conductance by an increase in intracellular
calcium, described by Meech (1974).

The intracellular concentration of Ca^{2+} involved in this action is extremely low (about 10^{-7} mol/l), indicating a very high specificity of the corresponding binding groups. This specificity can also be seen from the absence of the potentiating effect after the introduction of much higher amounts of other divalent cations (Ba^{2+}, Sr^{2+}). These groups probably occupy a very convenient position in the channel as they can react with Ca^{2+} ions coming both from the cell interior during perfusion and through the membrane during the action potential, even in the presence of Ca-chelating agents inside the cell.

The current-voltage characteristics of the TEA-resistant Ca-dependent outward current are in many respects similar to the current-voltage characteristics of currents produced by other electrically-operated ionic channels. They are shifted along the potential axis when extra- and intracellular Ca^{2+} concentrations are changed, indicating that their sensitivity to changes of the intramembrane electric field alters. It is therefore probable that Ca^{2+} ions in this case function only as a cofactor necessary for the maintenance of the channels in a state ready for activation; the immediate transition from closed to open state is produced by a gating mechanism responding to the electric field.

REFERENCES

Connor, J.A., Stevens, C.F., 1971, Voltage clamp studies of a transient outward membrane current in gastropod neural somata, J. Physiol. (Lond.), 213:21.

Doroshenko, P.A., Kostyuk, P.G., and Tsyndrenko, A.Ya., 1978, Separation of potassium and calcium channels in the somatic membrane of a nerve cell, Neurophysiology (Kiev), 10:645.

Doroshenko, P.A., Kostyuk, P.G., and Tsyndrenko, A.Ya., 1979, A study of the TEA-resistant outward current in the somatic membrane of perfused nerve cells, Neurophysiology (Kiev), 11: 460.

Heyer, C.B., and Lux, H.D., 1976, Control of the delayed outward potassium currents in bursting pace-maker neurones of the snail Helix pomatia, J. Physiol. (Lond.), 262:349.

Hille, B., 1972, The permeability of the sodium channel to metal cations in myelinated nerve, J. Gen. Physiol., 59:638.

Kostyuk, P.G., and Krishtal, O.A., 1977, Separation of sodium and calcium currents in the somatic membrane of mollusc neurones, J. Physiol. (Lond.), 270:545.

Kostyuk, P.G., Krishtal, O.A., and Doroshenko, P.A., 1975, Outward currents in isolated snail neurones. I. Inactivation kinetics, Comp. Biochem. Physiol., 51C:259.

Kostyuk, P.G., Krishtal, O.A., and Pidoplichko, V.I., 1975, Intracellular dialysis of nerve cells: effect of intracellular fluoride and phosphate on the inward current, Nature, 257, No5528, 691.

Kostyuk, P.G., Krishtal, O.A., Pidoplichko, V.I., and Shakhovalov, Yu. A., 1980, A spectral analysis of conductance fluctuations of calcium channels in a nerve cell membrane, Doklady Akad. Nauk SSSR (Moscow), 250:219.

Kostyuk, P.G., and Mironov, S.L., 1980, The application of three-barrier model to the description of the energy profile of the calcium channel in the membrane of mollusc neurones, Neuro-physiology (Kiev), 12, in press.

Kostyuk, P.G., Mironov, S.L., and Doroshenko, P.A., 1980, An energy profile of a calcium channel in a mollusc neuronal membrane, Doklady Akad. Nauk SSSR (Moscow), in press.

Krishtal, O.A., 1976, Blocking effect of cadmium ions on a calcium inward current in a nerve cell membrane, Doklady Akad. Nauk SSSR (Moscow), 231:1003.

Meech, R.W., 1974, The sensitivity of Helix aspersa neurones to injected calcium ions, J. Physiol. (Lond.), 237:259.

Neher, E., 1971, Two fast transient current components during voltage clamp in snail neurones, J. Gen. Physiol., 58:36.

Ponomaryov, V.N., Narushevichus, E., and Chemeris, N.K., 1980, Blocking effect of Ni^{2+}, Co^{2+}, Mn^{2+} and Mg^{2+} ions on the value of inward current through calcium channels of Limnea neurones, Neuro-physiology (Kiev), 12:211.

Thompson, S.H., 1977, Three pharmacologically distinct potassium channels in molluscan neurones, J. Physiol. (Lond.), 265:465.

Tsyndrenko, A.Ya., 1980, Comparative analysis of potassium channel characteristics in a membrane of spinal ganglion neurones and neuroblastoma cells, Neurophysiology (Kiev), 12:208.

Valeyev, A.E., 1979, Selectivity of calcium channels of a somatic membrane in Helix neurones for calcium, strontium and barium ions, Neurophysiology (Kiev), 11:371.

Veselovsky, N.S., and Fedulova, S.A., 1980, Revealing of calcium channels in a somatic membrane of spinal ganglion neurones of rats under an intracellular dialysis with cAMP, Doklady Akad. Nauk SSSR (Moscow), in press.

Veselovsky, N.S., Kostyuk, P.G., and Tsyndrenko, A.Ya., 1980, "Slow" sodium channels in a somatic membrane of spinal ganglion neurones in newborn rats, Doklady Akad. Nauk SSSR (Moscow), 250:216.

GLIAL CELLS AS POTASSIUM DETECTORS

R.K. Orkand, C-M. Tang and P.M. Orkand

Department of Physiology and Pharmacology, School of
Dental Medicine and Institute of Neurological Sciences,
University of Pennsylvania, Philadelphia,
PA 19104, U.S.A.

INTRODUCTION

The membrane potential of glial cells arises from the unequal distribution of K^+ across the membrane. The Nernst relation for K^+, $E_K = RT/F \ln [K^+]_o/[K^+]_i$ acurately predicts the membrane potential of glial cells in the mud puppy optic nerve when $[K^+]_o$ is between 1.5 and 115 mEq/l (Kuffler et al., 1966; for review see Orkand, 1977). This observation has led to the use of the glial membrane potential as an indicator of changes in K^+ in the extracellular clefts of the nervous system. The technique is analogous to that used by Frankenhaeuser and Hodgkin (1956) to measure the accumulation of K^+ in the periaxonal space of the squid giant axon following impulse activity. They measured the change in the after-hyperpolarization of the nerve impulse with repetitive activity and compared it to the change produced by increases in bath K^+. In the glial experiments, glial depolarization produced by trains of axon impulses was compared with the depolarization produced by increased $[K^+]_o$ (Orkand et al., 1966). The hypothesis that K^+ accumulation in the extracellular clefts depolarizes glial cells is consistent with the knowledge of the efflux of K^+ from unmyelinated axons during impulse activity and the size of the extracellular space as measured from electron micrographs. The early use of K^+-selective electrodes in the nervous system by Vyskočil, Kříž and Bureš (1972), Lux and Neher (1973), Krnjević and Morris (1972) and Vyklický, Syková, Kříž and Ujec (1972) provided decisive evidence for fluctuations of $[K^+]_o$ with neuronal activity.

In this brief review, we shall examine the application and limitations of the glial membrane as a K^+ electrode.

331

GLIAL MEMBRANE AS A POTASSIUM ELECTRODE

Temperature Effects

The Nernst relation predicts that for a 10 ^{o}C change in temperature the membrane potential should change by about 3 mV. When the temperature of the solution bathing the Necturus optic nerve was varied between 1 ^{o}C and 30 ^{o}C the glial membrane potential followed the Nernst relation (Bracho et al., 1975). Cooling depolarizes and warming hyperpolarizes the glial membrane. If a portion of the glial membrane potential was the result of active electrogenic ion transport or if the potential resulted from a combination of ionic conductances with temperature sensitive conductance ratios, as is the case in some neurons (Carpenter and Alving, 1968), the Nernst prediction would not be fulfilled. For example, electrogenic transport should be inhibited by cooling; if a portion of the membrane potential were dependent on pump activity a greater depolarization than that predicted by the Nernst relation would be observed. The temperature studies support the conclusion that the glial membrane potential is a K^+ diffusion potential. When the bathing solution was warmed to greater than 30 ^{o}C the glial membrane progressively depolarized. The effect could be reversed on cooling. At high temperatures the glial membrane loses its high selectivity for K^+.

Sodium Channels

There is no evidence that vertebrate glial cell membranes have sodium channels of the type found in electrically excitable membranes such as those of nerve and muscle cells. The voltage current relation of glial membranes is linear over a wide range (Kuffler et al., 1966); the conductance of the glial membrane is not voltage sensitive. Recently, radioactively labelled saxitoxin, which binds to sodium channels, and drugs which increase Na^+ conductance in excitable membrane were used in an attempt to detect sodium channels in mud puppy glial cells (Tang et al., 1979). Normal optic nerves show a suturable uptake of saxitoxin equivalent to a density of about 25 μm^{-2} of axon membrane. A couple of months following enucleation all the axons in the optic nerve degenerate and only glial cells remain. These 'glial' nerves show no significant saturable binding of saxitoxin. However, there is sufficient scatter in the data that some small saturable component to the binding cannot completely be ruled out. Normal nerves are depolarized by low (10^{-6} -10^{-5} mol/l) concentrations of veratridine. This depolarization is blocked by tetrodotoxin and appears to arise from the effect of veratridine to increase the population of open sodium channels in axons. By contrast, glial cells in glial nerves are not depolarized by low concentrations of veratridine but are depolarized by veratridine at 10^{-3} mol/l. This effect is not blocked by tetrodotoxin; its origin is unknown. Intracellular recordings from glial cells in normal nerves reveal that these cells are depolarized at low concentrations of veratridine. This depolarization is more transient than in the axons and is most likely the result of K^+ efflux from depolarized axons.

At low $[K^+]_o$ (below 1.5 mEq/l) the membrane potential of glial cells does deviate from that predicted for a K^+ electrode (Kuffler et al., 1966) and this might be the result of a significant permeability of other ions like Na^+. However, it might just as readily be the result of K^+ leak from neurons raising the cleft intracellular K^+ above that in the bathing solution (Frankenhaeuser and Hodgkin, 1956) or even an artifact of microelectrode recording. At low $[K^+]_o$ the glial membrane resistance would be increased and the shunt around the site of electrode penetration would lead to an underestimate of the actual membrane potential. Experiments involving prolonged soaking of glial cells in low $[K^+]_o$, indicate that Na^+ accumulates intracellularly under these conditions (Tang et al., 1980).Glial cells do have some small permeability of Na^+ either due to the presence of a low density of Na^+ channels or a low Na^+ permeability in the K^+ channel.

<u>Selectivity of Potassium Channel</u>

The relative permeability of the glial membrane to a number of monovalent cations was determined by comparing the depolarization produced by each with that resulting from a comparable increase in $[K^+]_o$ (Bracho et al., 1975). The selectivity sequence of permeable ions is as follows: $Tl^+2.2$; K^+1; $Rb^+0.55$; $Cs^+0.34$ and $NH_4^+ 0.16$. No significant permeability was found for Na^+, Li^+ or guanidinium. These results are essentially the same as that found for the K^+ channel in nerve. As Tl^+ has a larger unhydrated diameter than K^+ and NH_4^+ a smaller diameter than Rb^+, it is clear that the relative permeabilities do not simply reflect cation size.

<u>Sensitivity to Other Agents</u>

The glial membrane potential is not known to depend on the anion composition of the external solution. Even large changes in $[Cl^-]_o$, when replaced by $[SO_4^{2-}]$ did not produce significant changes in the glial membrane potential (Bracho et al., 1975).

The extracellular fluid in the central nervous system contains many other substances which might alter the membrane potential of the neuroglia. These include neurotransmitters, hormones, amino acids and peptides as well as metabolites (Davson, 1967). Such substances might depolarize glial cells either as a result of releasing K^+ from neurons or by direct effect on the glial membrane. As indicated above, low concentrations of veratridine appear to depolarize glial cells by releasing $K+$ from axons. By contrast, glutamate (10^{-3}-10^{-5}mol/1) has a direct depolarizing effect on glial cells (Tang and Orkand, unpublished observations). Glutamate depolarizes mud puppy optic nerve neuroglia either in the normal nerve or when the axons have all degenerated and the nerve consists solely of glial cells.

SPATIAL FACTORS

The electrical length constant, λ, for the glial cell syncytium in the Necturus optic nerve is about 0.8 mm (Tang, unpublished observation). This value was determined from square pulse analysis using independent intracellular voltage recording and current passing electrodes and assuming one dimensional geometry; comparable measurements have not been made on other glial cells. However, there is evidence for a considerable spread of potential in the glial cells in frog spinal cord. In the spinal cord it has been found with ion selective electrodes that following dorsal root stimulation there is a large increase in $[K^+]$ in the intermediate region of the cord and essentially no increase in the dorsal horn or motoneurone pool (Syková et al., 1976). In contrast, the glial depolarization resulting from K^+ accumulation following dorsal root stimulation is about the same throughout the spinal cord (Syková and Orkand, 1980). Such a result would be expected if the glial cells had a long length constant which spread the potential through the glial syncytium. Under these conditions, use of the glial cell membrane as a K^+ detector leads to an overestimate of $[K^+]_o$ in some regions of the spinal cord and an underestimate in others. Similar results were obtained in mammalian cortex (Futamachi and Pedley, 1976) but not in mammalian spinal cord (Lothman and Somjen, 1975). Therefore, in case where the glial cells form an electrical syncytium with a long electrical length constant, the glial cell membrane will only function as an accurate indicator of $[K^+]_o$ when the $[K^+]_o$ is uniform over a large volume of the tissue.

MEMBRANE POTENTIAL DURING ELECTROGENIC TRANSPORT

After a glial optic nerve is soaked in low $[K^+]$ Ringer at 5 $^\circ$C for a couple of hours, the recorded resting potential is much lower than normal. The depolarization presumably results from a loss of intracellular K^+ and gain of Na^+ under these conditions. If now, $[K^+]_o$ is increased to normal the membrane potential will either decrease much less than in a control glial cell(Tang et al., 1980) or even increase. The result reflects the activation of a hyperpolarizing electrogenic pump in the glial membrane by $[K^+]_o$. This conclusion is supported by the observation that the usual K^+ sensitivity of the glial membrane may be restored by pretreating the cells with strophanthidin or by substituting Li^+ for Na^+ in the bathing solution. Both these treatments block the activation of an electrogenic pump by raised K^+(DeWeer and Geduldig, 1973). In normal glial cells, an increase in $[K^+]_o$ does not appear to markedly stimulate the electrogenic pump. If it did, the known behavior of the glial membrane as a K^+ electrode would not be observed (Kuffler et al., 1966). It appears that the glial electrogenic pump is most sensitive to increases in $[Na^+]_i$. Substances which depolarize glial cells, such as high concentrations of veratridine produce a strophanthidin sensitive glial hyperpolarization after being washed out. The depolarization apparently is accompanied by an influx of Na^+ which is removed by electrogenic transport (Tang and Orkand, unpublished observations).

FUNCTIONAL CONSEQUENCES OF K^+ ELECTRODE BEHAVIOR

Two functional consequences of the depolarizing effect of K^+ on the glial membrane have been proposed. First, that K^+ induced glial depolarization serves to coordinate activity in neurons and glial cells. Second, that glial depolarization by K^+ plays a role in the intracellular clearance or redistribution of K^+ following K^+ efflux from active neurons.

Control of Glial Metabolism

The first hypothesis is supported by the observation that increases in $[K^+]_o$ alter the levels of reduced pyridine nucleotides in glial cells (P. Orkand et al., 1973) increases glucose uptake into glial cells (Salem et al., 1975) and stimulates the release of GABA from glial cells in rat dorsal root ganglia (Minchin and Iversen, 1974). At this time, however, there is no evidence to indicate whether these are effects of K^+ or of membrane depolarization.

Spatial Buffering

The second hypothesis, that differences in glial cell membrane potential due to local K^+ accumulation serve to produce current loops through the glial cytoplasm and intercellular clefts which disperses K^+ over relatively long distances, has received support from the experiments of Gardner-Medwin, Coles, Tsacopoulos, Dietzel, Heineman and Lux in a variety of systems (see discussion of these experiments in Nicholson, 1980 and elsewhere in this volume). The high selectivity of the glial membrane for K^+ would play an important role in this process. It assures that the currents entering and leaving the glial cell are carried by K^+ and it produces a maximum potential difference across the glial membrane due to a local rise in $[K^+]_o$.

SUMMARY

Under normal conditions the membrane of glial cells in the optic nerve of Necturus behaves as does an accurate K^+ electrode for changes in $[K^+]_o$ and temperature. Studies with saxitoxin binding and drugs which increase Na^+ permeability in excitable cells provide no evidence of Na^+ channels in glial membranes. The selectivity sequence of the K^+ channel is $Tl^+> K^+> Rb^+> Cs^+> NH_4^+ >> Cl^-, Li^+,$

Na^+ or guanidinium. Besides K^+ substances such as glutamate and veratridine depolarize glial cells. In some cases the depolarization is secondary to K^+ release from neurons; in others a direct effect on the permeability pattern of the glial membrane is implicated. The length constant of the glial syncytium in the optic nerve is about 0.8 mm. Thus, spatial variations in $[K^+]_o$ will produce a glial depolarization which reflects the 'average' $[K^+]_o$ within a few millimeters of the recording site. In Na^+ loaded glial cells, the glial membrane potential is affected by the activity of an electrogenic pump and is not a reliable indication of $[K^+]_o$. The sensitivity of the glial membrane to $[K^+]_o$ plays a role in the neuronal control of glial metabolism and in the redistribution of K^+ in the extracellular space following its local accumulation as a result of neuronal activity.

ACKNOWLEDGEMENT

This work was supported by U.S.P.H.S. Grant No. NS-12253.

REFERENCES

Bracho, H., Orkand, P.M., and Orkand, R.K., 1975, A further study of the fine structure and membrane properties of neuroglia in the optic nerve of Necturus, J. Neurobiol., 6:395.

Carpenter, D.O., and Alving, B.O., 1968, A contribution of an electrogenic Na^+ pump to membrane potential in Aplysia neurons, J. Gen. Physiol., 52:1.

Davson, J., 1969, Physiology of the Cerebrospinal Fluid., Churchill, London.

DeWeer, P., and Geduldig, D., 1973, Electrogenic sodium pump in squid giant axon, Science, 179:1326.

Frankenhaeuser, B., and Hodgkin, A.L., 1956, The after effects of impulse in the giant nerve fiber of Loligo, J. Physiol., 131:341.

Futamachi, K., and Pedley, T.A., 1976, Glial cells and potassium; their relationship in mammalian cortex, Brain Res., 109:31.

Krnjević, K., and Morris, M.E., 1972, Extracellular K^+ activity and slow potential changes in spinal cord and medulla, Can. J. Physiol. Pharmacol., 50:1214.

Krnjević, K., and Schwartz, S., 1967, Some properties of unresponsive cells in the cerebral cortex, Exp. Brain Res., 3:306.

Kuffler, S.W., Nicholls, J.G., and Orkand, R.K., 1966, Physiological properties of glial cells in central nervous system of amphibia, J. Neurophysiol., 29:768.

Lothman, E.W., and Somjen, G.G., 1975, The potential response in the spinal cord, J. Physiol., 252:115.

Lux, H.D., and Neher, E., 1973, The equilibration time course of K^+ in cat cortex, Exp. Brain Res., 17:190.

Minchin, M.C.W., and Iversen, L.L., 1974, Release of ^3H gamma-amino butyric acid from glial cells in rat dorsal root ganglia, J. Neurochem., 23:533.

Nicholson, C., 1980, Dynamics of the brain cell micro-environment, Neurosci. Res. Prog. Bull., 18:177.

Orkand, P.M., Bracho, H., and Orkand, R.K., 1973, Glial metabolism: alteration by potassium levels compatible to those during neural activity, Brain Res., 55:467.

Orkand, R.K., 1977, Glial Cells, in: "Handbook of Physiology, section 1: The Nervous System, Vol. 1 Cellular Biology of Neurons, part 2", Brookhart, J.M. et al., eds., American Physiological Society, Bethesda, Md.

Orkand, R.K., Nicholls, J.G., and Kuffler, S.W., 1966, Effect of nerve impulses on the membrane potential of glial cells in the central nervous system of amphibia, J. Neurophysiol., 29:788.

Salem, R.D., Hammerschlag, R., Bracho, H., and Orkand,R.K., 1975, Influence of potassium ions on accumulation and metabolism of ^{14}C glucose by glial cells, Brain Res., 86:499.

Syková, E., Shirayev, B., Kříž, N., and Vyklický, L., 1976, Accumulation of extracellular potassium in the spinal cord of frog, Brain Res., 106:413.

Syková, E., and Orkand, R.K., 1980, Extracellular potassium and transmission in frog spinal cord, Neurosci., 5:1421.

Tang, C-M., Cohen, M.W., and Orkand, R.K., 1980, Electrogenic pumps in axons and neuroglia and extracellular potassium homeostasis, Brain Res., 194:283.

Tang, C-M., Strichartz, G.R., and Orkand, R.K., 1979, Sodium channels in axons and glial cells of the optic nerve of Necturus maculosa, J. Gen. Physiol., 74:629.

Vyklický, L., Syková, E., Kříž, N., and Ujec, E., 1972, Post-stimulation changes of extracellular potassium concentration in the spinal cord of the rat, Brain Res., 45:608.

Vyskočil, F., Kříž, N., and Bureš, J., 1972, Potassium-selective microelectrodes used for measuring the extracellular brain potassium during spreading depression and anoxic depolarization in rats, Brain Res., 39:255.

THE ROLE OF CELLS IN THE DISPERSAL OF BRAIN

EXTRACELLULAR POTASSIUM

A.R. Gardner-Medwin

Department of Physiology
University College London
London, WC1E 6BT

What is the fate of potassium which is released into the extracellular space around active neurons? A lot of information relevant to this has appeared in the last ten years, much of it obtained through the use of K^+-selective microelectrodes. But there are many questions which remain unsettled and perhaps controversial (Gardner-Medwin, 1980). Potassium released into the extracellular (EC) space is ultimately restored to the neurons which have lost it; so one question centres round the time course of this restoration process and its relation to the dynamics of other processes. Potassium may also enter other cells temporarily, which thus act to 'buffer' the changes of K^+ concentration in the EC space. The extent and time course of such buffering processes are uncertain (Gardner-Medwin, 1980). A third type of process is that of dispersal to less affected regions of EC space, or to fluid ventricles: this may occur either by diffusion or by the action of currents flowing through cell membrane causing the cells (probably especially glial cells) to take up K^+ in one region and to release it elsewhere. This last process is known as the 'spatial buffer' mechanism and was originally suggested by Orkand, Nicholls and Kuffler in 1966. My own recent work in collaboration with various colleagues (Gardner-Medwin, 1977; Gardner-Medwin, and Nicholson, 1978; Gardner-Medwin et al., 1979; Gardner-Medwin and Coles, 1980) has suggested that the spatial buffer mechanism may be more important in relation to diffusion than was earlier appreciated. In this article I shall examine the consequences that the spatial buffer and uptake mechanisms may have in some of the situations that have been studied by other authors and in situations where it may be important for nervous systems to minimise a disturbance of EC K^+ concentration. We cannot straightforwardly turn these components of K^+ dynamics on and off in an experimental situation to determine their effect: but once we know or can guess at their parameters, we can do calculations to see what the effect of such a hypothetical experiment would be.

In order to calculate the changes of EC K^+ concentration which can be expected to occur in a particular experimental situation it is necessary to solve simultaneously the equations describing the various processes. These are the diffusion equations for flux in the EC space (incorporating terms to take account of the electrical as well as concentration gradients), the cable equations governing current flow and fluxes around the cells responsible for spatial buffering, and linear uptake equations to take account of processes of equilibration between the EC space and cytoplasm. These equations have been solved numerically for either 1-dimensional or 3-dimensional spherically symmetrical situations with various different parameters. In reality each process may involve several tissue compartments with different parameters. The calculations lump them all together with a single set of parameters. Various simplifying assumptions are also made and additional processes which are probably of less importance such as K^+ clearance into the bloodstream (Gardner-Medwin, 1980) are for the present ignored.

Parameters for the spatial buffer mechanism have been derived from experiments on rat brain (Gardner-Medwin, 1977; Gardner-Medwin and Nicholson, 1978; Gardner-Medwin et al., 1979), which suggest that it carries ca. 5 times more K^+ flux than EC diffusion over large distances, with an electrical space constant ca. 0.2 mm. These have been used to see what effects this mechanism would have on the K^+ concentration rises due to distributed sources. Assuming a net release of K^+ from, say, hyperactive nerve cells maintained steadily from time zero throughout a spherical region 0.8 mm diameter we can calculate the K^+ concentration rise at the centre of the region at various times. Inclusion of the spatial buffer equations leads this rise to be less than it would be with only EC dispersal and cytoplasmic equilibration by ca. 40 % after 1 minute, 60 % after 5 min and 70 % after 15 min. This illustrates one of the situations where a major advantage could result from the existence of spatial buffering: if prolonged periods occur with fairly widespread net release of K^+ from zones of neural tissue. If the source of K^+ is very localised there is little benefit close to the source due to spatial buffering. But at distances of 100 μm or more the K^+ elevation may be reduced by more than 50 %. We in fact know rather little about the size, duration and degree of synchrony of normal fluctuations of K^+ release in the brain. And we are also quite ignorant about the characteristics of EC concentration change which could lead to significant neural dysfunction. We are somewhat in the position of an engineer trying to assess whether the stabilising fins on a ship are any use, when he knows neither how rough a typical sea is or what kinds of ship movement would be disturbing to the passengers. But at least we know something of the circumstances in which this particular process tending to stabilise extracellular potassium may have an effect.

The spatial buffer mechanism also helps to speed the decline of EC K^+ concentration after a rise. The extremely rapid declines (taking a few seconds) observed after periods with brief stimulation (Vern et al., 1977; Cordingley and Somjen, 1978) are probably attributable more, however, to equilibration of EC fluid with cytoplasm than to dispersal processes (Gardner-Medwin, 1980). Somjen and Trachtenberg (1979) suggested that the spatial buffer contribution to K^+ clearance in this kind of situation was quite negligible, but unfortunately they seriously underestimated it due to a calculation error of 10^3 (p. 28, line 2). Once the calculation error is corrected, the spatial buffer contribution appears in fact to be possibly significant (Somjen, 1980). Experiments by Gardner-Medwin and Coles (1980) have invest-igated the role of the dispersal by spatial buffering of K^+ through glia in the retina of the honeybee drone. A calculation somewhat si-milar to that of Somjen and Trachtenberg suggests that in this prep-aration a large fraction of the K^+ released from photoreceptors may be dispersed by spatial buffer currents through the glia.

Two earlier experiments had led to the suggestion that EC diffusion might be the principal factor involved in K^+ movement in mammalian brain tissue. These both employed K^+-selective micro-electrodes to measure changes during artificial disturbances. Lux and Neher (1973) measured K^+ concentration changes close to an iontophor-etic point source of K^+, while Fisher et al., (1976) measured the changes beneath the cortical surface during superfusion with altered K^+ concentrations. It has already been pointed out elsewhere that there may be flaws in the interpretation of these experiments (Gardner-Medwin, 1978, 1980; Nicholson et al., 1979). The data differ from what should be expected if the added K^+ remained wholly in EC space. Related experiments using EC markers have been performed using iontophoresis (Nicholson et al., 1979) and superfusion of radioactive markers (Fenstermacher et al., 1974) and have produced different re-sults from those with K^+. Attempts have now been made to fit the published K^+ results with solutions of the equations for diffusion, spatial buffering and uptake. A satisfactory fit can be made with both these types of data if suitable parameters are chosen. It is necessary to invoke both cytoplasmic equilibration and spatial buffer-ing (carrying ca. 5 times as much K^+ flux as diffusion over large distances) to obtain a satisfactory fit. But the situation is not completely straightforward since the space constant that is required for the spatial buffer mechanism to fit the iontophoretic data is ca. 120 μm, that required for the superfusion data is ca. 450 μm, while that for my own data is ca. 200 μm. The reason for these dis-crepancies is not apparent. It is possible that the long space con-stant for the superfusion data might be due in part to shrinkage of the EC space in the relatively high (12 mmol/1) K^+ concentration employed. It is also possible that the factors involved in both these experiments are more complex than has been envisaged. Even if this is so, however, the data can no longer reasonably be regarded as supporting the idea that K^+ moves through brain tissue principally by EC diffusion, or as evidence against a contribution of the spatial buffer mechanism.

CONCLUSION

One of the contributions of ion-selective microelectrodes to brain physiology has been to provide data on the dynamics of extracellular potassium. The data indicate that potassium dispersal through glia and equilibration between cytoplasm and EC space are both likely to be important factors in the fate of K^+ released from nerve cells. The situation is not simply or principally one of release, extracellular diffusion and active reuptake as has been suggested. The involvement of glia so as to reduce the perturbations of EC potassium concentration suggests that such perturbations might be a cause of neural dysfunction. We still need further work to find out whether this is so or not.

REFERENCES

Cordingley, G.E., and Somjen, G.G., 1978, The clearing of excess potassium from extracellular space in spinal cord and cerebral cortex, Brain Res., 151:291.

Fenstermacher, J.D., Patlak, C.S.,and Blasberg, R.G., 1974, Transport of material between brain extracellular fluid, brain cells and blood, Fed. Proc., 33:2070.

Fisher, R.S., Pedley, T.A., and Prince, D.A., 1976, Kinetics of potassium transport in normal cortex, Brain Res., 101:223.

Gardner-Medwin, A.R., 1977, The migration of K^+ produced by electric current through brain tissue, J. Physiol., 269:32P.

Gardner-Medwin, A.R., 1978, The amplitude and time course of extracellular potassium concentration changes during potassium flux through brain tissue, J. Physiol., 284:38P.

Gardner-Medwin, A.R., 1980, Membrane transport and solute migration affecting the brain cell microenvironment, in: Neuroscience Res. Prog. Bull., 18 2 .

Gardner-Medwin, A.R., and Coles, J.A., 1980, Dispersal of potassium through glia, Proc. 28th Int. Congr. Physiol. Sci. Abstr. 1507, p. 427.

Gardner-Medwin, A.R., Gibson, J.L., and Willshaw, D.J., 1979, The mechanism of potassium dispersal in brain tissue, J. Physiol., 293:37P.

Gardner-Medwin, A.R., and Nicholson, C., 1978, Measurement of extracellular potassium and calcium concentration during passage of current across the surface of the brain, J. Physiol., 275:66P.

Lux,H.D., and Neher, E., 1973, The equilibration time course of $[K^+]_o$ in rat cortex, Exp. Brain Res., 17:190.

Nicholson, C., Phillips, J.M., and Gardner-Medwin, A.R., 1979, Diffusion from an iontophoretic point source in the brain: role of tortuosity and volume fraction, Brain Res., 169:580.

Orkand, R.K., Nicholls, J.G., and Kuffler, S.W., 1966, Effect of nerve impulses on the membrane potential of glial cells in the cns of amphibia, J. Neurophysiol., 29:788.

Somjen, G.G., 1980, in: The Application of Ion-Selective Electrodes, T. Zeuthen, ed., Elsevier/North Holland, Amsterdam.

Somjen, G.G., and Trachtenberg, M., 1979, in: Origin of Cerebral Field Potentials, E.J. Speckman and H. Caspers, eds., Thieme Verlag, Stuttgart.

MOVEMENT OF POTASSIUM INTO GLIAL CELLS IN THE RETINA

OF THE DRONE, Apis mellifera, DURING PHOTOSTIMULATION

J.A. Coles, M. Tsacopoulos, P. Rabineau
and A.R. Gardner-Medwin*

Experimental Ophthalmology Laboratory and
Physiology Department, Geneva University,
1211 Geneva 4, Switzerland, and
*Physiology Department, University College,
London, J.K.

Experiments on the drone retina have led to direct demonstrations of metabolic and ionic interactions between glial cells and sensory neurons. The tissue is composed of two essentially uniform populations of cells: photoreceptors and pigmented glial cells (Perrelet, 1970). The glial cells are not directly sensitive to light, but photostimulation of the photoreceptors causes an increase in glycogen turnover in the glial cells (Evequoz et al.1978). Measurements with intracellular, double-barrelled ion-sensitive electrodes have shown that light stimulation also causes potassium activity (a_K) in the photoreceptors to decrease by about 25 %, from a mean value of 79 mmol/1 to a mean of 67.5 mmol/1 (Coles and Tsacopoulos, 1979). Simultaneously, a_K in the glial cells rises from a mean of 52 mmol/1 to a mean of 66 mmol/1; since the total volume of the glia is greater than that of the photoreceptors, and the extracellular (e.c.) space fraction is thought to be less than 5 % (Shaw, 1977), the results can most readily be explained by supposing that K^+ ions leave the photoreceptors and enter the glia (see Coles and Tsacopoulos, 1979 for details). In the present paper we report that these ion movements are not accompanied by large changes in the volume of the e.c. space.

METHODS

The caudal part of the head of a drone (which is composed mainly of eye) was removed by a cut parallel to the axes of a layer of photoreceptors and the remaining rostral part was fixed in the floor of a perfusion chamber (Coles and Tsacopoulos, 1979). The cut surface

of the retina was superfused with an oxygenated Ringer solution of
composition (mmol/l): NaCl, 270; KCl, 3.2; $CaCl_2$, 1.6; $MgCl_2$, 10;
Na-MOPS buffer, 10, pH 7.3. Micropipettes were pulled from capillaries
with a double triangle section obtained from the Glass Company of
America, Inc., Bargaintown, N.J. 08232 (E. Dick and R.F. Miller,
personal communication). The pipettes were bevelled and the interior
of the active barrel was silanized with N,N-dimethyltrimethylsilylami-
ne (TMSDMA)(Kováts, 1980) in the apparatus described by Coles and
Tsacopoulos (1977). The silanization was carried out at 240-260 °C.
Two kinds of electrodes were prepared. Those sensitive to K^+ contained a valinomycin-based mixture in the active barrel (Wuhrmann et al.,
1979); those sensitive to tetraethylammonium (TEA) contained Corning
resin 477317 that had been equilibrated with 2 mol/l TEA Cl (Phillips
and Nicholson, 1979). The reference barrels contained Ringer solution
and the tips were very large: for the recordings shown in Fig. 1
the K^+ electrode had a tip diameter of 1.5 μm at the base of the bevel
and the TEA electrode had a diameter of 2.5 μm. Calibrations were
made in Ringer solutions in which Na^+ was partially replaced by the
ion of interest (Fig. 1c, d).

RESULTS

Following Phillips and Nicholson (1979), we introduced TEA into
the e.c. space and assumed that changes in its activity indicated
changes in the volume of the e.c. space. Fig. 1 shows records from
a TEA-sensitive electrode, and also a K^+sensitive electrode that was
used to check that the TEA did not significantly modify the K^+ movements normally observed during photostimulation (Coles and Tsacopoulos
1979). The two electrodes were advanced into the retina to a depth
of 135 μm while it was superfused with normal bee Ringer solution.
At first the electrodes were partly intracellular, but after 50 min
the reference barrels were recording stable e.c. responses to light
flashes (Baumann, 1974). The superfusate was than replaced by one
containing 1 mmol/l TEA Cl and when the output of the TEA electrode
reached a steady value the retina was stimulated with trains of 90
light flashes, at 1 Hz. The upper trace in Fig. 1a shows the response
of the K^+ electrode during photostimulation: the amplitude and time
course of the response were not detectably different from those observed before the addition of TEA so we assume that a_K in the glial
cells increased as it normally does during photostimulation (Coles
and Tsacopoulos, 1979). The lower trace is the simultaneous recording
from the TEA electrode and it is seen that there is a small, slow,
positive deflexion with a maximum amplitude of about 1.4 mV. In 7
other experiments in 6 retinas a similar slow positive deflexion was
observed and in every case its amplitude was less than that shown
here.

When the TEA electrode was initially advanced from the superfusate into the retina, a positive deflexion was observed. The elec-

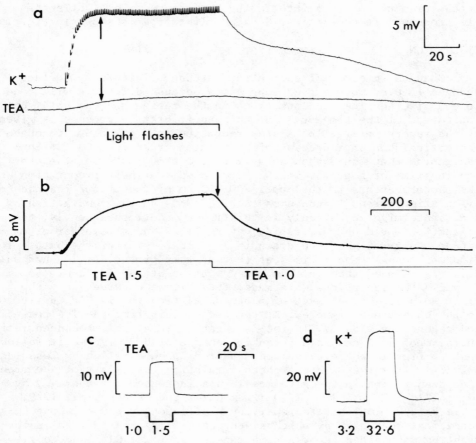

Fig. 1. The recordings show the difference in potential between
         the active and reference barrels of a K+ electrode and a
         TEA electrode. In a and b the electrode tips were in the
         retina, 135 μm from the superfused surface. Arrows are
         20s after the onset of photostimulation (a), or solution
         change (b). In c and d the electrodes were in a calibration
         chamber (Coles and Tsacopoulos, 1979). Concentrations are
         in mmol/l.

trode did not respond to light-induced changes in e.c. K+ concentration, so we suppose that there is an endogenous substance, other
than K+, to which Corning 477317 is sensitive see also Wuhrmann et
al.,(1979). This fact made it necessary to calibrate the electrode

in the presence of this interfering background, i.e., while the electrode was in the retina. Such a calibration is shown in Fig. 1b.

DISCUSSION

Changes in e.c. TEA concentration cannot faithfully reflect changes in e.c. volume over long times because diffusion will tend to equalize the TEA concentrations in the retina and the bath. An indication of the time scale of this equilibration process is given by the record in Fig. 1b: a step reduction in e.c. volume throughout the retina should produce an instantaneous rise in e.c. TEA concentration that would then decay with the time course of the descending limb of Fig. 1b. In the superfused, cut head preparation only the photoreceptors in the upper 200-300 μm of the tissue respond to light stimulation (Tsacopoulos et al., 1980) so the contraction of e.c. space might occur only in this region and, consequently, the relaxation would be more rapid, but still of the same order of magnitude. An arrow has been drawn in Fig. 1b 20 s after the bath solution was changed and it is seen that at this time diffusion had only slightly changed the e.c. TEA concentration at the depth of 135 μm at which the recordings were made. Thus, if we consider only the first 20 s after the onset of photostimulation in Fig. 1a, diffusion to the bath can be ignored. At the end of this time the TEA potential had changed by 0.84 mV. In the calibration (Fig. 1b), a concentration increase of 50 % caused a potential change of 8.75 mV, so it follows that in Fig. 1a the e.c. volume appeared to have fallen by less than 5 % 20 s after the onset of photostimulation. At this time the free K^+ concentration in the glial cells has increased, on average, by 10 mmol/1 (S.E. = 1.1 mmol/1) (from Coles and Tsacopoulos, 1979, Table 2, assuming that the activity coefficient y = 0.70). One hypothetical mechanism by which electroneutrality in the glial cells might be maintained is by a simultaneous entry of Cl^- (see, e.g., Gardner-Medwin, 1980). If we assume that the osmolarity of the glial cytoplasm remains constant then water must also enter the cell and cause the fractional volume change given by the following calculation: The osmolarity of the Ringer solution, taken as the sum of the concentrations of the particles, is 596 mOsm. Before stimulation, the glial cell has a volume V_1 and contains 75 mOsm of K^+ (Coles and Tsacopoulos, 1979) and hence (596 - 75) = 521 mOsm of other particles. 20 s after the onset of stimulation, let the volume increase to V_2: the osmolarity in the cell is then given by

$$(75 + 10)V_2 + (85\ V_2 - 75\ V_1) + 521\ V_1 \div V_2 = 596$$

where the three terms in the numerator represent the contribution of K^+, the additional Cl^- and the other particles, respectively. The solution of this equation is that the fractional increase in volume, $(V_2 - V_1)/V_1 = 20/426$. The ratio of the total volume of the glial cells to the volume of the e.c. space is estimated to be at least 57/5 (Coles and Tsacopoulos, 1979), so if the predicted in-

crease in volume of the glial cells were taken from the e.c. space
the volume of the latter would decrease to less than one half. This
seems to make the hypothesis that K^+ enters the glia in association
with Cl^- unattractive; in contrast, positive evidence exists for an
entry by spatial buffering (Gardner-Medwin and Coles, 1978) and by
Na^+/K^+ exchange (Tsacopoulos and Coles, 1978).

REFERENCES

Baumann, F., 1974, in: "The compound Eye and Vision of Insects",
    G.A. Horridge, ed., Clarendon, Oxford.
Coles, J.A., and Tsacopoulos, M., 1977, A method of making fine
    double-barreled potassium-sensitive micro-electrodes for intra-
    cellular recording, J. Physiol. (Lond.), 270:12-13P.
Coles, J.A., and Tsacopoulos, M., 1979, Potassium activity in photo-
    receptors glial cells and extracellular space in the drone
    retina: changes during photostimulation, J. Physiol. (Lond.),
    290:525.
Evequoz, V., Deshusses, J., and Tsacopoulos, M., 1978, The effect
    of photostimulation on glycogen turnover in the retina of the
    honey bee drone, Experientia, 34:897.
Gardner-Medwin, A.R., 1980, in: "Dynamics of the Brain Cell Micro-
    environment", C. Nicholson, ed., Neurosciences Res. Program
    Bull., 18:208.
Gardner-Medwin, A.R., and Coles, J.A., 1980, Dispersal of potassium
    through glia, Proc. intl. Union physiol. Sci.,14:427, free
    communications.
Kováts, E. sz., 1980, German patent P2930516.
Perrelet, A., 1970, The fine structure of the retina of the honey
    bee drone. An electronmicroscopical study. Z. Zellforsch.
    mikrosk. Anat., 108:530.
Phillips, J.M., and Nicholson, C., 1979, Anion permeability in
    spreading depression investigated with ion-sensitive micro-
    electrodes, Brain Res., 173:567.
Shaw, S.R., 1977, Restricted diffusion and extracellular space in
    the insect retina, J. comp Physiol., 113:257.
Tsacopoulos, M., and Coles, J.A., 1978, Inhibition by strophanthidin
    of the uptake of potassium by pigment cells in the drone retina,
    Experientia, 34:903
Tsacopoulos, M., Poitry, S., and Borsellino, A., 1980, Oxygen con-
    sumption by drone photoreceptors in darkness and during re-
    petitive stimulation with light flashes, Experientia, 36:702.
Wuhrmann, P., Ineichen, H., Riesen-Willi, U., and Lezzi, M., 1979
    Change in nuclear potassium electrochemical activity and puffing
    of potassium - sensitive salivary chromosome regions during
    Chironomus development, Proc. Natl. Acad. Sci. USA, 76:806.

INTRACELLULAR CALCIUM AND THE REGULATION OF NEURONAL MEMBRANE

PERMEABILITY

Forrest F.Weight and Stephen M. McCort

Laboratory of Preclinical Studies
National Institute of Alcohol Abuse and Alcoholism
12501 Washington Avenue
Rockville, Maryland 20852, USA

INTRODUCTION

Intracellular calcium ions (Ca^{2+}) are known to be important in several functions of excitable cells: for example, Ca^{2+} plays an essential role in muscle concentration, neurotransmitter release, and excitation-secretion coupling. The physiological function of intracellular Ca^{2+} in nerve cells, however, is less well understood. We have investigated the possible release of intracellular Ca^{2+} and its role in the regulation of membrane permeability in a vertebrate neuron.

METHODS

Intracellular recordings were made from "B" cells in the ninth or tenth paravertebral sympathetic ganglion of bullfrog (Rana Catesbeiana). Microelectrodes were filled with 3 M Kcl and had a tip resistance of 20-30 megohms. A Wheatstone bridge circuit was used for passing current through the recording microelectrode. The preparation was superfused with an oxygenated Ringer s solution, having the following composition : NaCl 100 mmol/1, $CaCl_2$ 1.8 mmol/1, KCl 2 mmol/1, $Tris^-Cl$ 16 mmol/1 (pH=7.2), glucose 1g/1.

RESULTS

Spontaneous Hyperpolarizations Induced by Theophylline

Previous investigations revealed that theophylline induces spontaneous activity in bullfrog sympathetic neurons (Busis and Weight, 1976; Weight et al.,1978). We report here a detailed investigation

351

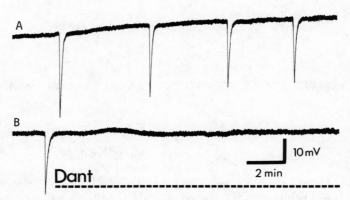

Fig. 1. A. Spontaneous hyperpolarizations induced by 5 mmol/1 theo-
         phylline. B. Effect of 0.056 mmol/1 dantrolene (dashed line).
         Record continuous with A.

of that phenomenon. Superfusion of the preparation with a Ringer's
solution containing 5 mmol/1 theophylline, depolarized the membrane
by 6-12 mV and induced spontaneous hyperpolarizations, which occurred
rhythmically every 1-5 minutes (Fig.1A). These rhythmic hyperpolarizations were observed in 68% (n =59) of the cells tested. The hyperpolarizations had an amplitude of 5-20 mV and a duration of 30-45 s.
Similar effects have also been observed with caffeine (Kuba and Nishi,
1976).

Ionic Mechanism of the Spontaneous Hyperpolarizations

Membrane resistance was tested using hyperpolarizing constant
current pulses. During the spontaneous hyperpolarizations, membrane
resist ance was markedly decreased. This decreased resistance is not
explained by anomalous rectification, since the current-voltage curve
was fairly linear with hyperpolarization.

Application of progressively increasing hyperpolarizing currents
progressively reduced the amplitude of both the rhythmic hyperpolarizations and the antidromic spike afterhyperpolarization. In a Ringer's
solution containing 8 mmol/1 K^+, progressive membrane hyperpolarization not only reduced, but also reversed both the spontaneous hyperpolarizations and the spike after-hyperpolarization. Both potentials reversed at approximately the same membrane potential.

Effect of Ca-free Ringer, Dantrolene, and D_2O on the Spontaneous Hyperpolarization

Table 1. The Effect of Ca-free Ringer, Dantrolene, and D_2O on the Spontaneous Hyperpolarizations

Ringer*	#of Neurons Tested	Total Block	Decreased Frequency	No Effect
Ca-free	12	67%	33%	0
Dantrolene	8	75%	25%	0
D_2O	6	33%	67%	0

*All Ringer's solutions contained 5 mmol/l theophylline

To study whether the increased conductance during the spontaneous hyperpolarizations might be a Ca-sensitive K^+ conductance (Meech, 1978), we tested the effect of a Ca-free Ringer's solution (1.8 mmol/l $MgCl_2$ replaced $CaCl_2$). The Ca-free Ringer either totally abolished or significantly reduced the frequency of the rhythmic hyperpolarizations (Table 1).

To evaluate whether an intracellular release of Ca^{2+} might be involved in the generation of the spontaneous hyperpolarizations, we tested the effect of dantrolene and deuterium oxide(D_2O). Dantrolene sodium (0.056 mmol/l) either totally blocked (Fig. 1) or significantly reduced the frequency of the spontaneous hyperpolarizations (Table 1). D_2O also either blocked or reduced the frequency of the rhythmic hyperpolarizations (Table 1).

DISCUSSION AND CONCLUSIONS

Theophylline (5 mmol/l) induced the generation of spontaneous hyperpolarizations in bullfrog sympathetic neurons. A decreased membrane resistance during the hyperpolarizations and a K^+ dependent reversal potential near E_K, provides evidence that the hyperpolarizations are generated by an increased K^+ permeability (conductance). The abolition of the rhythmic hyperpolarizations by a Ca-free Ringer's solution indicates that the K^+ conductance is Ca^{2+} sensitive. Since both dantrolene and D_2O block the intracellular release of Ca^{2+} in muscle fibers (Desmedt and Hainaut, 1977; Kaminer and Kimura, 1972; Eastwood et al., 1975), the abolition of the spontaneous hyperpolarizations by dantrolene and D_2O suggests that the rhythmic hyperpolarizations involve a periodic intracellular release of Ca^{2+}.

REFERENCES

Busis, N.A., and Weight, F.F., 1976, Spike after-hyperpolarization of a sympathetic neurone is calcium sensitive and is potentiated by theophylline, Nature, 263:434.

Desmedt, J.A., and Hainaut, K., 1977, Inhibition of the intracellular release of calcium by dantrolene in barnacle giant musle fibres, J. Physiol., 265:565.

Eastwood, A., Grundfest, H., Brandt, P., and Reuben, J.P., 1975, Sites of action of D_2O in intact and skinned crayfish muscle fibers, J. Membrane Biol., 24:249.

Kaminer, B., and Kimura, J., 1972, Deuterium oxide: Inhibition of calcium release in muscle, Science, 176:406.

Kuba, K., and Nishi S., 1976, Rhythmic hyperpolarizations and de-polarizations of sympathetic ganglion cells induced by caffeine, J. Neurophysiol., 39:547.

Meech, R.W., 1978, Calcium dependent potassium activation in nervous tissues, Ann. Rev. Biophys. Bioeng., 7:1.

Weight, F.F., Smith, P.A., and Schulman, J.A., 1978, Postsynaptic potential generation appears independent of synaptic elevation of cyclic nucleotides in symphatetic neurons, Brain Research, 158:197.

CNS AND Na-PUMP IN SITU MUSCLE

N. Akaike

Department of Pharmacology
Kumamoto University Medical School
Kumamoto 860, Japan

Recently, it has been demonstrated that the high $[Na]_i$ and low $[K]_i$ levels in in situ soleus muscle of the hypokalemic rat are the result of the direct inhibition of ouabain-sensitive Na-pump not by low plasma K^+ level but CNS (Akaike, 1979; 1980). Such a CNS-inhibition on Na-pump was eliminated by sectioning the peripheral nerve to soleus or by spinal transection at the cervical level. The activation of Na-pump following nerve section was not affected by pretreatment with curare, but was completely inhibited by the electrical stimulation (rectangular pulse with the duration of 0.05 msec at 10 Hz) of the sectioned nerve in the curarized hypokalemic rat. The muscle Na-pump was also activated in the presence of several adrenergic α-blockers without nerve section while β-blockers had no effects on the pump.

Therefore, it may be concluded that the inhibitory action of the central nervous system (CNS) on the pumping of the hypokalemic rat soleus muscle is maintained by the continuous release of norepinephrine (NE) from the sympathetic nerve terminal.

REFERENCES

Akaike, N., 1979, CNS effects on muscle Na/K levels in hypokalemia, Brain Research, 178:175.

SYMPOSIUM PARTICIPANTS

AKAIKE, N.
> Kumamoto University Medical School, Dept. of Pharmacology,
> Kumamoto 860, Japan.

ALVAREZ-LEEFMANS, F.J.
> Physiological Laboratory, Downing Street,
> Cambridge, CB2 3EG, Great Britain.

BERS, D.M.
> University Medical School, Dept. of Physiology, Teviot Place,
> Edinburgh EH8 9AG, Great Britain.

van BOGAERT, P.P.
> University of Antwerpen, Physiological Laboratory,
> Groenenboergerlaan 171, 2020 Antwerpen, Belgium.

ten BRUGGENCATE, G.
> Physiologisches Institut der Universität München,
> Pettenkoferstrasse 12, D 8000 München, Federal Republic Germany.

BUREŠ, J.
> Institute of Physiology, Czechoslovak Academy of Sciences,
> Vídeňská 1083, 142 20 Prague 4, Czechoslovakia·

COLES, J.A.
> Lab. d´ophtalmologie expérimentale, 22 rue Alcide Jentzer,
> 1211 Genève 4, Switzerland·

CORAY, A.
> 5 Bühlplatz, CH-3012 Berne, Switzerland.

CSILLAG, A.
> Semmelweis Univ.Med.School, 1st Dept. of Anatomy,
> 1450 Türolko utca 58, Budapest IX, Hungary·

DLOUHÁ, Hana
> Institute of Physiology, Czechoslovak Academy of Sciences,
> Vídeňská 1083, 142 20 Prague 4, Czechoslovakia·

EDWARDS, Ch.
> State University of New York at Albany, SUNYA, Dept.Biol. Sci.,
> 1400 Washington Avenue, Albany N.Y., 12222, U.S.A.

GALVAN, M.
> Physiologisches Institut d. Universität München,
> Pettenkofferstrasse 12, D 8000 München, Federal Republic Germany.

GARDNER-MEDWIN, A.R.
University College, Department of Physiology,
Gower Street, London WC1 E6BT, Great Britain.
GLITSCH, H.G.
Ruhr Universität, Institut f. Zellphysiologie,
Arbeitsgruppe Muskelphysiologie, Universitätsstrasse 150,
Postfach 10 21 48, 4630 Bochum-Querenburg, Federal Republic
Germany.
GUTNICK, M.J.
c/o Prof. D. Prince, Stanford University Medical Center,
Department of Neurology, Stanford, Calif. 94305, U.S.A.
HEINEMANN, U.
Max Planck Institute f. Psychiatrie, Kraepelinstrasse 2,
D 8000 München 40, Federal Republic Germany.
HNÍK, P.
Institute of Physiology, Czechoslovak Academy of Sciences,
Vídeňská 1083, 142 20 Prague 4, Czechoslovakia.
JANUS, J.
Physiologisches Institut I., Westring 6, D-4400 Münster,
Federal Republic Germany.
KELLER, O.
Institute for Postgraduate Medical Education,
Department of Neurology,
Vídeňská 800, 142 20 Prague 4, Czechoslovakia.
KHURI, R.N.
Faculty of Medicine, American University,
Department of Physiology, Beirut, Lebanon.
KORYTA, J.
Heyrovský Institute of Physical Chemistry and Electrochemistry,
Czechoslovak Academy of Sciences, Opletalova 25,
110 00 Prague 1 - Nové Město, Czechoslovakia.
KOSTYUK, P.G.
Institute of Physiology, Bogomoletz str. 4, Kiev 24,
252611 GSP, U.S.S.R.
KŘIVÁNEK, J.
Institue of Physiology, Czechoslovak Academy of Sciences,
Vídeňská 1083, Prague 4, Czechoslovakia.
KŘÍŽ, N.
Institue of Physiology, Czechoslovak Academy of Sciences,
Vídeňská 1083, Prague 4, Czechoslovakia.
KUNZE, Diana
University of Texas Medical Branch, Department of Physiology
and Biophysics, Galveston, Texas 77550, U.S.A.
LEE, C.O.
Cornell Univ. Medical College, Dept. of Physiology and
Biophysics, 1300 York Avenue, New York, N.Y., 10021, U.S.A.
LEHMENKÜHLER, A.
Physiologisches Institut d. Universität, Münster,
Federal Republic Germany.

LINDLEY, B.
    Case Western Reserve University, Department of Physiology,
    School of Medicine, Cleveland, Ohio 44106, U.S.A.
LUX, H.D.
    Max Planck Institute f. Psychiatrie, Kraepelinstrasse 2,
    D 8000 München 40, Federal Republic Germany.
MACHEK, J.
    Institute of Physiology, Czechoslovak Academy of Sciences,
    Vídeňská 1083, 142 20 Prague 4, Czechoslovakia.
McGUIGAN, J.
    5 Bühlplatz, CH-3012 Berne, Switzerland.
MELICHAR, J.
    Institute of Experimental Medicine, Czechoslovak Academy
    of Sciences, U nemocnice 2, 120 00 Prague 2, Czechoslovakia.
MORAD, M.
    University of Pennsylvania, The School of Medicine, A403
    Richards Bldg/G4, 37th & Hamilton Walk, Philadelphia 19104,U.S.A.
MORRIS, M.
    University of Toronto, 1 Kings College Circle, Room 4302,
    Med. Sci. Building, Toronto, Canada M5S, 1A8, Canada.
NICHOLSON, C.
    University Medical Center, School of Medicine, Dept. of
    Physiology and Biophysics, 550 First Avenue, New York, N.Y.
    10016, U.S.A.
O'DOHERTY, Josephine
    Indiana University, School of Medicine, Dept. of Physiology,
    1100 West Michigan Street, Indianapolis, Indiana 46223, U.S.A.
ORKAND, R.K.
    School of Dental Medicine, Dept. of Physiology and Pharmacology,
    Univ. of Pennsylvania, 4001 Spruce Street A1, Philadelphia,
    Pa 19104, U.S.A.
PAYNE, Ruth
    Marischal College, Dept. of Physiology, Aberdeen, AB 1AS,
    Scotland.
PRINCE, D.A.
    Stanford University Medical Center, Depart. of Neurology,
    Stanford, California 94305, U.S.A.
PUSCH, H.
    Ruhr Universität, Institut f. Zellphysiologie, Arbeitsgruppe
    Muskelphysiologie, Universitätsstrasse 150, Postfach 10 21 48,
    4630 Bochum-Querenburg, Federal Republic Germany.
ROITBAK, A.
    Institute of Physiology, Georgian Academy of Sciences,
    L. Gotua 14, Tbilisi 380060, U.S.S.R.
SIMON, W.
    Eidgenossische Technische Hochschule, Lab. f. Organische
    Chemie, Universitätsstrasse 16, CH 8092 Zürich, Switzerland.
SMITH, D.O.
    University of Wisconsin, Department of Physiology,
    470 North Charter Street, Madison 53706, Wisc., U.S.A.

SOMJEN, G.G.
    Duke University, Dept. of Physiology and Pharmacology,
    Durhan N.C. 27710, U.S.A.
SONNHOF, U.
    I. Physiologisches Institut d. Univ. Heidelberg,
    Im Neuenheimer Feld 326, D 6900 Heidelberg, Federal Republic
    Germany.
SYKA, J.
    Institute of Experimental Medicine, Czechoslovak Academy
    of Sciences, U nemocnice 2, 120 00 Prague 2, Czechoslovakia.
SYKOVÁ, Eva
    Institute of Physiology, Czechoslovak Academy of Sciences,
    Vídeňská 1083, 142 20 Prague 4, Czechoslovakia.
UJEC, E.
    Institute of Physiology, Czechoslovak Academy of Sciences,
    Vídeňská 1083, 142 20 Prague 4, Czechoslovakia.
VEJSADA, R.
    Institute of Physiology, Czechoslovak Academy of Sciences,
    Vídeňská 1083, 142 20 Prague 4, Czechoslovakia.
VYKLICKÝ, L.
    Institute of Physiology, Czechoslovak Academy of Sciences,
    Vídeňská 1083, 142 20 Prague 4, Czechoslovakia.
VYSKOČIL, F.
    Institute of Physiology, Czechoslovak Academy of Sciences,
    Vídeňská 1083, 142 20 Prague 4, Czechoslovakia.
WALKER, J.L.
    The University of Utah, Dept. of Physiology, College of
    Medicine, 410 Chipeta Way, Room 156, Research Park,
    Salt Lake City, Utah 84108, U.S.A.
WEIGHT, F.
    Laboratory of Preclinical Studies, NIAAA, 12501 Washington
    Avenue, Rockville, Md. 20852, U.S.A.
WEINGART, R.
    Universität Bern, Physiologisches Institut, 3012 Bern,
    Bühlplatz 5, Switzerland.
WOODY, C.
    UCLA Medical Center, 760 Westwood Plaza, Los Angeles,
    Calif. 90024, U.S.A.

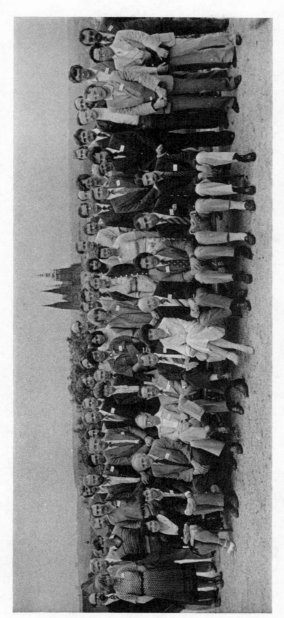

The participants of the ISM Symposium, with the Prague Castle in the background.

INDEX